Minimally Invasive Musculoskeletal Pain Medicine

Minimally Invasive Procedures in Orthopedic Surgery

Series Editors

Alexander R. Vaccaro
Rothman Institute
and
Thomas Jefferson University Hospital
Philadelphia, Pennsylvania, U.S.A.

Christopher M. Bono
Boston University Medical Center
Boston, Massachusetts, U.S.A.

Minimally Invasive Musculoskeletal Pain Medicine

Edited by

Mitchell K. Freedman
Thomas Jefferson University Hospital
Philadelphia, Pennsylvania, U.S.A.

William B. Morrison
Thomas Jefferson University Hospital
Philadelphia, Pennsylvania, U.S.A.

Marc I. Harwood
Thomas Jefferson University Hospital
Philadelphia, Pennsylvania, U.S.A.

informa
healthcare

New York   London

Informa Healthcare USA, Inc.
270 Madison Avenue
New York, NY 10016

WE
140
M665
2007

© 2007 by Informa Healthcare USA, Inc.
Informa Healthcare is an Informa business

No claim to original U.S. Government works
Printed in the United States of America on acid-free paper
10 9 8 7 6 5 4 3 2 1

International Standard Book Number-10: 0-8493-7256-9 (Hardcover)
International Standard Book Number-13: 978-0-8493-7256-8 (Hardcover)

Visit the Informa Web site at
www.informa.com

and the Informa Healthcare Web site at
www.informahealthcare.com

Preface

The subspecialty of pain management has advanced considerably over the last 20 years. Once considered the domain of anesthesiology, it has now become an integral part of many specialties. This is reflected in the opening of the subspecialty board in pain medicine to multiple disciplines. The "fourth vital sign" concept has advanced pain medicine one step further to the point that it is a basic part of medical management. This book is a compilation of chapters regarding interventional pain management from a variety of subspecialties. It is our hope that the management of pain continues to grow in a multidisciplinary direction. There are a variety of interventional and noninterventional pain management techniques. The critical issue is not that any one mode of treatment is employed consistently by any certain physician, but that the correct strategy or combination of strategies is employed for the individual patient.

We have collected a number of experts in the field of musculoskeletal intervention and pain management, in a cooperative effort from the disciplines of physical medicine and rehabilitation, sports medicine, and radiology. The chapters in this book discuss the topics of pharmacology, office-based injections, viscosupplementation, trigger point injection, acupuncture, botulinum treatment, joint injection, and bone biopsies using image guidance, ultrasound-guided interventions, thermoablation, epidural injections, zygapophyseal joint intervention, and discography.

Imaging guidance plays an important role in many musculoskeletal interventions. Fluoroscopy, computed tomography, ultrasound, and magnetic resonance imaging can be used as tools to safely and accurately position needles, biopsy devices, radiofrequency probes, and other instruments in the optimal location. Proper selection of the guidance modality and approach requires knowledge of indications and contraindications of each as well as relevant anatomy. Proper technique is essential to ensure success, patient safety, and comfort. This book discusses the basics of many such image-guided procedures, and the chapters herein provide the reader with a framework for this practice. However, reading is not a substitute for hands-on training with an experienced practitioner. Furthermore, success with the most effective intervention must complement appropriate patient selection based on comprehensive evaluation and teleological thinking about the goal of any given procedure.

Mitchell K. Freedman
William B. Morrison
Marc I. Harwood

Contents

Contributors

Kenneth P. Botwin   Florida Spine Institute, Clearwater, Florida, U.S.A.

Zach Broyer   Rothman Institute, Thomas Jefferson University Hospital, Philadelphia, Pennsylvania, U.S.A.

Theodore D. Conliffe, Jr.   Rothman Institute, Thomas Jefferson University Hospital, Philadelphia, Pennsylvania, U.S.A.

Jeffrey W. R. Dassel   Thomas Jefferson University Hospital, Philadelphia, Pennsylvania, U.S.A.

Michael J. DePalma   Department of Physical Medicine and Rehabilitation, Virginia Commonwealth University/Medical College of Virginia, Richmond, Virginia, U.S.A.

M. Dholakia   Thomas Jefferson University Hospital, Philadelphia, Pennsylvania, U.S.A.

Damian E. Dupuy   Department of Diagnostic Imaging, Brown University Medical School, Rhode Island Hospital, Providence, Rhode Island, U.S.A.

Guy W. Fried   Thomas Jefferson University Hospital, Philadelphia, Pennsylvania, U.S.A.

Carmine A. Grieco   Department of Diagnostic Imaging, Brown University Medical School, Rhode Island Hospital, Providence, Rhode Island, U.S.A.

Geoffrey Gustavsen   Sports Medicine, University of Delaware, Newark, Delaware, U.S.A.

Syed A. Hasan   Department of Physical Medicine and Rehabilitation, and The Penn Spine Center, Hospital of the University of Pennsylvania, Philadelphia, Pennsylvania, U.S.A.

Gene Hong   Drexel University College of Medicine, Philadelphia, Pennsylvania, U.S.A.

Leonard B. Kamen   Moss Rehabilitation Hospital, Albert Einstein Healthcare Network, Temple University Hospital, Philadelphia, Pennsylvania, U.S.A.

Vishal Kancherla   Florida Spine Institute, Clearwater, Florida, U.S.A.

Eoin Kavanagh   Department of Musculoskeletal Radiology, University of Pittsburgh Medical Center, Pittsburgh, Pennsylvania, U.S.A.

Ira Kornbluth   Center for Pain Management, Glen Burnie, Maryland, U.S.A.

Mendel Kupfer   Thomas Jefferson University Hospital, Philadelphia, Pennsylvania, U.S.A.

William B. Morrison   Thomas Jefferson University Hospital, Philadelphia, Pennsylvania, U.S.A.

E. Anthony Overton   Rothman Institute, Thomas Jefferson University Hospital, Philadelphia, Pennsylvania, U.S.A.

Luis E. Palacio   Thomas Jefferson University, Philadelphia, Pennsylvania, U.S.A.

Beth Palmisano   Florida Spine Institute, Clearwater, Florida, U.S.A.

Gregory R. Saboeiro   Weill Medical College of Cornell University, Hospital for Special Surgery, New York, New York, U.S.A.

Adam L. Schreiber   Thomas Jefferson University Hospital, Philadelphia, Pennsylvania, U.S.A.

Jeremy Simon   Orthopedic and Spine Specialists, Physical Medicine and Rehabilitation, Bowie, Maryland, U.S.A.

Curtis W. Slipman   Department of Physical Medicine and Rehabilitation, and The Penn Spine Center, Hospital of the University of Pennsylvania, Philadelphia, Pennsylvania, U.S.A.

Carolyn M. Sofka   Weill Medical College of Cornell University, Hospital for Special Surgery, New York, New York, U.S.A.

Peter C. Vitanzo   Rothman Institute, Thomas Jefferson University, Philadelphia, Pennsylvania, U.S.A.

1   Pharmacology of Low Back Pain

Leonard B. Kamen
Moss Rehabilitation Hospital, Albert Einstein Healthcare Network, Temple University Hospital, Philadelphia, Pennsylvania, U.S.A.

Adam L. Schreiber
Thomas Jefferson University Hospital, Philadelphia, Pennsylvania, U.S.A.

INTRODUCTION

Treating low back pain (LBP) with pharmacological agents is first and foremost a limited proposition. Despite an estimated $26 billion per year (1998) spent on treating LBP in the United States, with $3.9 billion for pharmaceuticals alone, there is a lack of evidence-based studies demonstrating any singular or collective advancements in our medical or surgical treatment of this common malady (1,2). To effectively provide a pharmaceutical treatment plan to a collection of spinal disorders, the practitioner must conceptualize the broad scope of structural, physiologic, and psychological pathologies that contribute to acute and chronic pain of spinal etiology. When the right medication is chosen, based on this sifting of information, rewards are reaped by improvement in pain and function.

This chapter will provide a practical review of the pharmaceutical agents used to treat acute and chronic pain secondary to spinal disorders. It is the intent of the authors to construct a rationale for use of pharmacologic agents based on the knowledge of the pathology contributing to pain of spinal origin as well as a working knowledge of how these agents may modulate the many factors that contribute to and sustain a pain syndrome. Evidence-based material is cited whenever it is available.

Conceptual Models of Low Back Pain

Pain perception has been likened to a multidimensional holograph with projection of multiple constructs known as qualia composed of sensory and memory components into each individual's pain experience (3). This spectrum of acute to chronic LBP conditions exists at three hierarchical levels: a sensory-discriminatory component, that is, acute lumbar sprain, a motivational-affective component, that is, work-related lumbar disc herniation, and a cognitive-evaluative component, that is, failed spinal surgery syndrome. The accepted time frame for this evolution from acute to chronic stages is stated by the International Association for the Study of Pain (IASP) as "...pain that has persisted beyond the normal tissue healing time (usually taken to be 3 months)." These models must be considered and determined on initial presentation of the patient in order to discern the impact of acute to chronic pain on each individual. Primary and secondary pain generators (i.e., degenerative disc disease leading to radiculopathy with weakness and fear of collapse on weight bearing) need to be elicited during initial patient interviews.

1

TABLE 1 Anatomical Models of Low Back Pain Which May Be Employed as a Foundation for Pharmaceutical Intervention

Anatomical pain generator model	Examples of structural components	Pharmacological agents with potential for modulation at this site
Anterior spinal elements	Vertebral body compression, discal pathology, infection, tumor, or dysvascular state in bone or disc	nsNSAIDs, biphosphonates, salmon calcitonin, opioids, and antibiotics
Posterior spinal elements	Facet joint hypertrophy with degenerative joint disease, spondylosis, spondylolithesis, and spinal stenosis	nsNSAIDs, steroidal agents, opioids, glucosamine, and chondroitin sulfate
Soft tissue structures	Spinal ligaments, bursae, muscle groups surrounding spine and pelvis	Muscle relaxants, AEDs, and NSAIDs
Neuropathic pain generators	Nerve root compression, ischemia, and metabolic neuropathies	AEDs, alpha-2 blockers, opioids, single- and dual-action antidepressants
Visceral pain generators	Referred renal lithiasis pain, abdominal organ disturbances, infections, and tumors	Opioids, cathartics, cholinergic agents, antibiotics, and chemotherapeutic agents

Abbreviations: AED, antiepileptic drug; NSAID, nonsteroidal anti-inflammatory drug; nsNSAID, nonselective nonsteroidal anti-inflammatory drug.

An anatomical view of LBP generators and medication classes typically employed for treatment is presented in Table 1. With an integrated knowledge of the anatomy, physiology, chronology, and functional categories of LBP, the practitioner can best decide what pharmaceutical, physical medicine, or surgical tools may then be used to modify the nociceptive pathways that evolve into our patient's perception of pain.

Targeting Sites of Pharmaceutical Action

Clinical examination of LBP is a stepwise interpretation of presenting symptoms and physical signs. Underlying this assessment is a biologically driven change in physiology at a histochemical and neuroanatomical level. Low back pain represents a continuum of peripheral nociception to central perception. Behavioral response to this perception is the summation of this individual's experience of pain. Each step along the way represents an opportunity for pharmacological modification. A schematic listing of sites of neuroanatomical processes, reactions, and behavioral responses to spinal pain is presented in Table 2. Pharmacological agents from one or more of these classes listed in Table 3 may be considered in order to target these processing sites in the treatment of LBP.

PHARMACEUTICAL AGENTS EMPLOYED IN THE TREATMENT OF ACUTE LOW BACK PAIN

The World Health Organization (WHO) ladder of analgesic (Table 4, WHO 1986) management of cancer pain has provided a graphic algorithm for stepwise application of analgesics to malignant pain syndromes. Nonmalignant conditions such as LBP have been widely applied to this model. This graduated approach to

TABLE 2 Nocioceptive Mechanisms at the Peripheral to Central Nervous System Level

Nocioceptive process	Localization	Comments
Transduction	Cellular level in peripheral to axial musculoskeletal system including pain-sensitive lumbo-sacral spine and associated structures.	Release of nocioceptor chemicals: bradykinin, glutamate, calcitonin, gene-reactive proteins
Transmission	Primary afferents, A delta and unmyelinated C fibers	Chemical, thermal, or mechanical pain signals transmitted to dorsal root ganglion
Translation	Dorsal horn of spinal cord	Peripheral to central sensitization, wind-up occurring in rexed layers of dorsal horn
Transmission	Ascending spinal cord, spino-thalamic tracts	Activation of spinal cord transmission pathways
Perception	Thalamic and peri-aqueductal gray areas of cerebrum	Registration of peripheral nocioceptive stimulation in central nervous system
Descending inhibition	Dorsal lateral funiculus to dorsal horn	Inhibition mediated via serotonergic or possibly norepinephrine neurotransmitters
Cognitive-behavioral response	Higher cortical levels	Response to threat of either acute pain or persistence of chronic pain

chronic pain has served as a standard of care. The WHO model has been revised and adapted by many in the ensuing two decades but has come under some criticism for not being aggressive enough in the early stages of an acute pain syndrome threatening to become a chronic condition (4,5).

An additional model of stepwise introduction of analgesics for acute LBP was promoted by the Agency for Health Care Policy and Research (AHCPR) in 1994 (6). This federally funded agency with a mission to develop evidence-based health care standards underwent a name change to become the current Agency for Healthcare Research and Quality (AHRQ). The AHCPR Clinical Practice Guideline for acute LBP was an evidence-based meta-analysis of literature authored by a

TABLE 3 Classes of Pharmacologic Agents (Commonly Known as Adjuvants Except Opioids) with Potential to Treat Low Back Pain and Potential Sites of Activity

	Transduction	Transmission	Perception	Behavior
Alpha-2 blockers		✓		
Antidepressants			✓	✓
Antiepileptic drugs		✓	✓	
Antipsychotics				✓
Antispasticity agents		✓		
Anxiolytics				✓
Botulinum toxins	✓			
Capsaician	✓			
Corticosteroids	✓			
COX-2 inhibitors	✓		✓	
Local anesthetics		✓		
nsNSAIDs	✓			
Opioids	✓	✓	✓	✓

Abbreviations: COX-2, cyclo-oxygenase-2; nsNSAIDs, nonselective nonsteroidal anti-inflammatory drugs.

TABLE 4 Three-Step Analgesic Ladder (WHO) Caps

Step	Pain	Medication
III	Moderate to severe pain	Nonopioids plus strong opioids[a]
II	Mild to moderate pain	Nonopioids plus opioids for moderate pain[a]
I	Mild pain	Nonopioids

[a]In each step, adjuvants should be prescribed according to the clinical situations.

multidisciplinary group of practitioners and researchers. Ultimately, from a field of several thousand articles on acute LBP management, 360 references were scored as valid for inclusion in this project. This guideline became mired in controversy as practices of treating and medicating acute back pain varied widely on a regional, specialty orientation, and perhaps individual bases. The AHRQ now discredits this report based on evolution of new treatments and medications but likely because of this public controversy as well. Nevertheless, there is statistical power to this review. The AHRQ has not redone this analysis. However, with regard to acute LBP, and pharmacological treatment, many of the recommendations are applicable today and therefore included here with the caveat that no major changes in medications cited have occurred to date. Recommendations of the 1994 AHCPR for acute LBP are considered in Table 5. These findings are based on the following strength of evidence criteria established by this panel.

Additional statements were made by the AHCPR group regarding the lack of measured efficacy of colchicine and antidepressant medications for the treatment of acute LBP. This material is dated by the aforementioned development of new agents such as the cyclo-oxygenase selective inhibitors (COX-2) and dual mechanism antidepressants marketed for treatment of diabetic and postherpetic neuropathic (PHN) pain. However, neither of these agents is specifically indicated or demonstrated as clinically more effective than the existing traditional nonselective nonsteroidal anti-inflammatory drugs (nsNSAIDs) or antidepressants available in the 1990s for treatment of acute LBP. Tramadol was not available for use in the 1994 meta-analysis. Several studies have demonstrated that this nonscheduled mild opioid has been found to be effective in treatment of acute to chronic LBP (7). Statements regarding use of opioids and muscle relaxants remain valid today for treatment of acute LBP. Oral steroids may have a role in acute sciatic pain for rapid induction of anti-inflammatory effect and edema reduction (8).

CHRONIC LOW BACK PAIN MEDICATION OVERVIEW

In the rationale selection of medication, chronic LBP presents a challenge to even the most experienced practitioner. Eliciting a careful history, especially with regard to previous medication use, yields the most valuable information with regard to treatment decisions. Identifying pertinent medical comorbidities with potential for negative drug interactions is an essential part of today's defensive medicine strategy. Treating chronic LBP without a diligent medical review is tantamount to missing the trees when viewing the forest.

Red flags, with regard to pharmacological treatment of chronic pain, are usually found in the medical history. This would likely demonstrate failure of prior medication owing to poor compliance, too rapid titration, and timing with regard to layering of medications. Starting treatment with a potent opioid and then expecting efficacy with weaker opioids alone may be better managed by

TABLE 5   AHCPR Panel Ratings of Available Evidence Supporting Guideline Statements

NSAIDs: panel findings and recommendations
1. Acetaminophen is reasonably safe and is acceptable for treating patients with acute low back problems (Strength of evidence = C)
2. NSAIDs, including aspirin, are acceptable for treating patients with acute low back problems (Strength of evidence = B)
3. NSAIDs have a number of potential side effects. The most frequent complication is gastrointestinal irritation. The decision to use these medications can be guided by comorbidity, side effects, cost, and patient and provider preference (Strength of evidence = C)
4. Phenylbutazone is not recommended based on an increased risk for bone marrow suppression (Strength of evidence = C)

Muscle relaxants: panel findings and recommendations
1. Muscle relaxants are an option in the treatment of patients with acute low back problems. While probably more effective than placebo, muscle relaxants have not been shown to be more effective than NSAIDs (Strength of evidence = C)
2. No additional benefit is gained by using muscle relaxants in combination with NSAIDs over using NSAIDs alone (Strength of evidence = C)
3. Muscle relaxants have potential side effects, including drowsiness in up to 30% of patients. When considering the optional use of muscle relaxants, the clinician should balance the potential for drowsiness against a patient's intolerance of other agents. (Strength of evidence = C)

Opioid analgesics: panel findings and recommendations
1. When used only for a time-limited course, opioid analgesics are an option in the management of patients with acute low back problems. The decision to use opioids should be guided by consideration of their potential complications relative to other options (Strength of evidence = C)
2. Opioids appear to be no more effective in relieving low back symptoms than safer analgesics, such as acetaminophen or aspirin or other NSAIDs (Strength of evidence = C)
3. Clinicians should be aware of the side effects of opioids, such as decreased reaction time, clouded judgment, and drowsiness which lead to early discontinuation by as many as 35% of patients (Strength of evidence = C)
4. Patients should be warned about potential physical dependence and the danger associated with the use of opioids while operating heavy equipment or driving (Strength of evidence = C)

Oral steroids: panel findings and recommendations
1. Oral steroids are not recommended for the treatment of acute low back problems (Strength of evidence = C)
2. A potential for severe side effects is associated with the extended use of oral steroids or the short-term use of steroids in high doses (Strength of evidence = D)

Note: A = strong research-based evidence (multiple relevant and high-quality scientific studies). B = moderate research-based evidence [one relevant, high-quality scientific study or multiple adequate scientific studies (met minimal formal criteria for scientific methodology and relevance to population and specific method addressed in guideline statement)]. C = limited research-based evidence (at least one adequate scientific study in patients with low back pain). D = panel interpretation of information that did not meet inclusion criteria as research-based evidence.
Abbreviations: AHCPR, Agency for Health Care Policy and Research; NSAID, nonsteroidal anti-inflammatory drug.

using a daily NSAID or COX-2 agent and then sequentially adding a weaker opioid. Using an analgesic to treat an anxiety syndrome or sleep disturbance is often fraught with frustration, misunderstanding, and failure to achieve the goals of pharmaceutical intervention.

The following statements are provided as a review of the most current medications used in the pharmacological management of chronic LBP. All medication doses have been reviewed but require careful individualization by each prescribing physician and are subject to changes as knowledge and applications develop demanding a disclaimer with regard to doses stated by the authors.

Nonsteroidal Anti-inflammatory Drugs

Introduction

A large percentage of the population presenting to a physician's office with LBP already self-medicate with over-the-counter (OTC) NSAIDs. Once a patient with back pain has seen a doctor, there is an increased likelihood that they will be prescribed a NSAID (9).

With this class of medication used so commonly, it is imperative to have a strong working knowledge of indications and more recently published contraindications for use of NSAIDs including the more controversial COX-2 inhibitors.

Mechanism of Action

The primary property of this class of drugs is inhibition of COX. There are two major classes of COX enzymes. Cyclo-oxygenase-1 is expressed in most tissues, whereas COX-2 is elicited during inflammation. Both enzymes use arachidonic acid to generate the prostaglandin H_2 (PGH_2). A number of enzymes further modify this product to generate bioactive lipids (prostanoids) such as prostacyclin, thromboxane A_2, and prostaglandins D_2, E_2, and F_2, which influence several different organ systems.

Nonselective COX inhibition (i.e., ibuprofen and naproxen) block both COX-1 and COX-2 enzymes providing anti-inflammatory relief but carry the risk of erosive gastritis and gastrointestinal (GI) bleeding. Selective COX-2 inhibitors were developed to minimize GI toxicity because of the relative small expression of COX-2 enzymes in the GI tract and their abundant role in the inflammatory process.

Indications

Both traditional NSAIDs and selective COX-2 inhibitors have analgesic, anti-inflammatory, and antipyretic activity. There is strong evidence for the efficacy of NSAIDs in acute back pain, but only moderate support in chronic back pain (10). In randomized trials, the differences in pain after a patient has taken any NSAID as compared with placebo have generally been minimally detectable (11). Particularly, there are marginal improvements documented with use of a COX-2 inhibitor over placebo in chronic back pain (12). Despite this disarming information, a discussion of this class of drugs is warranted by the common use of these agents.

In selecting NSAID therapy, it should be noted that there is interindividual variation among patients in their response to a specific choice of drug. If a patient with chronic LBP does not respond to one NSAID, there is an equal likelihood that the patient may respond to another NSAID (Table 6) (13).

Contraindications

Nonselective NSAIDs (nsNSAIDs) inhibit platelet aggregation through inhibition of COX-1; therefore anticoagulation, coagulopathy, and thrombocytopenia are relative contraindications to their use. Gastrointestinal side effects, such as dyspepsia, ulceration, bleeding, and perforation are most commonly associated with the older nsNSAIDs. The addition of proton pump inhibitors or the synthetic prostaglandin analog misoprostol can provide some protection (14).

Risk factors for development of NSAID-associated gastroduodenal ulcers are advanced age, history of ulcer, concomitant use of corticosteroids, use of multiple NSAIDs, concomitant use of anticoagulants, and serious systemic disorders. Possible risk factors include infection with *Helicobacter pylori*, cigarette smoking, and alcohol consumption (15). There are some nsNSAIDs that are preferential to

TABLE 6   Nonopioid Oral Analgesics for Use in Chronic Low Back Pain

Medication	Average adult dose (mg)	Dose interval (hr)	Maximal daily dose (mg)	Comments
Acetaminophen	500–1000, 1250 in extended doses	4–6, extended 8-hr dose available	4000	Renal and hepato-toxicity considerations
Salicylates Aspirin	500–1000	4–6	4000	Avoid in children <12 with viral illness
Nonacetylated choline magnesium trisalicylate	1000–1500	12	2000–3000	No increase in bleeding time
Classes of NSAIDs				
Propionic acids				
Ibuprofen	200–400	4–6	2400	Available OTC
Naproxen	250–500	6–8	1500	OTC
Ketoprofen	25–50	6–8	300	OTC
Oxaprozin	600	12–24	1200	
Indolacetic acids				
Indomethacin	25–75	8–12	200	High incidence of GI and CNS intolerance
Etodolac	300–400	8–12	1000	
Enolic acids				
Meloxicam	7.5–15	24	15	Nonselective
Piroxicam	20–40	24	40	anti-inflammatories with both Cox-1 and Cox-2 associated risks
Napthylalkanlone				
Nabumetome	500–750	8–12	2000	More alkaline
COX-2				
Celecoxib	200–400	12–24	400	Additional cardiovascular considerations

Note: All doses are oral.
Abbreviations: CNS, central nervous system; COX-2, cyclo-oxygenase selective inhibitions; GI, gastrointestinal; NSAIDs, nonsteroidal anti-inflammatory drugs; OTC, over-the-counter.

COX-2 inhibition that have less incidence of GI injury (nebumetone, etodolac, and meloxiam) (16–18).

COX-2 inhibitors are thought of as having a better safety profile with regard to adverse GI effects (19), although there is some contradictory evidence to this concept (20). Either selective or nsNSAIDs can induce renal insufficiency, especially with underlying renal disease. All NSAIDs can cause an increase in blood pressure or water retention. Celecoxib cannot be used with people having sulfa allergy.

Considerations

With the limited evidence regarding NSAIDs versus placebo in treating LBP and the risk factors associated with nonselective and selective classes, what should physicians and their patients do? Current evidence and standards of care indicate that whether a nsNSAID or COX-2 inhibitors are used for treating chronic LBP, medical risk factors from the patient's history need to be carefully documented and calculated.

Without Concomitant Risk Factors

Adult patients with no known cardiovascular, hepatic, or renal disease may be started on either an nsNSAID or a COX-2 agent with medical oversight for two to four weeks. Symptoms should dictate the continuation of the agent based on the response of the patient to the medication. Potential intolerance to GI, hepatic, or renal side effects may be medically monitored with appropriate testing. Adverse symptoms alone should not be the sole factor in making a decision as to whether or not to discontinue the medication. Periodic re-evaluation of both positive (i.e., less back pain) and negative parameters (i.e., peripheral edema or GI intolerance) should be documented for those continuing therapy for more than 8 to 12 weeks. In the elderly, with no active cardiovascular, GI, or renal risk factors, an nsNSAID or COX-2 agent with a proton pump inhibitor or misoprostol may be used even for short-term (<10 days) therapy (21). Addition of a cyto-protective agent and cardiovascular risks of this class of medication should be discussed with patients and documented in the medical record.

Gastrointestinal Risk Factor

If anti-inflammatory treatment with a known healed gastroduodenal ulcer is necessary, concomitant administration of a COX-2 inhibitor with misoprostol or proton pump inhibitor is preferred (22). COX-2 inhibitors remain a rational choice for patients with low cardiovascular risk who have had serious GI events, especially from NSAIDs in the past (23).

Cardiovascular Risk Factors

With cardiovascular risk factors or chronic renal insufficiency, NSAIDs and the COX-2 agent celecoxib may be used cautiously with monitoring of clinical signs, symptoms, and laboratory values (24–27). A Federal Drug Agency (FDA)-sponsored joint meeting of the Arthritis Advisory Committee and the Drug Safety and Risk Management Committee in February 2005 recognized the relative risks and benefits of the COX-2 inhibitors, with pragmatic conclusions using available data (28). Cardiovascular risks of the available COX-2 medication were not deemed adverse when used in lower doses (i.e., 200 mg daily for celecoxib). Higher doses of these agents when used for long durations in high-risk individuals were discouraged. The cardiovascular effects of both COX-2 inhibitors and nsNSAIDs should be considered and prioritized in the total health picture for each individual. These agents should be used at the lowest dose for a limited duration and carefully reassessed for efficacy and safety in back pain patients (29).

These recommendations are far from straightforward, nor conclusive. Reviews of the literature strongly suggest a need for a reappraisal of the role of these agents with regard to different categories of LBP. Patients with mechanically inflamed or arthritic-related lumbar dysfunction may have greater pain relief from NSAIDs. Adverse events may likewise be minimized by a diligent medical history and clinical examination.

Muscle Relaxants

Introduction

Up to 80% of patients seeking a physician's consultation for LBP will receive a prescription for some type of medication. One-third of these patients will be prescribed some form of muscle relaxant, usually in concert with an NSAID (30). Evidence available from the acute pain population studies for use with chronic LBP will be helpful in determining whether your patient will benefit from this class of drugs.

Mechanism of Action
"Muscle relaxants" are a heterogeneous group of medications that can be used to treat LBP. This group of drugs covers several specific classes of medications. The two main categories are antispasmotics and antispasticity medications (Table 7).

Antispasmotics are used to reduce muscle spasm in painful LBP. In this category, there are benzodiazepines and nonbenzodiazepines. Benzodiazepines are used in many different areas of medicine to treat conditions such as anxiety, seizures, and for the purposes of our discussion on skeletal muscle relaxants. Typically for this class of medication, diazepam (Valium®, Hoffman-La Roche, Nutley, New Jersey, U.S.A.) is utilized extensively. Diazepam's mechanism of action is by facilitating postsynaptic effects of gamma aminobutyric acid (GABA)-A, resulting in an increase in inhibition at the presynaptic level. This benzodiazepine acts indirectly with a GABA-mimetic effect when GABA transmission is functional (31).

Nonbenzodiazepines are a class of sedative drugs working at the brain stem or spinal cord. The mechanism of action within the central nervous system is not well understood. Cyclobenzaprine (Flexeril®, McNeil, Fort Washington, Pennsylvania, U.S.A.) has structural similarities to tricyclic antidepressants with some antimuscarinic effects. Carisoprodol (Soma®, Medpointe, Somerset, New Jersey, U.S.A.), which metabolizes to meprobamate, has a moderate antispasmotic effect. Orphenadrine (Norflex®, 3M Pharmaceuticals, St. Paul, Minnesota, U.S.A.), similar to cyclobenzaprine, has anticholinergic activity but may more specifically function as an antagonist in N-methyl-D-aspartic acid (NMDA) channel pain mechanisms (32). Other common medicines include: metaxalone (Skelaxin®, King Pharmaceuticals, Bristol, Tennessee, U.S.A.) and methocarbamol (Robaxin®, Schwarz Pharma, Milwaukee, Wisconsin, U.S.A.).

Tizanidine (Zanaflex®, Acorda, Hawthorne, New York, U.S.A.) has spasmolytic actions as an alpha-2-adrenoreceptor agonist, similar to clonidine with fewer effects on blood pressure. It acts at both pre- and postsynaptic inhibition at the spinal cord. It also inhibits nociceptive transmission at the dorsal horn in animal models (33). Interestingly, it has gastroprotective effects, which may make it synergistic with NSAIDs (34). Antispasticity medications work at several places as well. Dantrolene sodium (Dantrium®, Procter & Gamble, Cincinnati, Ohio, U.S.A.) blocks calcium release from the sarcoplasmic reticulum, which interferes with excitation and contraction (actin–myosin interaction) coupling in skeletal muscle. Baclofen (Lioresal®, Novartis, Basel, Switzerland) is a presynaptic inhibitor; it is an analog of GABA (35). This acts as a neurotransmitter at the GABA B receptor. This agonist activity inhibits calcium influx into presynaptic terminals and suppresses release of excitatory neurotransmitters (36).

Indications
Several studies show that nonbenzodiazepine muscle relaxants are effective for acute LBP (37–41). There is limited evidence of any skeletal muscle relaxant being efficacious in chronic LBP. The only study found showed limited evidence effect with tetrazepam, which is not available in the United States (42).

TABLE 7 Muscle Relaxants

Classes	Generic (brand name)	Average adult dosage	Mechanism of action	Comments
Antispasmotics				
Benzodiazepines				
	Diazepam (Valium®)	2–10 mg, tid–qid	Postsynaptic effects of GABA-A, resulting in increase in inhibition at, the presynaptic level. It acts indirectly with GABA-mimetic effect when GABA transmission in functional	Drowsiness confusion, and hepatotoxicity
Nonbenzodiazepines				
	Cyclobenzaprine (Flexeril®)	5–10 mg/tid, max 60 mg/day	Structural similarities to tricyclic antidepressants with some antimuscarinic effects	Drowsiness, confusion, dry mouth, and transient hallucinations
	Carisoprodol (Soma®),	350 mg, tid and qhs	Metabolizes to meprobamate, has a moderate antispasmotic effect	Drowsiness, confusion, psychological and physical dependence; contraindicated in acute intermittent porphyria
	Chlorzoxazone (Eze D.S.®, Paraflex®, Parafon Forte DSC®, Relaxazone®, Remular®, Remular-S®, and Strifon Fort®)	500 mg, q6–8 h; daily max 3000 mg	Acts at the spinal cord and subcortical levels	Drowsiness and confusion
	Orphenadrine (Norflex®)	100 mg, q12 h	Similar to cyclobenzaprine; has anticholinergic activity but may more specifically function as an antagonist in NMDA channel pain mechanisms	Drowsiness, confusion, and dry mouth
	Metaxalone (Skelaxin®)	800 mg, tid–qid	Central acting, less sedation reported	Drowsiness and confusion

	Dosage	Mechanism	Side effects
Methocarbamol (Robaxin®)	1500 mg qid	CNS depression	Drowsiness and confusion
Tizanidine (Zanaflex®)	4–8 mg, q6-24 h; daily max 36 mg	Spasmolytic actions as an alpha-2 adrenoreceptor agonist, similar to clonidine with fewer effects on blood pressure. It acts at both pre and postsynaptic inhibition at the spinal cord. It also inhibits nociceptive transmission at the dorsal horn	Drowsiness, confusion, hypotension, dry mouth, headaches, and asthenia
Antispasticity			
Dantrolene sodium (Dantrium®)	25 mg bid, up to 100 mg bid–qid	Blocks calcium release from the sarcoplasmic reticulum, which interferes with excitation contraction (actin–myosin interaction) coupling in skeletal muscle	Drowsiness, confusion, cause muscle weakness, hepatotoxicity, and sudden death
Baclofen (Lioresal®)	5–20 mg, q8 h (start low, titrate); daily max 80 mg	Presynaptic inhibitor; analog of GABA. This acts as a neurotransmitter at the GABA B receptor. This agonist activity inhibits calcium influx into presynaptic terminals and suppresses release of excitatory neurotransmitters.	Drowsiness and confusion, must be withdrawn slowly

Abbreviations: CNS, central nervous system; GABA, gamma aminobutyric acid; NMDA, N-methyl-D-aspartic acid.

Contraindications/Side Effects
In this class of drugs, the benefit of muscle relaxation, which may compliment rehabilitation efforts, is offset by frequent sedating side effects. Of course, many sleep-deprived individuals may respond well to this sedation although quality of sleep on these agents has not been well studied. Some of the more common toxicities are included in Table 7. There may be some concern about abuse and dependency with all of the skeletal muscle relaxants (43). From a functional perspective, they may increase risk of falls and impair ability to drive automobiles or operate heavy machinery.

Considerations
Nonsteroidal anti-inflammatory drugs and muscle relaxants are widely used medications for back pain (44). Muscle relaxants have more side effects than traditional NSAIDs and do not show superior efficacy (45–48). Generally, they are not used as a monotherapy; usually these agents are taken with NSAIDs or opiates (49). Although as many as 40% of patients use muscle relaxants for greater than a year, there is little evidence-based medicine to support these prescription practices as being beneficial (50). Empirically, the authors have found that clinicians tend to prescribe these drugs as a once-a-day bedtime medication, but the manufacturer's package insert literature generally recommends that the medication be taken up to two to three times a day.

Opioids

Introduction
Opioids used to treat chronic LBP have created controversy in the clinical practice of pain medicine just as they have been controversial in the treatment of cancer pain worldwide (51). The use of opium, and subsequently its derivatives (opiates are semisynthetic opium alkaloids and opioids are synthetic preparations), for medicinal purposes goes back over 3000 years (52). Barriers to the use of opioids in LBP include fear of addiction or abuse, side effects including respiratory depression, lack of education in long-term management, that is, awareness of opioid rotation, and legal repercussions of prescribing a highly regulated and controlled substance. Nevertheless, opioids for chronic LBP remain in the current clinical treatment paradigm of severe nonmalignant back pain. There is growing data on the contribution of opioids to quality of life but not necessarily productivity or return to work with a chronic LBP impairment (53,54).

Mechanism of Action
Opioid receptors (mu, kappa, and delta) are glycoproteins identified at several sites of the peripheral nervous system, GI tract, bladder, and cardiopulmonary system to the central nervous tracts through the dorsal spinal column to the brain (55). Activation of these receptors endogenously or by exogenous opioids causes inhibition of pain impulses at any of these sites. Stimulation of opioid receptors is associated with hyperpolarization, causing reduction of excitatory neurotransmitter release. Agonist activity has a stabilizing effect making the cell membrane less susceptible to neurotransmitters. The action of morphine at selected opioid receptors is mediated by a second messenger G-protein (56). Equivalent oral doses of common opioids and half-life information is included in Table 8 with estimated ratios of morphine to equianalgesic doses of oral or transdermal opioid.

TABLE 8 Oral Estimated Equivalents

Opioid	Estimated oral/ transdermal 20−30 mg of morphine to equianalgesic relative potency	Duration of activity expected/plasma half life (hrs)	Comments
Morphine	20−30 mg (1 : 1)	4−7/1.5−4.5	Sustained release morphine available in variety of formulas with 8−24-hr duration
Codeine	200 mg (1 : 0.1)	3−6/2.5−3.5	With or without APAP ($\pm$)
Tramadol	100−150 mg (1 : 0.2)	4−6/6	Inhibits 5HT and NE reuptake
Hydromorphone	7.5 mg (1 : 5)	3−4/2.5	Short acting only
Oxycodone	10−20 mg (1 : 2)	3−6/3.5	APAP ($\pm$)
Oxycodone CR	20 mg (1 : 2)	12	Same as above
Levorphanol	4 mg (1 : 5)	3−6/12−16	Half-life sustained
Methadone	10−20 mg (1 : 5−10)	4−8/8−75	Accumulates in tissues with high volume of distribution and protein binding
Fentanyl	25−50 mcg patch (1 : 150)	72/22	Steady state after 36−48 hr

Abbreviations: 5HT, serotonin; APAP, acetaminophen; CR, controlled release; NE, norepinephrine.
Source: From Ref. 56.

Indications

Use of opioids has traditionally been associated with the loss of hope for recovery. On the contrary, opioids in the context of chronic LBP rehabilitation may provide a window of opportunity. These agents may facilitate renewed efforts at physical exertion that would otherwise be painfully improbable. Randomized, double blind trials of morphine in doses up to 120 mg a day in the treatment of musculoskeletal pain was shown to convey analgesic benefit with limited risk of addiction after nine weeks (57). However, psychological and functional improvements were less likely to be measured positively in this same study. Transdermal fentanyl was equal to oral sustained release morphine in a study demonstrating significant relief of chronic LBP (58). Breakthrough opioid pain medications are utilized to keep pace with the day-to-day fluctuations in pain thresholds. Maintaining a chronic LBP patient on the lowest daily dose of a combination of sustained and immediate release opioids is a goal of chronic pain management schemes. Short-acting opioids were recognized by the AHCPR as having a limited role in treatment of acute back pain. Short-acting agents alone without a sustained opioid may suffice for individual circumstances of chronic pain allowing a reduction in total daily dosage of potent opioid agents (59).

Contraindications

Opioid use was associated with greater self-reported disability and poorer function in both women and men with chronic spine pain (60). The frequently stated caveats of prescribing opioids often begin with the dictum "balance risks and benefits." High-risk individuals are identified by a careful medical history and in particular a careful medication history. Previous substance use and addiction behavior raises red flags as does rapid self-titration of medications previously prescribed. A history of hepatitis raises the specter of intravenous drug abuse now or in the past. Any of these scenarios set the stage for further investigations as to the risks and benefits of opioid prescription.

Considerations
Opioids for the treatment of a nonmalignant condition have suffered pendulum swings of patients' demands and societal concerns over the years. The pain practitioner working in the realm of LBP is frequently faced with the dilemma of choosing the medical agent that will rapidly address the suffering of a LBP patient. Opioids fit the bill for many but create a new dilemma for a significant few. Portnoy has said there is "no litmus test" for the use of opioids in any pain condition (61). At present, we are treating the behavior of pain, which varies considerably, without guidelines based on the objective pathology of lumbar spine dysfunction (62). Development of an entrance and exit strategy for the introduction and eventual weaning from opioids for these patients must be constructed by the responsible pain practitioner. This includes patient education and narcotic agreements. Documentation and opioid-oriented progress notes are required to substantiate legitimate use of these controlled substances. Without the support of informed office staff members and the ability to meet documentation criteria, this prescription practice should be deferred to pain specialists who have demonstrated their capacity to meet these regulations.

Adjunctive Pharmaceutical Agents for the Treatment of Chronic Low Back Pain
Over the last decade, there has been a burgeoning off-label practice of treating chronic pain (63). In 2003 when total U.S. prescription-drug spending was about $216 billion, studies found that off-label use accounted for 40% to 50% of all prescriptions (64). Studies supporting the off-label medical management of LBP have been extensively reported. Nevertheless, FDA approval for the use of antineuropathic pain agents such as the antiepileptic drugs (AEDs) in the treatment of chronic radicular nerve pain from lumbar stenosis or other compressive spinal lesions is lacking. A review of the most frequently prescribed albeit "off-label" agents employed in the treatment of LBP is therefore provided for use at the reader's discretion.

Topical Agents
Topical agents have always had an appeal to the patient who could self apply a focal treatment and the practitioner in the avoidance of many systemic side effects of pain medications. Topical lidocaine 5% in the form of an adhesive patch (Lidoderm®, Endo Pharmaceuticals, Chadds Ford, Pennsylvania, U.S.A.) has been demonstrated in the treatment of LBP. In an effort to supplant the loss of COX-2 agents, a head-to-head study with lidocaine patches 5% and celecoxib for LBP patients ($n = 36$) was conducted by Endo. Fifty percent of the patients receiving topical lidocaine reported a 30% or greater improvement in daily pain intensity compared with 42% of the celecoxib group. Both groups also reported an improvement in mood, walking ability, and sleep after four weeks of treatment (65).

Antidepressants
Antidepressants have long been employed for treatment of chronic pain. LBP has responded to tricyclic antidepressants (imipramine, desipramine, and doxepin) in placebo-controlled studies (66,67). Questions remain regarding the role of these agents as singularly antinociceptive without the mechanism of the antidepressant

effect. The advent of dual action, norepinephrine and serotonergic venlaflaxin (Effexor®, Wyeth, Madison, New Jersey, U.S.A.), and duloxitine (Cymbalta®, Lilly, Indianapolis, Indiana, U.S.A.) reuptake inhibitors appears to offer an advantage over single neurotransmitter active agents for treatment of pain. Duloxitine has been FDA approved for both depression and painful diabetic neuropathy (PDN) and PHN. There are frequent mentions in the marketing literature for these agents regarding somatic pain complaints associated with depression. Logic would lead us to conclude that neuropathic pain from PDN or PHN may be similar enough to painful lumbar radiculopathy or lumbar spinal arachnoiditis to apply this pharmaceutical class of agents to these conditions. However, there are no convincing studies to date that support this line of thought (68).

Antiepileptic Drugs
These are increasingly used in the treatment of neuropathic pain as indicated by the U.S. FDA for trigeminal neuralgia (carbamazepine), PHN (gabapentin and pregabalin), and PDN (pregabalin) seen in Table 9. The second and most recent generation of AEDs created a firestorm of professional and public attention in part because of their documented effectiveness (69) and owing to alleged marketing of "off-label" uses. Both first- and second-generation AEDs target the transmission pathways referred to earlier in this chapter in Tables 1 and 2. These agents are thought to limit neuronal excitation and enhance inhibition (70). Relevant sites of action include voltage-gated ion channels (i.e., sodium and calcium channels), ligand-gated ion channels, the excitatory receptors for glutamate and N-methyl-D-aspartate, and the inhibitory receptors for GABA and glycine (71). Despite the opportunity for employing these agents in the neuropathic component of acute or chronic low back with sciatic nerve symptoms, there are no randomized, placebo-controlled, cross-over studies that support monotherapy or a protocol for combined therapy in treatment of these disorders (72).

ESTABLISHING OUTCOMES OF PHARMACOLOGIC TREAMENT OF LOW BACK PAIN

As in all medication decisions, establishing goals and determining outcome measures for medication treatment is fundamental to any rehabilitative approach. Gathering functional information at the onset of therapy sets a foundation for measuring the success or failure of a particular pharmaceutical agent. A core set of information for outcome measurement includes a patient perception of quality of pain via a verbal or visual analog scale. This may evaluate pain at the moment of the interview or in general over the preceding days or weeks. A skilled practitioner will sometimes be challenged to draw out even these basic concepts from patients who may not have the language to describe their very personal experience of pain.

Standards have been established for quality of life measures in the assessment of chronic LBP that are reasonably easily implemented in most office settings. The Oswestry, Rowland-Morris, McGill, and other validated LBP-oriented questionnaires are in the public domain requiring no special permissions for reproduction (73–75). Justification for instituting pharmaceutical management with long-term implications on each individual's health increasingly demands this level of documentation. Comparison of this type of quantitative data set often spells the difference to insurers and third parties who may have to foot the bill for expensive long-term pharmacotherapy.

TABLE 9 Antiepileptic Drugs as Proposed Off-Label Adjuncts in Treatment of Low Back Pain with Neuropathic Features

Antiepileptic medications[a]	Typical dosages for neuropathic low back pain	Proposed mechanism of action	Comments
First-generation agents			
Carbamazepine	200 mg/day × 7 days up to 1200 mg/day in divided doses	Blockade of sodium channels	Therapeutic serum levels may be obtained. Side effects include: dizziness, diplopia, nausea, and aplastic anemia
Phenytoin	100 mg at bedtime; increase weekly up to 500 mg/day	Decrease high-frequency repetitive firing of action potentials by enhancing sodium-channel inactivation	Therapeutic serum levels may be obtained. Side effects include: dizziness, nystagmus, ataxia, nausea, rash, hematologic dyscrasias, and hepatotoxicity
Second-generation agents			
Gabapentine	100–300 mg at bedtime; increase by 100–300 mg increments every three days to 1800 mg in 3–4 divided doses	Blockade of sodium and calcium channels	Somnolence, dizziness, GI symptoms, peripheral edema, and weight gain
Pregabalin	50–150 mg up to twice daily	Blockade of ligand-gated sodium and calcium channels	Somnolence, dizziness, GI symptoms, peripheral edema, and weight gain
Lamotrigine	50 mg per day; increase by 50 mg every two weeks up to 400 mg daily in divided doses	Blockade of calcium channels	Dizziness, ataxia, constipation, nausea, and rarely life-threatening rashes

[a]Titrate each agent to efficacy and tolerance of side effects.
Abbreviation: GI, gastrointestinal.

ADVANCES IN ANALGESIC MEDICATIONS USED IN TREATMENT OF CHRONIC LOW BACK PAIN

The major classes of analgesic agents available to treat chronic LBP have not changed much over the last decade (76,77). Analgesics (narcotic and non-narcotic), anti-inflammatories, muscle relaxants, and adjuvants are applied to the problem of LBP countless times each day despite the lack of evidence-based studies in this important area. In the last 10 years, the pharmaceutical industry has focused on repackaging more than producing commercially available alternatives to the standards of the WHO analgesic ladder. Opioids have been reformulated to provide extended-release packaging. This does allow more potent doses in time released delivery systems. Although this strategy is deemed effective for analgesia, it is fraught with controversy and potential for misuse (78). Transdermal, transmucosal, intranasal, and proposed effervescent delivery systems for opioids have been devised. Another key area in the pharmacological treatment armamentarium of chronic LBP will be the intrathecal delivery of novel antinocioceptive agents such as ziconotide, a conotoxin derived from a sea snail. These developments were not covered in this chapter, which focused on available oral or transdermal compounds. Because of the ubiquitous penetration of LBP in society, the allure of this market to scientists, clinicians, and pharmaceutical companies will no doubt produce new, effective, and hopefully ever safer analgesics, anti-inflammatories, muscle relaxants, and adjunctive medications.

In conclusion, LBP, whether it is acute or chronic, appears to be an inherent part of the human experience. For this, there is no cure. Back pain must be recognized and treated as a multifaceted disease not an anatomical aberration that can be simply ablated by procedural intervention. Perhaps the best tincture to apply to this condition is the proverbial ounce of prevention. To date, we have yet to reach an evidence-based consensus as to what a more specific prevention or pharmaceutical pathway should entail. This chapter should provide the reader with the stem cells of information regarding the pharmacological treatment of LBP from a multidimensional perspective. Utilizing medication, based on the outlines provided here in the context of the hologram of pain, can be a mutually and reasonably satisfying experience for the patient with LBP as well as the clinician.

REFERENCES

1. Kolata G. With Costs Rising, Treating Back Pain often Seems Futile. NY Times. http://query.nytimes.com/gst/fullpage.html?sec = health&res = 9 A04EFDF173AF93AA35751C0A9629C8B63 (accessed January 2006).
2. Xuemei L, Pietroban R, Sun SX, et al. Estimates and patterns of direct health care expenditures among individuals with back pain in the United States. Spine 2003; 29(1):79–86.
3. Ray AL. Pain perception in the older patient: using the pain hologram to understand neck and shoulder pain. Geriatrics 2002; 57:22–26.
4. Jadad AR, Browman GP. The WHO analgesic ladder for cancer pain management: stepping up the quality of its evaluation. JAMA 1995; 274:1870–1873.
5. Eisenberg E, Marinangeli F, Birkhahn J, et al. Time to modify the WHO analgesic ladder? Pain Clinical Updates, Int Assoc Study Pain 2005; 8(5):1–4.
6. Bigos S, Bowyer O, Braen G, et al. Acute Low Back Problems in Adults. Clinical Practice Guideline No. 14. AHCPR Publication No. 95-0642. Rockville, MD: Agency for Health Care Policy and Research, Public Health Service, U.S. Department of Health and Human Services. December 1994. Available at http://www.ncbi.nlm.nih.gov/books/bv.fcgi?rid = hstat6.chapter.25870 (accessed January 2006).
7. Schnitzer TJ, Gray WL, Paster RZ, et al. Efficacy of tramadol in treatment of chronic low back pain. J Rheumatol 2000; 27(3):772–778.
8. Green, LN. Dexamethasone in the management of symptoms due to herniated lumbar disc. J Neurol Neurosurg Psychiatry 1975; 38:1211–1217.
9. Cherkin DC, Wheeler KJ, Barlow W, et al. Medication use for low back pain in primary care. Spine 1998; 23:607–614.
10. Van Tulder MW, Koes BW, Bouter LM. Conservative treatment of acute and chronic non-specific low back pain: a systemic review of randomized controlled trial of the most common interventions. Spine 1997; 22:2128–2156.

11. Van Tulder MW, Scholten RJ, Koes BW, et al. Nonsteroidal anti-inflammatory drugs for low back pain: a systemic review within the framework of the Cochrane Collaboration Back Review Group. Spine 2000; 25:2501–2513.
12. Coats TL, Borenstein DG, Nangia NK, et al. Effects of valdecoxib in the treatment of lower back pain: results of a randomized, placebo-controlled trial. Clin Ther 2004; 26:1249–1260.
13. Ashburn MA, Lipman AG, Carr D, et al. Principles of Analgesics Use in the Treatment of Acute Pain and Cancer Pain. 5th ed. Glenview, IL: American Pain Society, 2003.
14. Graham DY, Agrawal NM, Campbell DR, et al. Ulcer prevention in long-term users of nonsteroidal anti-inflammatory drugs: results of double-blind randomized, multicenter, active- and placebo-controlled study of misoprostol versus lansprazole. NSAID-Associated Gastric Ulcer Prevention Study Group. Arch Intern Med 2002; 162:169–175.
15. Wolfe MM, Lichtenstein DR, Singh G. Medical progress: gastrointestinal toxicity of non-steroidal anti-inflammatory drugs. N Engl J Med 1999; 24:1888–1899.
16. Roth SH, Tindall EA, Jain AK, et al. A controlled study comparing the effects of nabume-tone, ibuprofen, and ibuprofen plus misoprostol on the upper gastrointestinal tract mucosa. Arch Intern Med 1993; 153:2565–2571.
17. Schattenkirchner M. An Updated safety profile of etodolac in several thousand patients. Eur J Rheumatol Inflamm 1990; 10:56–65.
18. Distel M, Mueller C, Bluhmki E, et al. Safety of meloxicam: a global analysis of clinical trials. Br J Rheumatol 1996; 35(S):68–77.
19. Simon L, Lipman A, Caudill-Slosberg M, et al. Guidelines for the Management of Pain in Osteoarthritis, Rheumatoid Arthritis and Juvenile Chronic Arthritis. 2nd ed. APS Clinical Practice Guidelines Series, No. 2. Glenview, IL: American Pain Society, 2002.
20. Chan FK, Hung LC, Suen BY, et al. Celecoxib versus diclofenic and omeprazole in redu-cing the risk of recurrent ulcer bleeding in patients with arthritis. N Eng J Med 2002; 347:2104–2110.
21. Kaplan, RJ. Current status of nonsteroidal anti-inflammatory drugs in physiatry. Am J Phys Med Rehabil 2005; 84:885–894.
22. Wolfe MM, Lichtenstein DR, Singh G. Medical progress: gastrointestinal toxicity of non-steroidal anti-inflammatory drugs. N Engl J Med 1999; 24:1888–1899.
23. Fitzgerald GA. Coxibs and cardiovascular disease. N Engl J Med 2004; 351:1709–1719.
24. Reig E. Tramadol in musculoskeletal pain: a survey. Clin Rheumatol 2002; 21(suppl): S9–S11.
25. Podichetty VK, Mazanec DJ, Biscup RS. Chronic non-malignant musculoskeletal pain in older adults: clinical issues and opioid intervention. Postgrad Med J 2003; 79:627–633.
26. Gambaro G, Perazella MA. Adverse renal effects of anti-inflammatory agents: evaluation of selective and nonselective cyclooxygenase inhibitors. J Inter Med 2003; 253:643–652.
27. Bleumink GS, Feenstra J, Sturkenboom MC, et al. Nonsteroidal anti-inflammatory drugs and heart failure. Drug 2003; 63:524–534.
28. American College of Rheumatology: Hot Line: The Safety of COX-2 Inhibitors Delibe-rations from the February 16–18, 2005 FDA Meeting. Available at: http//www.rheumatology.org/publications/hotline/0305NSAIDs.asp (accessed January 2006).
29. Bennett JS, Daugherty A, Herrington D, et al. The use of nonsteroidal anti-inflammatory drugs (NSAIDs): a science advisory from the American Heart Association. Circulation 2005; 111:1713–1716.
30. Cherkin DC, Wheeler KJ, Barlow W, et al. Medication use for low back pain in primary care. Spine 1998; 23:607–614.
31. Miller RD, Katzung BG. Skeletal muscle relaxants. In: Basic & Clinical Pharmacology. 8th ed. New York: McGraw Hill Publishing, 2001:457–511.
32. Sureda FX, Gabriel C, Pallas M, et al. In vitro and in vivo protective effects of orphena-drine on glutamate neurotoxicity. Neuropharmacology 1999; 38(5):671–677.
33. Nance PW, Young RR. Antispasticity medications. Phys Med Rehabil Clin NA 1999; 10(2):337–355; Philadelphia: WB Saunders.
34. Sirdalud Terelin Asian Pacific Group. Efficacy and gastroprotective effects of tizanidine plus diclofenac versus placebo and diclofenac in patients with painful muscle spasms. Curr Ther Res 1998; 59:13–22.

35. Katz RT, Dewald J, Schmit BD. Spasticity. In: Braddom RL, ed. Physical Medicine and Rehabilitation. 2nd ed. Philadelphia: WB Saunders, 2000:592–615.

36. Price CW, Wilkin GP, Turnbull MJ, Bowery NG. Are baclofen sensitive GABA$_B$ receptors present on primary afferent terminals of the spinal chord? Nature 1984; 307:71–74

37. Baratta RR. A double-blind study of cyclobenzaprine and placebo in the treatment of acute musculoskeletal conditions of the low back. Curr Ther Res 1982; 32:646–652.

38. Berry H, Hutchinson DR. Tizanidine and ibuprofen in acute lower-back pain: results of a double-blind muticentre study in general practice. J Int Med Res 1988; 16:83–91.

39. Casale R. Acute lower back pain: symptomatic treatment with a muscle relaxant drug. Clin J Pain 1988; 4:81–88.

40. Dapas F, Hartman SF, Martinez L, et al. Baclofen for the treatment of acute low-back syndrome: a double blind comparison with placebo. Spine 1985; 10:345–349.

41. Hindle TH. Comparison of carisoprodol, butabarbital, and placebo in the treatment of the low back syndrome. Calif Med 1972; 117:7–11.

42. Arbus L, Fajadet B, Aubert D, et al. Activity of tetrazepam (myolastin) in low back pain: a double blind trial v. placebo. Clin Trials J 1990; 27:258–267.

43. Elder NC. Abuse of skeletal muscle relaxants. Am Fam Physician 1991; 44:1223–1226.

44. Hart LG, Deyo RA, Cherkin DC. Physician office visits for lower back pain: frequency, clinical evaluation, and treatment patterns from the U.S. national survey. Spine 1995; 20:11–19.

45. Deyo R. Drug therapy for back pain: which drugs help which patients? Spine 1996; 21:2840–2849.

46. Bernstein E, Carey TS, Garrett JM. The use of muscle relaxant medications in acute low back pain. Spine 2004; 29:1346–1351.

47. Van Tulder MW, Scholten RJ, Koes BW, et al. Nonsteroidal anti-inflammatory drugs for low back pain: a systemic review within the framework of the Cochrane Collaboration Back Review Group. Spine 2000; 25:2501–2513.

48. Van Tulder, Touray T, Furlan AD, et al. Muscle relaxants for nonspecific lower back pain: a systemic review within the framework of Cochrane collection. Spine 2003; 28: 1978–1992.

49. Dillon C, Paulose-Ram R, Hirsch R, et al. Skeletal muscle relaxants use in the US: data from the Third National Health and Nutrition Examination Survey (NHANES III). Spine 2004; 29:892–896.

50. Cherkin DC, Wheeler KJ, Barlow W, et al. Medication use for low back pain in primary care. Spine 1998; 23:607–614.

51. Selva C. International control of opioids for medical use. Eur J Palliat Care 1997; 4(6):194–198.

52. Loeser JD. Opiophobia and opiophilia. In: Meldrum M, ed. Opioids and Pain Relief: A Historical Perspective. Progress in Pain Research and Management. Vol. 25. Seattle: IASP Press, 2003:1–4.

53. Fillingim RB, Doleys DM, Edwards RR, et al. Clinical characteristics of chronic back pain as a function of gender and oral opioid use. Spine 2003; 28:143–150.

54. Moulin DE, Iezzi A, Amireh R, et al. Randomized trial of oral morphine for chronic non-cancer pain. Lancet 1996; 347:143–147.

55. Sweeney C, Bruera E. Opioids. In: Melzack R, Wall PD, eds. Handbook of Pain Management. A clinical companion to Wall and Melzak's Textbook of Pain. Edinburgh: Churchill Livingstone, 2003:377–396.

56. Twycross RG. Opioids. In: Wall PD, Melzack R, eds. Textbook of Pain. 4th ed. London: Churchill Livingston Harcourt, 1999:1187–1214.

57. Moulin DE, Iezzi A, Amireh R, et al. Randomized trial of oral morphine for chronic non-cancer pain. Lancet 1996; 347:143–147.

58. Allan A, Ute R, Simpson K, et al. Transdermal fentanyl versus sustained release oral morphine in strong-opioid naïve patients with chronic low back pain randomized trial. Spine 2005; 30(22):2484–2490.

59. Simon S. Opioids and Treatment of Chronic Pain: Understanding Pain Patterns and the Role for Rapid-Onset Opioids. MedGenMed 2005, 7 (4):54. http://www.medscape.com/viewprogram/4756_pnt (accessed January 2006).

60. Fillingim RB, Doleys DM, Edwards RR, et al. Clinical characteristics of chronic back pain as a function of gender and oral opioid use. Spine 2003; 28:143–150.

61. Portenoy RK. Opioid therapy for nonmalignant pain. In: Fields HL, Liebeskind JC, eds. Progress in Pain Research and Management. Vol. 1. Seattle: IASP Press, 1994:247–287.

62. Turk DC, Okifuji A. What factors affect physicians' decisions to prescribe opioids for chronic noncancer pain patients? Clin J Pain 1997; 13(4):330–336.

63. Angarola RT, Joranson DE. Off-label uses of prescription drugs in pain management. APS Bull 1995; 5(1):14–15.

64. Armstrong D, Mathews AW. Wall Street J, May 14, 2004; Page B1.

65. Nicholson B, Galer B, Oleka N, et al. A randomized, open-label study comparing the efficacy and safety of lidocaine patch 5% with celecoxib 200 mg in patients with chronic axial low-back pain. Am Coll Rheum Ann Sci Semin 2005; poster session C, 1384-poster section 160.

66. Jenkins DG, Ebbut AF, Evans CD. Tofranil in the treatment of low back pain. J Int Med Res 1976; 4(suppl 2):28–40.

67. Egbunike IG, Chaffee BJ. Antidepressants in the management of chronic pain syndromes. Pharmacotherapy 1990; 10:262–270.

68. Salerno SM, Browning R, Jackson JL. The effect of antidepressant treatment on chronic back pain: a meta-analysis. Arch Intern Med 2002; 162(1):19–24.

69. Backonja M, Beydoun A, Edwards KR, et al. Gabapentin for the symptomatic treatment of painful neuropathy in patients with diabetes mellitus; a randomized controlled trial. JAMA 1998; 280:1831–1836.

70. Macdonald RL, Kelly KM. Antiepileptic drug mechanisms of action. Epilepsia 1995; 36(suppl):S2–S12.

71. Maizels M, McCarberg B. Antidepressants and antiepileptic drugs for chronic non-cancer pain. Am Fam Physician 2005; 71(3):483–494.

72. Gilron I, Bailey JM, Tu D, et al. Morphine, gabapentin, or their combination for neuropathic pain. N Engl J Med 2005; 352:13–31.

73. Melzack R. The McGill pain questionnaire: major properties and scoring methods. Pain 1975; 1:277–299.

74. Fairbank JC, Couper J, Davies JB, et al. The Oswestry low back pain disability questionnaire. Physiotherapy 1980; 66:271–273.

75. Roland M, Morris R. A study of the natural history of back pain: part I: development of a reliable and senback pain. Spine 1983; 8:141–144.

76. Malanga GA, Nadler SF, Lipetz JS. Pharmacological treatment of low back pain. Phys Med Rehab: State of the Art Reviews, Philadelphia, Hanley and Belfus 1999; 13(3):531–549.

77. Robinson JP, Brown PB. Medication in low back pain. Phys Med Rehabil Clin NA 1991; 2(1):97–126.

78. Bartleson JD. Evidence for and against the use of opioid analgesics for chronic non-malignant low back pain. Pain Med 2002; 3(3):260–271.

2 Office-Based Aspiration and Injection of Joints and Soft Tissues

Jeffrey W. R. Dassel
Thomas Jefferson University Hospital, Philadelphia, Pennsylvania, U.S.A.

Gene Hong
Drexel University College of Medicine, Philadelphia, Pennsylvania, U.S.A.

INTRODUCTION

This chapter reviews general principles and proper techniques of aspiration and injection of joints and soft tissues. Indications and contraindications, preparation and materials, interpretation of aspirate fluid, postprocedural care, and possible side-effects are also discussed.

Aspiration and injection of joints and soft tissues are important adjunctive or, at times, definitive diagnostic and therapeutic procedures. The diagnosis of infectious or crystal-induced arthritis is made upon synovial fluid analysis, and aspiration of a tensely swollen joint may immediately relieve discomfort. Both the immediate and long-term response to a properly placed injection can further support a diagnosis and guide management, while a corticosteroid injection can provide dramatic pain relief. Inflammatory and crystal-induced arthritides, bursitis, and other conditions typically respond very well to corticosteroid injections. Corticosteroid or hyaluronic acid injections are also considered for degenerative conditions when other measures have failed to provide adequate relief or return of function (1).

With appropriate knowledge of anatomy and procedural technique, aspiration and injection of joints and soft tissues can be easily and safely performed. Despite this, many primary practitioners complete residency feeling uncomfortable performing these procedures. A study by Nelson et al. (2) found that 65% of practicing general internists in the United States felt that they needed more training in performing arthrocenteses. Overall, 35% did not perform this service. This statistic has been replicated internationally, demonstrating that only 54% to 68% of primary care providers perform aspiration or injection of joints or soft tissues. Among the most commonly cited barriers was a lack of practical training or confidence in skills (3–5).

HISTORY

The diagnosis and treatment of musculoskeletal and rheumatic disorders date to the time of Hippocrates. A review by Rodnan details writings by Hippocrates, Celsus, Galen, and others that describe synovial fluid, and the anatomy and physiology of joints and synovial membranes (6). Diagnostic aspiration began to be practiced with increasing frequency in the early twentieth century, with texts describing the procedure first being published at this time. Initial attempts at using injection

TABLE 1   Joint and Soft Tissue Disorders Amenable to Office-Based Aspirations or Injections

Osteoarthritis
Inflammatory arthritis/synovitis
   Crystal-induced arthropathies
   Rheumatoid arthritis, juvenile rheumatoid arthritis
   Collagen vascular disorders (systemic lupus erythematosus, mixed connective tissue disorder)
   Sarcoidosis
   Seronegative spondyloarthropathies (psoriatic arthritis, Reiter's syndrome, inflammatory bowel
   disease, ankylosing spondylitis)
   Traumatic
Hemarthrosis
Tendonitis/tenosynovitis
   Supraspinatus, bicipital tendonitis
   de Quervain's, digital flexor (trigger finger), intersection tenosynovitis
Epicondylitis
   Medial (golfer's elbow), lateral (tennis elbow) epicondylitis
Bursitis
   Subacromial, olecranon, trochanteric, ischiogluteal, prepatellar, pes anserine bursitis
Adhesive capsulitis
Plantar fasciitis
Entrapment neuropathies
   Carpal, cubital tunnel syndromes
Ganglion/synovial cysts
Myofascial pain syndromes/trigger points
Morton's neuroma

Source: From Refs. 7, 18, 21, 22, 33, 42, 107.

therapy to ameliorate symptoms and halt or reverse disease progression had poor results, often with significant side-effects. Agents used early on included formalin, glycerin, lipiodol, lactic acid, liquid petrolatum, and autologous liquefied fat (7). Since then, many other agents, such as intra-articular salicylates, antibiotics, phenylbutazone, gold, and orgotein superoxide dismutase, have been tried (8). Local anesthetics demonstrated temporary relief, but it was not until corticosteroids were injected in the 1950s that a medication providing substantial benefit was found (7).

Thorn was first credited with intra-articular injection of steroids in 1950 (9). The first cortisone intra-articular injections, performed in rheumatoid arthritis patients, showed disappointing, inconsistent results. In 1951, Hollander injected its active metabolite, hydrocortisone into the knees of rheumatoid arthritis sufferers and noted dramatic, prolonged relief (10). Numerous publications have since chronicled the response of hundreds of thousands of patients to intra-articular and soft-tissue corticosteroid therapy and demonstrated the beneficial effect of these medications on the many inflammatory and noninflammatory conditions listed in Table 1. Hyaluronic acid viscosupplementation has been the most recently developed class of widely used intra-articular therapy. It has been used in Europe for several decades, and was approved for use in the United States in 1997.

GENERAL PRINCIPLES
Aspiration
Any joint, either with or without effusion, should be aspirated if synovial fluid analysis will assist in determining the etiology of an arthropathy. Aspirate analysis

TABLE 2 Indications/Contraindications to Aspiration

Indications
Undiagnosed arthritis with or without effusion
Suspected septic arthritis (may be repeated for as part of treatment course)
Suspected ligamentous injury or occult intra-articular fracture
Symptomatic relief of tense effusion or hemarthrosis
Improve effect of corticosteroid or hyaluronic acid injections
Determination if laceration communicates with joint space
Relative contraindications
Overlying cellulitis, psoriasis, or abraded skin
Bacteremia
Bleeding disorder
Joint prosthesis
Joint anatomically inaccessible without imaging
Noncooperative patient

Source: From Refs. 7, 15, 22, 74, 108.

will clarify if an arthropathy is inflammatory or not, definitively diagnose crystal-induced and septic arthridites, and support the diagnosis of traumatic ligamentous injury or prove occult intra-articular fracture. Aspiration of an effusion frequently relieves pain of a tensely swollen joint, and is commonly performed prior to injection of corticosteroids or hyaluronic acid. This practice has been demonstrated to improve response and duration in various arthridites (11–13). Some have proposed that aspiration of hemarthrosis prevents possible adhesion or band formation, but it has been noted that a single occurrence of hemarthrosis in an otherwise healthy knee will spontaneously reabsorb, and does not cause long-term joint damage (14–16).

Contrary to injection, there are no absolute contraindications to aspiration. Indications and relative contraindications, and the interpretation of various synovial fluid properties are presented in Tables 2–4. Of particular note, aspiration is considered to be relatively safe even in the presence of anticoagulation therapy or bleeding disorders. Thumboo et al. (17) have estimated the risk of significant hemarthrosis in patients receiving warfarin therapy within international normalized ratio (INR) values up to 4.5 to be less than 10%.

Complications encountered in aspiration are very rare, but do include iatrogenic infection, articular cartilage injury, bleeding and hemarthrosis, injury to soft tissue or neurovascular structures, vaso-vagal episodes, and hypersensitivity to cleansing solutions or anesthetics. Rates of these complications parallel those noted for corticosteroid injection in Table 5.

Local Anesthetics
Local anesthetics are used alone in diagnostic injections, or in combination with corticosteroids for therapeutic injections. As a diagnostic modality, the response to a properly administered local anesthetic can be used to either support or refute a tentative diagnosis. A common example would be injecting the subacromial bursa to discern intrinsic shoulder pathology from extrinsic causes of shoulder pain (15). As a therapeutic modality, local anesthetics serve to provide immediate relief from pain, to dilute the corticosteroid and ensure widespread dispersion within the joint or tissue, and to confirm proper placement (18). Typically used local anesthetics are 1% lidocaine without epinephrine and 0.5% bupivicaine.

TABLE 3 Aspirate Analysis

Synovial fluid characteristics	Normal	Arthropathy			
		Noninflammatory	Inflammatory	Septic	Traumatic
Volume	Normal	Often increased	Often increased	Often increased	Often increased
Color	Clear to straw yellow	Straw yellow to xanthochromic	Xanthochromic to white	Variable	Sanguineous
Clarity	Transparent	Transparent	Translucent to opaque	Opaque	Translucent to opaque
Viscosity	High	High	Low	Variable	Variable
Leukocyte count (mm^3)	<200	<2000	2,000–100,000	>50,000	Equal to blood
PMNs	<25%	<25%	>50%	>75%	Equal to blood
Gram stain	Negative	Negative	Negative	Positive or negative	Negative
Culture	Negative	Negative	Negative	Positive or negative	Negative
Glucose	Approximately equal to blood	Approximately equal to blood	Often lower than blood	Often <50% blood	Equal to blood
Crystals	None	Rare	Present	None	None

Note: A negative Gram stain and culture do not specifically rule out septic arthritis.
Abbreviation: PMN, polymorphonuclear neutrophils.
Source: From Refs. 8, 15, 18, 26, 76.

TABLE 4 Crystal Analysis

Crystal	Length	Appearance	Birefringence
Monosodium urate (gout)	0–20 μm	Needle-shaped	Strongly negative
Calcium pyrophosphate dihydrate (pseudo-gout)	3–15 μm	Rod or rhomboid-shaped	Weakly positive
Calcium hydroxyapatite (osteoarthritis, nonspecific synovitis)	0–5 μm	Individual crystals may not be seen by light microscopy; clumps may appear as amorphous, globular matter	Nonrefringent

Source: From Refs. 15, 107, 109.

As both anesthetics have onset within two to five minutes, the principal difference is duration of action. Lidocaine provides effective local anesthesia for one to two hours, whereas the effects of bupivicaine last between four and six hours (19,20).

Adverse reactions to local anesthetics are rare, occurring in 0.1% to 0.4% of patients, and may include allergic or toxic reactions. Most allergic reactions are due not to the anesthetic, but rather the paraben preservatives found in multidose vials (20,21). Allergic reactions should be handled as per common practice. Toxic reactions are especially rare with the relatively low doses used in musculoskeletal procedures. Symptoms that would be most likely encountered include tongue numbness or metallic taste, lightheadedness or dizziness, tinnitus, sweating, or pallor. The patient should be reclined, reassured, and offered cool compresses. Most symptoms resolve within a few minutes. Intravascular injection should be avoided. Symptoms occurring with intravascular administration at higher doses include drowsiness, slurred speech, respiratory depression, seizures, cardiovascular collapse, and cardiac arrest. Toxicity resulting in these symptoms requires expedient monitoring and treatment (19,20).

TABLE 5 Adverse Reactions to Corticosteroid Injections

Abnormal uterine bleeding/disturbance of menstrual cycle	May be as high as 50%
Soft-tissue atrophy	1–14%, may occur 1–6 mo later
Steroid flare	1–6%
Steroid arthropathy	0.8%
Tendon rupture	<1%
Facial flushing	<1%
Hypopigmentation	<1%, may occur 1–6 mo later
Hypersensitivity reaction	<1%
Iatrogenic septic joint	1:10,000–50,000
Local nerve damage	Rare
Transient paresis of injected extremity	Rare
Avascular necrosis	Rare[a]
Hyperglycemia	Not documented
Suppression of hypothalamic-pituitary-adrenal axis	Not documented
Vaso-vagal reaction	Not documented

[a]Case reports are of patients also on systemic corticosteroids.
Source: From Refs. 7, 19, 22, 107, 111.

Corticosteroids

Corticosteroids provide powerful pain-relieving effects and are the most potent class of anti-inflammatory medications; however, corticosteroid injections should always be considered an adjuvant therapy to systemic treatment, physical therapy, and lifestyle or activity modification. Corticosteroid injections should never be performed without a working diagnosis and a specific treatment plan. Indiscriminate injection of corticosteroids places a patient at an increased risk of complications (22).

The mechanism of action of corticosteroids is complex and not completely known. Corticosteroids inhibit the production of prostaglandins, interleukins, thromboxane, and proteolytic enzymes (8,23–26). They also appear to inhibit neutrophil chemotaxis and phagocytosis, decrease synovial membrane permeability to leukocytes, and stabilize lysosomal membranes (8,26–32). Effects seen on synovial fluid include an increase in viscosity and hyaluronic acid concentration, and decreased leukocyte counts (26,32,33). How these mechanisms of action may relieve pain in chronic tendinopathy or bursitis is unclear, as histology shows no inflammation. It is possible that corticosteroids interact with nociceptive receptors, substance P, and chondroitin sulfate (34).

Indications for corticosteroid injection are wide-ranging. Corticosteroids provide prompt, efficient, and long-lasting relief in inflammatory conditions, and may be disease-modifying (35–40). Their effect on noninflammatory arthropathies or soft-tissue disorders is much more variable. Clinical experience and many studies show that corticosteroids often provide substantial relief, but the duration is often short-lived. In these instances, injections are of benefit to patients with conditions failing noninvasive treatment, or to allow participation in adjunctive therapies. Compared with aspiration, there are several absolute contraindications to corticosteroid injection. A list of indications and contraindications are presented in Table 6.

Despite the amount of literature discussing corticosteroid injection use, no available data substantively clarifies the most efficacious or safest choice and dose of corticosteroid (18). As no evidence-based consensus exists, choice and dose of corticosteroid largely depends upon practitioner training. Dosages are chosen by joint or structure size. The authors prefer triamcinolone or betamethasone to be used for injections because they are less soluble and, hence, longer acting. Dexamethasone is another longer acting agent that may be used in practice. For soft-tissue injections, shorter acting, more soluble corticosteroids, such as methylprednisolone, is also appropriate. Tables 7 and 8 compare a variety of steroids used in joint and soft tissue injections, and provide recommended dosages.

In general, it is recommended to avoid exceeding four injections per year, and to wait six to eight weeks between injections (19,33,41,42). Response to previous injections should be considered in deciding whether or when to proceed with a repeat injection (43). Repeat injections should not be performed if there has been neither relief nor functional improvement after two injections by the same practitioner. Injections repeated without benefit may place a patient at risk for adverse reactions or side-effects. Intratendinous or peritendinous injections of weight-bearing tendons, such as the patella and Achilles tendons should be avoided or performed with caution—there may be an increased risk of rupture following injection.

Adverse reactions are uncommon, but can be quite severe. The most commonly occurring side-effects are postinjection "steroid flare," hypopigmentation, subcutaneous atrophy, and menstrual irregularities (7,8,44,45). Steroid flare is a

TABLE 6 Indications/Contraindications to Medication Injections

Indications
  Local anesthetics
    To facilitate examination or establish diagnosis
    To dilute corticosteroids and confirm accurate placement
  Corticosteroids
    Mono- or oligoarticular inflammatory arthritides
    Inflammatory soft-tissue disorders
    Noninflammatory joint or soft-tissue conditions failing conservative treatment
    Patients unable to tolerate systemic treatments
    To facilitate participation in other treatment modalities
    Flexion deformities accompanying joint inflammation
  Hyaluronic acid
    Knee arthritis failing conservative treatment

Absolute contraindications
  Infection
    Septic joint, periarticular cellulitis, adjacent osteomyelitis, and bacteremia
  Hypersensitivity
  Osteochondral fracture
  Joint prosthesis
  Uncontrolled coagulopathy
  Injection into weight-bearing tendons (Achilles, patellar)
  Overlying abraded skin or psoriasis
  Noncooperative patient
  Anatomically inaccessible without imaging

Relative contraindications
  Joint instability
  Poorly controlled diabetes
  Minimal/lack of efficacy following two injections
  Internal derangement of knee
  Hemarthrosis
  Distant chronic foci of infection
  Surrounding osteoporosis
  Skeletal immaturity

Source: From Refs. 7, 8, 15, 18, 19, 22, 26, 76, 107, 110.

synovitis that begins shortly after injection, and may persist for 24 to 48 hours. The joint swells and becomes painful, erythematous, and warm, mimicking a septic joint. It occurs much more commonly than iatrogenic infection (commonly reported to occur in 2% vs. 1:10,000 to 50,000 of patients, respectively) (46–48), and may be difficult to differentiate. Surrounding regional or systemic complaints, such as lymphangitis, fever, or malaise, do not occur with steroid flare and should raise concern of a septic joint. Any concern of septic arthritis requires immediate evaluation.

    The most concerning adverse events include the aforementioned iatrogenic infection, tendon rupture, and the controversial entity called steroid arthropathy. The incidence of steroid-associated tendon rupture is difficult to accurately ascribe, but has been reported—most frequently in weight-bearing tendons, such as the Achilles and patellar tendons (49–59). Steroid arthropathy is a Charcot-like arthropathy, involving gradual destruction of the joint. Anecdotal case reports were described in the 1950s and 1960s involving patients usually receiving 10 to hundreds of steroid injections over many years. It is postulated that

TABLE 7 Relative Potencies of Corticosteroid Preparations

Generic name	Proprietary name	Relative anti-inflammatory potency	Concentration (mg/mL)	Approximate equivalent dose (mg)
Short-acting preparations				
Cortisone acetate	Cortone® (Merck, Westpoint, Pennsylvania, U.S.A.)	0.8	50	25
Hydrocortisone				
Acetate	Hydrocort-AC® (Merck, Westpoint, Pennsylvania, U.S.A.)	1	25, 50	20
Sodium phosphate	Hydrocortone® (Merck, Westpoint, Pennsylvania, U.S.A.)	1	50	20
Intermediate-acting preparations				
Prednisolone				
Sodium phosphate	Hydeltrasol® (Merck, Westpoint, Pennsylvania, U.S.A.)	4	20	5
Tebutate	Hydeltra® (Merck, Westpoint, Pennsylvania, U.S.A.)	4	20	5
Methylprednisolone				
Acetate	Depo-Medrol® (Pfizer, New York, New York, U.S.A.)	5	20, 40, 80	4
Sodium succinate	Solu-Medrol® (Pfizer, New York, New York, U.S.A.)	5	40, 125	4
Long-acting preparations				
Triamcinolone[a]				
Acetonide	Aristospan® (Merck, Westpoint, Pennsylvania, U.S.A.)	5	10, 40	4
Diacetate	Aristocort® (Merck, Westpoint, Pennsylvania, U.S.A.)	5	25, 40	4
Hexacetonide	Kenalog® (Bristol-Myers Squibb, Princeton, New Jersey, U.S.A.)	5	5, 20	4
Dexamethasone[a]				
Sodium phosphate	Decadron® (Merck, Westpoint, Pennsylvania, U.S.A.)	25	4, 24	0.75
Acetate	Decadron-LA® (Merck, Westpoint, Pennsylvania, U.S.A.)	25	8	0.75
Betamethasone[a]				
Phosphate/acetate	Celestone® (Schering, North Wales, Pennsylvania, U.S.A.) Soluspan® (Schering, North Wales, Pennsylvania, U.S.A.)	25	6	0.75

Note: Relative anti-inflammatory potency derived from systemic administration, and does not necessarily equate to intrasubstance or intra-articular potency.
[a]Fluorinated.
Source: From Refs. 8, 22, 33.

TABLE 8 Recommended Corticosteroid Dosages per Anatomic Site

Corticosteroid	Concentration (mg/mL)	Soft tissues (mg)	Small joints (mg)	Medium joints (mg)	Large joints (mg)
Short-acting preparations					
Hydrocortisone		10–50	10–25	25–50	50–100
Acetate	25, 50				
Sodium phosphate	50				
Intermediate-acting preparations					
Prednisolone		5–40	2–10	10–40	20–80
Sodium phosphate	20				
Tebutate	20				
Methylprednisolone		5–40	2–10	10–40	20–80
Acetate	20, 40, 80				
Sodium succinate	40, 125				
Long-acting preparations					
Triamcinolone		N/A[a]	2–10	5–30	20–80
Acetonide	10, 40				
Diacetate	25, 40				
Hexacetonide	5, 20				
Dexamethasone		N/A[a]	1–3	2–4	4–16
Sodium phosphate	4, 24				
Acetate	8				
Betamethasone		N/A[a]	1–3	3–6	6–12
Phosphate/acetate	6				

Note: Small joints refer to joints within the fingers or toes. Medium joints refer to the elbow, wrist, and ankle. Large joints refer to the knee and shoulder.
[a]Long-acting corticosteroids are not recommended for injection into soft-tissue structures.
Source: From Refs. 8, 15, 19, 22, 24, 26, 33, 76.

steroid-mediated pain reduction prevents a patient from recognizing injury to the joint, and that repeated corticosteroid injection may have a deleterious effect on bone. There is conflicting evidence, however, as it has never been demonstrated in primate models. It is also difficult to discern joint destruction attributed to steroid arthropathy from that associated with the natural progression of degenerative disease (39,40,47,60–68). A complete list of adverse reactions is presented in Table 5. For a more detailed discussion, please refer to the chapter on corticosteroids.

Viscosupplementation

Hyaluronic acid is an important component of synovial fluid. It has both viscous and elastic properties that are shear force-dependent. With high shear forces, it has increased elasticity and lowered viscosity, hence serving as a shock absorber. Its characteristics are opposite with low shear forces, increasing its lubricating ability. In addition, it serves to provide nutrients to, and remove waste products from, the articular cartilage, and exhibits anti-inflammatory effects. In arthritides, the concentration of hyaluronic acid is decreased which impairs its functioning (21,26). Viscosupplementation with exogenous hyaluronic acid appears to restore some of its intra-articular function and provide symptomatic relief. It may also stimulate endogenous production of healthy synovial fluid (21). A Cochrane Database review suggests that viscosupplementation provides short-term pain relief and improved functioning, but that it has not been shown to halt disease progression (69). In the United States, viscosupplementation is currently approved only for knee injections. Adverse reactions are similar to those presented for aspiration. For a more detailed discussion, please refer to the chapter on viscosupplementation.

GENERAL TECHNIQUE

Any attempt at aspiration or injection requires knowledge of the targeted anatomy, the techniques of the procedure, and medications used. Verbal or signed consent should be obtained, and the patient then situated such that the area of interest is supported, the tissue or joint is positioned to facilitate entry, and the patient safe-guarded against possible vaso-vagal events. Most procedures can be performed with the patient sitting in a chair, or lying supine or prone. As with all medical pro-cedures, preparation is important. All materials should be within easy reach, including items to address possible complications. Some practitioners find it con-venient to have an arthrocentesis tray prepared in advance. Materials that should be included in such a tray are listed in Table 9.

Aseptic technique should be observed to avoid introduction of bacteria into the joint or tissue. Once the entry site is palpated and marked by pressing with needle cap, the skin should be cleansed. Traditionally, this has involved one or two appli-cations of povidone-iodine solution, allowing this to dry, and then wiping twice with isopropyl alcohol starting from the injection site and circling outward. Studies, however, have demonstrated that the use of alcohol alone is sufficient. While Glaser et al.'s study (70) demonstrated the introduction of skin tissue into the knee joint in almost all arthrocenteses, Hollander's review (48) of 250,000 patients and Gray et al.'s review (47) of 100,000 patients injected with alcohol-based aseptic techniques demonstrated only 18 and two incidences of septic arthritis, respectively. Finally, a controlled study by Cawley et al. (71) showed that a comparison of a chlor-hexidine preparation and a preparation using only isopropyl alcohol demonstrated no difference in outcomes (71).

TABLE 9   Equipment Tray Contents for Joint/Soft-Tissue Injection or Aspiration

Povidone-iodine (Betadine®, Purdue, Stamford, Connecticut, U.S.A.) wipes
Alcohol wipes
Disposable gloves (need not be sterile)
Sterile drapes
25- to 30-gauge, 0.5- to 1-inch needle for local skin anesthesia
18- to 20-gauge, 1.5-inch needle for aspirations
22- to 25-gauge, 1- to 1.5-inch needle for injections
3-inch spinal needle for large knee or hip aspirations or injections
1 mL- to 10 mL-syringe for injections
3 mL- to 60 mL-syringe for aspirations
Local anesthetic (1–2% lidocaine without epinephrine or ethyl chloride vapo-coolant)
Corticosteroid preparation
Plain test tubes for culture and chemistry tests
Test tubes w/liquid anticoagulant (purple or green top) for cell count and crystal
   analysis
Hemostat (if joint is to be aspirated and then injected using same needle)
Adhesive bandage/dressing

Universal precautions should be followed, but if the needle tip and injection site are not touched, the gloves need not be sterile. Sterile gloves and drapes may be used as per the discretion of the physician. Local anesthesia may be achieved by either injecting 1% lidocaine without epinephrine subcutaneously via a 25-gauge needle to form a wheal, or spraying a vapo-coolant, such as ethyl chloride. Vapo-coolants have been shown not to contaminate the sterile field (72). In some instances, particularly with children, sedation or general anesthesia may be required for a safe and accurate aspiration or injection.

When aspirating an effusion, the seal of the syringe should be broken prior to the procedure. Several syringes should be at hand in case the volume of the effusion is greater than the capacity of the syringe, and a hemostat should be available to facilitate exchanging syringes without necessitating removal of the needle. If aspiration is performed for diagnostic purposes, the aspirate should be sent to the lab in citrate (blue-topped), ethylenediaminetetraacetic acid (EDTA, purple-topped), or heparin (green-topped) tubes to prevent coagulation of inflammatory fluids for accurate cell counts and crystal analysis. Plain tubes may be used for chemistries. Aspirate for gram stain and culture should be sent in a sterile tube. If less than 2 mL is sent, it should be performed in a bacterial culture bottle. Two milliliter or more of aspirate has been shown to maintain bacterial viability for 24 hours at standard temperatures. It should not be refrigerated (21).

If an effusion is detected, but no or minimal fluid is obtained with aspiration, several problems could exist. Tissue may be obstructing the needle bore, the needle may be up against the bone or not in the target cavity, or the needle may not be of a sufficient gauge. A hemarthrosis may be coagulated, tensed muscles may be obstructing flow, or soft-tissue swelling may have been mistaken for true intra-articular or intrabursal fluid. Attempts to correct this may be made by rotating or flushing the needle, slightly advancing or withdrawing the needle, withdrawing and redirecting the needle, ensuring the patient has relaxed the surrounding musculature, and sometimes replacing the needle with a larger bore (lower gauge).

If injection of local anesthetic or corticosteroid is to follow aspiration, it may easily be performed by leaving the needle in the joint or tissue space. The needle hub is grasped with a hemostat, and the aspirating syringe carefully removed. The syringe with the local anesthetic or corticosteroid is attached, and after gentle aspiration has ensured the needle has not migrated into a vessel, the solution is injected. All injections should be without significant resistance. If significant resistance or patient discomfort is encountered, it suggests that the needle is improperly placed. Agitation of a corticosteroid and local anesthetic mixture immediately prior to injection will help prevent layering, and ensure full corticosteroid deployment and more equal dispersion within the space.

Postprocedural care involves applying direct pressure after the removal of the needle. This should be done until hemostasis is achieved, followed by an adhesive bandage or other dry sterile dressing. The authors instruct the patient to ice the site for 15 to 20 minutes three times a day for at least three days. Relative rest for 24 to 48 hours may be recommended and has been shown to improve both degree and duration of relief (73). The patient should be instructed about both the possibility of steroid flare and iatrogenic infection. Any warmth, erythema, and swelling that persists for greater than 24 hours, is increasing, or that is accompanied by lymphangitis, fevers, or chills, should be immediately evaluated.

REGIONAL ASPIRATION AND INJECTION TECHNIQUES

The proceduralist needs to decide on several items: the approach to the site, the corticosteroid and dose, the syringe size, and the needle gauge and length. Most approaches are based on ease of anatomic access and avoiding important neurovascular structures. Practitioner preference of one approach over another usually depends on training, as most evidence is anecdotal; few studies comparing various approaches exist. When material does exist, this will be noted.

The authors use 40 mg/mL triamcinolone preparations, as this is a commonly used steroid with a long intra-articular duration and great intra-articular potency. The authors prefer 0.5% bupivicaine for the local anesthetic because of its longer half-life. As noted before, there is no one standard corticosteroid or dosage for any of these procedures. Alternate corticosteroids and suggested dosages are listed in Table 8. It is not necessary to know all of the drugs listed, but rather be comfortable with one or two preparations. Ten cubic centimeter syringes are used most commonly for injections, with 3 and 5 cc syringes used for smaller joints. Sixty cubic centimeter syringes are used for aspiration of large joints (e.g., knee), and 20 or 33 cc syringes for aspiration of medium joints (e.g., elbow) or bursae.

What follows is a description of a number of aspiration and injection approaches, with the authors' preferred method emphasized. It is by no means meant to be an exhaustive list of possible injections or approaches, but rather a practical how-to guide for the busy practitioner.

Shoulder
Glenohumeral Joint
The glenohumeral joint may be approached by either an anterior or a posterior approach. A 22-gauge 1.5-inch needle is used along with 40 to 80 mg of triamcinolone and 2 to 6 mL of local anesthetic (7,8).

Anterior Approach
The patient should be seated. External rotation of the arm may further open the joint space. Mark a spot just medial to the head of the humerus and 1 to 2 cm lateral and inferior to the coracoid process. The needle is directed posteriorly and slightly upward and laterally. Entry into the joint space is usually made after approximately 2 cm in normal-sized individuals (7,8,15,21,42,74).

Posterior Approach (Authors' Preferred Method)
The patient should be seated and the arm internally rotated with the forearm across the chest or resting in the lap. The needle is inserted two to three fingerbreadths below the posterolateral corner of the acromion, at the level of the mid-humeral head. The needle is directed anteriorly and slightly superiorly toward the coracoid process. The joint space is entered after the needle is advanced 2 to 3 cm (7,8,21,74). This approach is easy to perform and poses less risk of damaging neurovascular structures (Fig. 1) (42).

Acromioclavicular Joint
The acromioclavicular joint is a superficial joint that can be palpated at the lateral end of the clavicle. Most commonly, a depression can be felt, but soft-tissue swelling, dislocation, or arthritic changes may alter the landmarks. Palpation of the contralateral acromioclavicular joint may facilitate proper positioning. Entering the

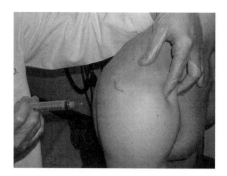

FIGURE 1 Glenohumeral joint injection—posterior approach. The posterolateral corner of the acromion is identified with the injection site marked three fingerbreadths below. Notice that the practitioner has identified the coracoid process with his index finger and is directing the needle toward it.

joint with the needle takes practice and patience. An arthritic joint may have a tough fibrous capsule, joint hypertrophy, and joint space collapse, making an intra-articular injection challenging. The joint is entered from directly superior with a 25-gauge 1-inch needle (8,19). If the joint space is not initially entered, "walk" the needle tip down the clavicle laterally until it slips into the joint. It should not be necessary to advance much more than one-half inch to enter the joint. Ten to twenty milligrams of triamcinolone with 1 mL of local anesthetic may be injected into the joint (Fig. 2) (7,21,24,75).

Subacromial Space
Rotator cuff tendonopathy and subacromial bursitis are conditions along the same spectrum, for which corticosteroid injection may be an important adjunctive therapy. The bursa lies just superior to the supraspinatus tendon, and inflammation usually involves both the bursa and tendon. Corticosteroid injected into the subacromial space will diffuse into both the bursa and rotator cuff, and because of the ease in injecting the space, this method is generally recommended (21,24,76). Several approaches, all utilizing a 22-gauge 1.5-inch needle, are possible. The patient should be seated for each. Forty to eighty milligrams of triamcinolone with 5 to 9 mL of local anesthetic may be injected (1,7,19).

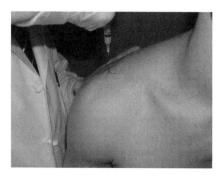

FIGURE 2 Acromioclavicular joint injection. The borders of the acromion and the distal clavicle are identified, and the needle is inserted perpendicularly to the joint.

Anterior Approach

With the patient's arm resting in the lap, insert the needle over the depression palpable inferior and lateral to the coracoid process and medial to the head of the humerus (19).

Lateral Approach

Enter the sulcus between the midpoint of the lateral acromion and the superior aspect of the humeral head. Direct the needle anteromedially as the bursa lies under the anterior–inferior aspect of the acromion (8,21,24,76).

Posterior Approach (Authors' Preferred Method)

The needle is inserted one fingerbreadth below the posterolateral corner of the acromion and directed anteriorly. In a posterior to anterior orientation, the acromion angles upward with the subacromial space superior to the injection site. As such, once the needle is underneath the acromion, the practitioner's hand is dropped, directing the needle superiorly and slightly medially. The needle should be advanced 2 to 3 cm to its hilt (19,42). If the injection is not free flowing, the needle tip may be against the underside of the acromion. The needle should then be withdrawn slightly and redirected (Fig. 3).

Bicipital Tendon

Injection into a tendon sheath may be performed in two manners. The first technique involves advancing the needle into the substance of the tendon and then slightly withdrawn, attempting to leave the needle within the sheath (1). If properly positioned, the solution should be injected easily. The injection may also be infiltrated in a fan-like distribution along the outer surface of the tendon sheath (21). The area of maximal tenderness within the bicipital groove is targeted, but the injection should not be intratendinous (18,19).

With the arm internally rotated 20°, the groove and tendon lie directly anterior (8). Its location may easily be palpated, and confirmed by rolling the tendon underneath one's finger, or by internally and externally rotating the arm and feeling the groove pass beneath (7,21,76,77). The walls of the groove can be used to guide the course of the injection. Twenty to forty milligrams of triamcinolone and 2 to 4 mL of local anesthetic are infiltrated via a 22-gauge, 1.5-inch needle. One-third is injected at the site of maximal tenderness, with the other two-thirds injected just superior

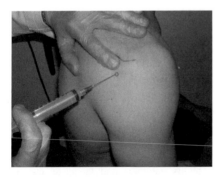

FIGURE 3 Subacromial space injection—posterior approach. The posterolateral corner of the acromion is identified with the injection site marked one fingerbreadth below. Once the needle passes the acromion border, the needle should be angled superiorly.

and inferior along the course of the tendon (19). Rarely, the short head of the biceps requires injection at the coracoid process. The needle should be advanced to the bone, withdrawn 1 to 2 mm, and injected (21).

Elbow
Elbow Joint
The elbow is easily entered with the patient lying prone, the elbow flexed 90°, and the forearm pronated and hanging over the table's edge. If this position is difficult for the patient, the patient may be seated with the palm resting on the patient's lap, or laid supine with the palm on the abdomen. The olecranon, lateral epicondyle, and radial head form a triangle, the center of which is the target site for aspiration or injection (7,8,15,21,74). An 18-gauge, 1.5-inch needle is used for aspirations, while a 22-gauge needle is used for injections. The needle is positioned perpendicularly to the skin and parallel to the surface of the radial shaft, and advanced 1 to 2 cm toward the hand (7,74,75). Forty to eighty milligrams of triamcinolone may be injected with 6 to 8 mL of local anesthetic. An alternative approach is to insert the needle superior to the olecranon process just laterally to the triceps tendon (74). A medial approach is not recommended because of concern for the ulnar nerve and superior ulnar collateral artery (Fig. 4) (15).

Medial and Lateral Epicondylitis
Controlled studies have demonstrated that corticosteroid injections performed for the treatment of recalcitrant medial and lateral epicondylitis provide significant relief, but that it is short-lived. Stahl et al. (78) showed that corticosteroid injection for medial epicondylitis was superior to placebo at six weeks, but that by three months, there was no difference in symptoms or function.

    Approaches for both medial and lateral epicondylitis are similar. The elbow is flexed to 45° or 90° and supported by a table. A 22-gauge, 1.5-inch needle is inserted in the area of maximal tenderness over the insertion of the flexor or extensor tendons, respectively (7,19,42). This area is typically at the distal of the epicondyle. The needle enters the skin perpendicularly, advanced until bone is encountered, and then withdrawn 1 to 2 mm (21). A combination of 40 to 80 mg of triamcinolone and 4 to 8 mL of local anesthetic are distributed in a stellate distribution (Fig. 5) (1,7,19,24). Some experts advocate repetitive insertion to bone and withdrawal as the solution is injected, or "needling" of the tendon (1,7).

    Care must be taken when injecting either medial or lateral epicondylitis to avoid injuring the ulnar or radial nerves. The ulnar nerve lies behind the medial

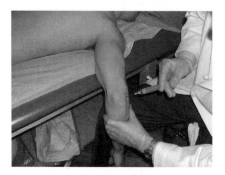

FIGURE 4 Elbow joint aspiration and injection. The olecranon, lateral epicondyle, and radial head form a triangle identifying the region easily entered for aspirations or injections.

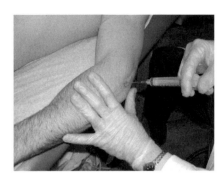

FIGURE 5 Lateral epicondylitis injection. The margins of the lateral epicondyle are identified and the area of maximal tenderness is injected repeatedly in a stellate pattern.

epicondyle in the cubital tunnel and the radial nerve lies posterior to the lateral epicondyle. These nerves or their branches may be inadvertently anesthetized. Both procedures carry a greater risk of subcutaneous atrophy and hypopigmentation owing to the tissue's superficial nature. Repeated injections may predispose the tendons to rupture (76); however, this may be of little clinical significance.

Olecranon Bursa

The olecranon bursa is located just under the skin over the tip of the olecranon process. As such, it is predisposed to infection and, while this occurs infrequently, the olecranon is the most common site of septic bursitis (21). Most patients with septic bursitis have risk factors including diabetes, chronic alcohol abuse, gout, uremia, or immunosuppression (19). Overlap with inflammatory bursitis may exist, but painful range of motion and a surface temperature greater than 2.2°C compared with the contralateral surface typically differentiates the clinical picture of septic bursitis (79,80). If there is a concern for septic bursitis, the aspirate should be sent for gram stain and culture. The role of empiric oral antibiotics is controversial. Septic bursitis should not be injected with corticosteroids.

Aseptic bursitis may resolve spontaneously, but if it is large and particularly inflamed, corticosteroids have been shown to speed resolution and decrease the incidence of recurrence at six months (81). Corticosteroid injection may also be considered for chronic or recurrent cases of aseptic bursitis.

When indicated, the olecranon bursa is easily aspirated and injected. The elbow may be flexed to 90° and is supported on a table (1,19,42). For aspiration, an 18-gauge, 1.5-inch needle is positioned parallel to the surface of the olecranon, and after insertion, as much fluid as possible is aspirated (7). If injection is to be performed, a 22-gauge needle, 20 mg of triamcinolone, and 2 mL of local anesthetic are used (7,19). Following aspiration or injection, ice should be applied and an elastic compressive dressing should be worn for five to seven days. If required, a second injection may be performed in one to three months (1,18,19).

Wrist and Hand

The wrist is a complex articulation involving the radioulnar, radiocarpal, ulnocarpal, and intercarpal articulations. Most of these articulations communicate freely with one another. The wrist and hand are sites commonly involved in inflammatory arthritides, such as rheumatoid arthritis—the second most common arthritis in the United States. Noninflammatory arthritis, several well-known tenosynovitides, and nerve impingement syndromes commonly occur at the wrist or hand. Some of the most satisfying results to corticosteroid injection are experienced when treating these conditions.

Wrist Joint

The wrist should be approached from the dorsal aspect. Positioning it on a table in 20° to 30° of flexion with a rolled-up towel beneath it, and in slight ulnar deviation will facilitate entry of the radiocarpal joint (15,74). A 25-gauge, 1-inch needle is inserted perpendicularly to the skin just distal to the dorsal radial tubercle (Lister's tubercle) and on the ulnar side of the extensor pollicis longus (8,15,21,42). Traction may facilitate entry (15). Alternately, the ulnocarpal joint may be accessed dorsally, just distal to the ulnar styloid with the wrist in radial deviation (8,74). When injecting either site, the needle should be advanced approximately 1 cm (74). Ten to twenty milligrams of triamcinolone may be injected along with 1 to 2 mL of local anesthetic (7). The anatomic snuff box located radially to the extensor pollicis longus should be avoided, as the radial artery, radial nerve, or musculocutaneous nerves contained within may be injured (15).

de Quervain's Tenosynovitis

The abductor pollicis longus and extensor pollicis brevis travel together through the first extensor compartment on the dorsal aspect of the wrist. Injection with cortico-steroid can provide dramatic and long-lasting relief in a majority of patients, and should be considered as first line treatment once symptoms interfere with activities of daily living. A collection of studies has demonstrated 83% to 91% resolution of symptoms with one to two injections. Only 10% failed treatment and required surgery (82–84).

A 25-gauge, 1-inch needle with 10 mg of triamcinolone and 0.5 mL of local anesthetic should be angled 30° and introduced at the point of maximal tenderness, usually 1 cm distal to the radial styloid (7,19,42,76). The solution should be injected peritendinously within the first extensor compartment (24). Ideally, the injection can be seen traveling along the tendon sheath. A generous volume of local anes-thetic may help dispersal of the corticosteroid (19). A thumb spica splint may be considered for the next several weeks, but some evidence exists that it may worsen outcomes (84). While it is usually recommended to wait eight weeks until reinjection with corticosteroid, some experts recommend repeat injection within one week if there is not a significant initial response (Fig. 6) (76).

Intersection Syndrome

This is another tenosynovitis that is similar to, and may be confused with, de Quervain's tenosynovitis. Anatomically, this is inflammation or compression of the second dorsal compartment of the wrist, which houses the extensor carpi radialis longus and brevis tendons (85). Tenderness, edema, and occasionally cre-pitus occur about 4 to 8 cm proximal to the radial styloid (19). If two to three weeks of conservative therapy does not relieve symptoms, 10 mg of triamcinolone and 0.5 to 1 mL of local anesthetic may be administered to the site of maximal tenderness in a fashion otherwise similar to that for de Quervain's tenosynovitis. Corticosteroid injection provides relief in approximately 60% of the patients (19).

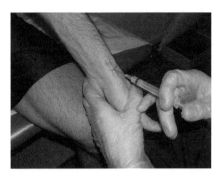

FIGURE 6 de Quervain's tenosynovitis injection. The first extensor compartment containing the abductor pollicis longus and extensor pollicis brevis tendons is identified. The injection is peritendinous at the site of maximal tenderness.

Carpal Tunnel

Corticosteroid and local anesthetic injection into the carpal tunnel may provide significant relief of pain and paresthesias, and may obviate the need for a surgical release. A study by Gelberman et al. found that, with one injection of corticosteroids and three weeks of splinting, 76% of patients had complete resolution of symptoms by six weeks. By 12 months, however, only 22% remained asymptomatic. Patients with recurrent symptoms were more likely to have initially exhibited severe symptoms with atrophy, weakness, and sensory deficits that were present for greater than one year (86). If severe symptoms are absent, several attempts at achieving permanent relief may be attempted before ultimately referring to surgery (87). Coincidentally, an initial positive response to injection has been found to be a positive prognosticator of response to release, if ultimately required. Injection may safely be performed despite the presence of nine flexor tendons, the median nerve, and superficial vasculature within the carpal tunnel.

Authors' Preferred Method

The forearm should be placed on a table with the forearm supinated and the wrist in 30° of extension and resting on a towel. A 22-gauge, 1.5-inch needle with 20 to 40 mg of triamcinolone and 1 to 2 mL of local anesthetic is used (1,7,8,19). The approach is at the volar surface between the second and third distal creases of the wrist, on the ulnar side of the palmaris longus tendon to avoid the median nerve. The palmaris longus tendon may be identified by having the patient oppose the thumb and little finger, and flex the wrist. In 15% of the people, palmaris longus is absent making the injection more difficult in these patients. The needle is angled 45°, directed toward the tip of the middle finger, and advanced 1 to 2 cm before injection (Figs. 7 and 8) (7,19,21,42).

Alternative Methods

Alternately, the needle may be inserted: (*i*) perpendicularly through the flexor retinaculum and directly into the median nerve space, (*ii*) immediately radial to the pisiform bone and pointed dorsally and distally to pass beneath the transverse carpal ligaments and enter the carpal tunnel, or (*iii*) more obliquely at an angle of 10° to 20° from the skin surface, but at 4 cm proximal to the wrist crease, and

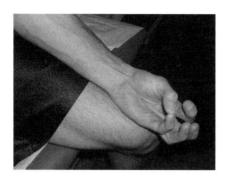

FIGURE 7 Palmaris longus tendon. The palmaris longus tendon is identified by having the patient oppose the thumb and little finger and flex the wrist.

between the palmaris longus and radial flexor tendon. It has been claimed that this last approach may minimize chance of injury to the nerve (21). In all cases, if the patient experiences increased pains or paresthesias in a median nerve distribution, the needle should be withdrawn and redirected.

First Carpometacarpal Joint

The first carpometacarpal joint is frequently involved in osteoarthritis, and is amenable to local injection. Long-lasting and significant relief has been documented with corticosteroid injection of this joint. Aspiration is seldom possible, and rarely indicated (7).

The thumb should be flexed across the palm and the wrist ulnarly deviated to open the dorsal aspect of the joint. Traction provided by an assistant may further ease this procedure (15). A 25-gauge, 1-inch needle with 5 to 10 mg of triamcinolone and 0.25 to 0.5 mL of local anesthetic is inserted dorsally, just radial to the abductor pollicis longus tendon (7,8). Using an approach from the radial side, and avoiding the anatomic snuff box to the ulnar side of the abductor pollicis longus, minimizes risk to the radial artery (8,15). If the carpometacarpal (CMC) joint is not easily appreciable, "walk" the needle tip down the metacarpal to enter the joint (Fig. 9).

Metacarpophalangeal and Interphalangeal Joints

These joints are also commonly affected by inflammatory and noninflammatory arthritides. Approach is to either side of the extensor tendon mechanism on the dorsal surface, but avoiding the nerves and vessels, which run laterally along the digits (7,8,21,76). Flexing the joint 15° to 20°, and having an assistant either apply traction

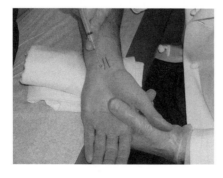

FIGURE 8 Carpal tunnel syndrome injection. The injection is performed to the ulnar side of the palmaris longus tendon between the second and third wrist creases and directed toward the middle finger.

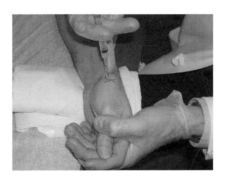

FIGURE 9 First carpometacarpal joint injection. The base of the first metacarpal is identified and the needle is inserted perpendicularly on the radial side of the abductor pollicis longus tendon.

distally or pressure on the joint line opposite the intended insertion site may further open the joint space and facilitate entry (15,74). Five milligrams of triamcinolone and 0.25 to 0.5 mL of local anesthetic are injected with a 25-gauge, 1-inch needle (7,8). It is not always possible to enter the joint space, but subcutaneous or pericapsular deposition should allow rapid dissemination into the joint (76).

Trigger Finger (Tenosynovitis of the Digital Flexor Tendon)
Triggering occurs most commonly at the metacarpophalangeal joint at the level of the A1 tendon pulley. Swelling, induration, and tenderness can be palpated. Corticosteroids offer 60% to 65% of patients significant and long-lasting relief (vs. 16–20% for placebo) when injected after a trial of noninvasive measures fails. Repeated injections can be performed after two weeks. Patients are most likely to derive benefit when symptoms have been present less than four months (88–90). Patients may be referred for surgical evaluation if one to three injections do not provide relief (19).

   To inject, the forearm should be supported and the palm supinated. A 25-gauge, 1-inch needle is introduced at a 45° angle proximal to the finger flexion crease directed at the level of the A1 tendon pulley (or A2 if the PIP joint is involved). The needle should parallel the course of the tendon toward the swelling (7,8,21,24,76). Ten milligrams of triamcinolone and 0.25 to 0.5 mL of local anesthetic can be injected within the sheath after the needle has been advanced about one-half inch (7,19).

Ganglion Cysts
Ganglion cysts grow slowly and rarely cause pain or disability. They are most commonly found dorsally, arising from the scapholunate joint. Other locations include volar ganglia over the distal radius, and flexor tendon sheath ganglia. In the case that a ganglion cyst causes discomfort, or if the patient is unhappy with its appearance, aspiration and injection often provide resolution. Studies show that 69% resolve with a single aspiration, and that an additional 19% resolve if the aspiration is repeated once or twice. Only 12% required surgery, and 6% to 50% of ganglion recur after the surgery (91,92).

   Aspiration may be attempted with an 18- or 22-gauge, 1-inch needle and 5-cc syringe. Even if no fluid is obtained, the puncture itself often causes gradual expulsion of the contents. Corticosteroid injection can further improve the rate of resolution (92). Injection of 5 to 10 mg of triamcinolone and 0.25 to 0.5 mL of local anesthetic is used (1,7,19,76).

Back
Trigger Points
The most common sites of muscle spasms and trigger points are the cervicothoracic and lumbosacral areas. Commonly involved muscles include the trapezius, parascapular, and paravertebral muscles. When other noninvasive methodologies have not provided relief, trigger point injections may be considered (76). This procedure has been noted to provide up to 95% immediate relief with a 75% permanent reduction in pain (1).

A 25-gauge, 1.5-inch needle is used to administer 20 mg of triamcinolone and 5 mL of local anesthetic. The needle should be passed repeatedly through the muscle belly in a stellate pattern while the mixture is injected (1,76). This procedure should be viewed as an adjunct to physical therapy and home exercise programs.

Hip and Pelvis
Femoral-Acetabular Joint
Aspiration and injection of the hip is essentially a blind process. Two approaches—an anterior and lateral—exist, but a cadaver study by Leopold et al. (93) found that rates of success are poor for both (60% and 80% success, respectively). Additionally, the anterior approach resulted in insertions neighboring the femoral neurovascular bundle. As such, fluoroscopic or ultrasound guidance by an experienced practitioner is recommended (7,8,74). If an aspiration must be attempted (e.g., to rule out a septic joint), and imaging is not available, the two approaches are listed subsequently. Both utilize an 18- to 22-gauge, 3-inch spinal needle.

Anterior Approach
The patient is supine with the hip extended and externally rotated. The insertion point is at the intersection of the line drawn vertically from the anterior superior iliac spine (ASIS) with the line drawn horizontally from the proximal aspect of the greater trochanter. This point should be approximately 2 to 3 cm inferior to the ASIS and at least 2 to 3 cm lateral to the femoral pulse. The needle is angled at 60° in a posteromedial direction (toward the umbilicus) and inserted until bone is felt. The needle is withdrawn slightly and aspirated (7,8,74,75).

Lateral Approach
The patient is supine with the hip extended and internally rotated—knees apart and toes touching. The needle is inserted anterior to the proximal tip of the greater trochanter and directed medially and slightly cephalad to a point below the middle of the inguinal ligament between the symphysis pubis and the ASIS. Once bone is encountered, the needle is withdrawn slightly and aspirated (7,8,74).

Iliotibial Band Syndrome/Trochanteric Bursa
The iliotibial band (ITB) runs from the pelvic crest down along the lateral thigh, past the knee and inserts on Gerdy's tubercle on the proximal lateral tibia. The point of maximal tenderness in ITB syndrome is usually at the level of the greater trochanter. Several bursae are also located around the greater trochanter. Which is principally irritated is not important to the injection technique as the 22-gauge, 1.5-inch needle is inserted at the point of maximal tenderness (most often posterior to the greater trochanter) (7,8,19). The patient should lie on the unaffected side with the hips and knees slightly flexed, and the greater trochanter of interest exposed.

The needle is inserted perpendicularly and advanced until bone is felt. It is then withdrawn 2 to 3 mm, and 40 to 80 mg of triamcinolone with 6 to 10 mL of local anesthetic is injected in a wide stellate pattern (19,21). A study by Shbeeb et al. (94) demonstrated 77% improvement after injection, with 61% demonstrated continued improvement at 26 weeks. As such, injection may play an important role in facilitating patient participation in physical therapy designed to address the lumbar spine, pelvis, and hip muscle group deficiencies and imbalances that typically accompany these disorders (19,24).

Ischiogluteal Bursa
The ischiogluteal bursa may be directly palpated over the ischial tuberosity as the patient lies on the opposite side with knees fully flexed. It is more easily palpated when the gluteus muscles are displaced from the area. If other etiologies of lumbrosacral pain have been excluded, injection with 20 to 40 mg of triamcinolone and 6 to 10 mL of local anesthetic may be performed. A 22-gauge, 1.5-inch needle is inserted horizontally at the area of maximal tenderness. It is advanced until bone reached, slightly withdrawn, and the solution is injected (7,19). Care should be taken to avoid the sciatic nerve (24).

Knee
Knee Joint
The knee is a very accessible joint, and there are many satisfactory approaches to aspiration and injection. An 18-gauge 1.5-inch needle is used for aspiration, while a 22-gauge needle is used for injection. Corticosteroids play an important role in both inflammatory and noninflammatory arthritides of the knee; however, successful sustained relief is more common in inflammatory arthritides. A Cochrane Database review found that, for osteoarthritis, corticosteroids provided relief for four to six weeks, but that they were not better than placebo at later times (95). Factors associated with better response to corticosteroid injection in osteoarthritis include less severe radiographic changes, presence of an effusion, and successful aspiration of that effusion prior to injection (7). As such, any substantial effusion should be drained prior to corticosteroid or hyaluronic acid administration (12,13). If corticosteroids are to be administered, 40 to 80 mg of triamcinolone are usually injected with 4 to 6 mL of local anesthetic (1,7).

Authors' Preferred Method for Aspiration
Aspiration should be performed with the knee in extension. With the knee in extension, either patellofemoral facet can be accessed anywhere along its course (7,8,15,74,76). The authors recommend entering laterally, approximately one-third the distance down the patella. The needle should be directed posteromedially along the undersurface of the patella, toward the superior pole of the patella. Gently externally, rotating the leg or placing a small roll behind the knee may help the patient relax their leg and open the retropatellar space. If there is minimal or no effusion and joint fluid is necessary to establish a diagnosis, this approach is most likely to provide an aspirate (96). Jackson et al. (97) demonstrated that the lateral mid-patellar approach had a first attempt success rate of 93% in entering the joint (Fig. 10).

If there is a substantial effusion, an approach preferred by many is to access the suprapatellar pouch located superior and posterior to the patella. With the knee extended, the needle is introduced perpendicularly to the skin at a point 2

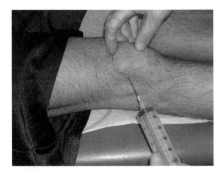

FIGURE 10 Knee joint aspiration—lateral patellar facet approach. The lateral patellar facet is identified with the aspiration site approximately one-third the distance down the patella. The needle is directed under the patella toward its superior pole.

to 3 cm posterior to the superior pole of the patella. It is directed medially just above the superior edge of the patella (75). When this is performed, rather than entering solely through a skin wheal, the entire tract should first be anesthetized with a separate 25-gauge 1.5-inch needle and local anesthetic. This approach is often better tolerated, and may allow more fluid to be aspirated.

Authors' Preferred Method for Injection

Injection can be performed with the knee in either extension or flexion. In extension, the method is the same as for aspiration. The authors, however, prefer injecting the knee in flexion. The patient may either be seated or lying supine with the knee flexed 90°. Injection is performed inferior to the patella in the recess lateral to the patellar tendon. The needle should be inserted parallel to the tibial plateau, and angled toward the center of the knee, behind the patellar tendon (74,75). Despite one study by Jackson et al. (97) questioning correct intra-articular placement with this approach, many practitioners—including the authors—find this approach technically easy and well tolerated by patients. If the injection is performed without significant resistance and without the patient experiencing significant discomfort, the practitioner should feel comfortable in its proper placement. Either resistance encountered with injection or pain felt by the patient suggests injection into an intra-articular structure, such as the infrapatellar fat pad or plicae (8). If this occurs, the needle should be slightly withdrawn and redirected (Fig. 11).

Prepatellar Bursa

Prepatellar bursitis is readily differentiated from a knee effusion, and is usually easily aspirated. An 18- to 22-gauge 1.5-inch needle is used for this. With the patient supine and knee extended, the needle is advanced from the side toward the center of the bursa in a manner parallel to the surface of the patella (21). The bursa may be multilocular, and milking the bursa may facilitate more complete aspiration (19). While uncommon overall, this site—like the olecranon bursa—is predisposed to septic bursitis (98). If a minimal fluid collection is present and only injection is planned, a 25-gauge 1.5-inch needle may be used to instill 20 to 40 mg of triamcinolone and 2 to 4 mL of local anesthetic (7,19).

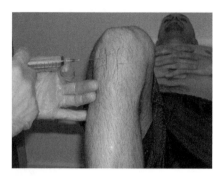

FIGURE 11   Knee joint injection—anterolateral approach. The knee is flexed 90° and the recess inferior to the patella and lateral to the patellar tendon is identified. The needle is angled toward the center of the knee and behind the patellar tendon.

Pes Anserine Bursa

Aspiration of the pes anserine bursa is generally not performed. Injection is typically reserved for failure of noninvasive measures (8). With the patient supine, the knee may be kept in extension or flexed to 90°. A 22-gauge, 1.5-inch needle is inserted perpendicularly to the skin at the area of maximum tenderness and advanced to the bone. It is then withdrawn 2 to 3 mm and 20 to 40 mg of triamcinolone and 2 to 4 mL of local anesthetic are injected (1,7,19). Efficacy may be variable, although an injection can be useful in conjunction with other modalities.

Ankle and Foot

Ankle (Tibiotalar) Joint

Aspiration or injection is usually performed at one of two locations, either medial to the tibialis anterior tendon and lateral to the medial malleolus (the medial malleolar sulcus), or just lateral to this between the extensor hallucis longus and tibialis anterior tendons (7,8,15,42,74,75). These tendons may be identified by having the patient extend the great toe and dorsiflex the foot, respectively. Arthrocenteses should be performed with the patient supine and the foot positioned at 90°, with the insertion site immediately proximal to the talus (7,15).

A 22-gauge, 1.5-inch needle needs to be advanced approximately 2 to 3 cm before entering the joint, at which time 10 to 20 mg of triamcinolone and 2 to 4 mL of local anesthetic can be injected (1,7,8,99). If the superior aspect of the talus cannot be palpated, radiographs may be of assistance in estimating its position.

Lateral and Anterior Ankle Impingement

Lateral and anterior ankle impingement typically occurs from repetitive injury to the ankle, and is characterized by chronic pain located below the lateral malleolus or along the anterior ankle joint line. Increasing valgus positioning of the heel or dorsiflexion of the foot exacerbates the pain.

Impingement can be caused by the accumulation of scar tissue or osteophytes. Impingement symptoms related to scar tissue are frequently improved by corticosteroid injections performed as an adjuvant treatment to physical therapy. Symptoms related to osteophytes, however, are typically less responsive. Injection and infiltration of the soft tissue along the lateral gutter or anterior ankle joint line

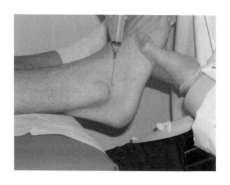

FIGURE 12 Lateral ankle impingement injection. The inferior border of the lateral malleolus is identified and the lateral gutter below is infiltrated.

utilizes a 22-gauge, 1.5-inch needle with 40 mg of triamcinolone and 1 to 2 mL of local anesthetic. This procedure can be repeated once or twice at four-week intervals (Fig. 12).

Sinus Tarsi Syndrome

The sinus tarsi are an anatomical space on the lateral aspect of the ankle bounded by the talus, navicular, and calcaneus. Trauma to the foot or ankle can injure the deep soft tissues within the tarsi, resulting in sinus tarsi syndrome. Complaints of chronic pain localized to this area and tenderness to palpation of the sinus tarsi are two clinical findings. Injection of the sinus tarsi can provide substantial relief (100), and should be performed in the palpable depression located just anteroinferior to the anterior talofibular ligament. A 22-gauge, 1.5-inch needle is used to inject 20 mg of triamcinolone and 1 mL of local anesthetic (Fig. 13).

Retrocalcaneal Bursa

As this bursa may communicate with the Achilles tendon sheath, it is recommended that it not be injected with corticosteroids. Intra- and peritendinous corticosteroid injections have been associated with reports of Achilles tendon ruptures (55). If an aspiration or diagnostic injection needs to be performed, a 25-gauge, 1-inch needle may be passed perpendicularly through the skin just anterior to the Achilles tendon (7). If, after carefully consideration, a corticosteroid injection is still thought to be necessary, 10 to 20 mg of triamcinolone with 1 to 2 mL of local anesthetic may be injected (7,19).

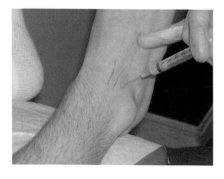

FIGURE 13 Sinus tarsi syndrome injection. The palpable depression located anteroinferior to the anterior talofibular ligament is identified and the needle is inserted perpendicularly to the skin.

Plantar Fascia

If plantar fasciitis pain persists after a comprehensive noninvasive treatment program, corticosteroid injection into the origin of the plantar fascia may be considered (24). This treatment has been reported to have a 70% success rate in relieving symptoms and improving functioning, however there is a risk of plantar fascial rupture and fat pad atrophy (101). The risk of rupture is thought to be greatest in athletic individuals receiving repeated injections (102).

A 22-gauge, 1.5-inch needle is inserted perpendicularly to the medial aspect of the heel, and directed to the area of maximal tenderness below the midpoint of the calcaneus at the plantar fascia insertion (19,21). Ten to twenty milligrams of triamcinolone and 1 to 2 mL of local anesthetic are injected in several passes through the area (19).

First Metatarsophalangeal Joint

The first metatarsophalangeal joint is a commonly involved site for gout, rheumatoid arthritis, osteoarthritis, or bunion. Any aspirate should be examined for crystals (76). With the patient supine, the toe is flexed 15° to 20°, traction is applied, and a 25-gauge, 1-inch needle is inserted just medial to the extensor hallucis longus tendon (15). Five to ten milligrams of triamcinolone with 0.5 to 1 mL of local anesthetic is injected (7). If the joint line is obscured by swelling, the other foot may be compared with the estimated correct placement (Fig. 14).

Metatarsophalangeal and Interphalangeal Joints

As with the fingers, these joints are approached from the extensor surface either just medial or lateral to the extensor tendons. The patient is supine, and the toe is flexed 15° to 20°. Traction facilitates entry into the joint space via a perpendicularly directed, 25-gauge, 1-inch needle. Five to ten milligrams of triamcinolone and 0.5 to 1 mL of local anesthetic may be introduced (7,8,15,75).

Morton's Neuroma

This condition is most commonly encountered in individuals exhibiting a hypermobile forefoot and excessive pronation. Pain is located between the second and third, or third and fourth metatarsal heads, and can cause significant pain and disability. Injection may provide substantial relief, and is most easily performed from the dorsal aspect. A 25-gauge, 1.5-inch needle is inserted 1 to 2 cm proximal to the affected web space (7,21). The needle is oriented perpendicularly to the skin and, after

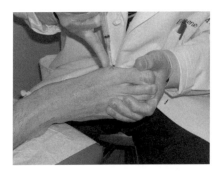

FIGURE 14 First metatarsophalangeal joint injection. The head of the first metatarsal is identified and the needle is inserted perpendicularly on the medial side of the extensor hallucis longus tendon.

advancing 0.5 to 1 in to the level of the metatarsal heads, 10 to 20 mg of triamcinolone and 0.5 to 1 mL of local anesthetic are injected (7).

SUMMARY

The management goals of a patient with a musculoskeletal or sports medicine condition owing to injury or illness are to relieve discomfort and preserve, restore, and maximize function. As with all conditions, accurate diagnosis is the precursor to optimal management. In the case of musculoskeletal and sports medicine, accurate diagnosis and optimal management frequently depend on competently and judiciously performed aspirations and injections.

In the future, these skills will likely become even more important. Various studies are using biologic agents or genetic manipulation to target distinct biological processes in inflammatory and noninflammatory arthritides. Insulin-like growth factor, transforming growth factor-β, interleukin receptor antagonists, and tumor necrosis factor inhibitors may prevent inflammation and bony destruction, and promote healing or growth of articular cartilage (103–105). It is possible that these agents may eventually be injected into joints and soft tissues, or that the development of a safe and effective vector may allow delivery to, and incorporation of, these genes into synovial membranes (106). Being comfortable with performing these procedures will enable a practitioner to skillfully make use of this ever-growing armamentarium.

REFERENCES

1. Scott WA. Injection techniques and use in the treatment of sports injuries. Sports Med 1996; 22:406–416.
2. Nelson RL, McCaffrey LA, Nobrega FT, et al. Altering residency curriculum in response to a changing practice environment: Use of the mayo internal medicine residency alumni survey. Mayo Clin Proc 1990; 65:809–817.
3. Chaytors RG, Szafran O, Crutcher RA. Rural-urban and gender differences in procedures performed by family practice residency graduates. Fam Med 2001; 33:766–771.
4. Gormley GJ, Corrigan M, Steele WK, Stevenson M, Taggart AJ. Joint and soft tissue injections in the community: questionnaire survey of general practitioners' experiences and attitudes. Ann Rheum Dis 2003; 62:61–64.
5. Roberts C, Adebajo AO, Long S. Improving the quality of care of musculoskeletal conditions in primary care. Rheumatology (Oxford) 2002; 41:503–508.
6. Rodnan GP, Benedek TG, Panetta WC. The early history of synovia (joint fluid). Ann Intern Med 1966; 65:821–842.
7. Wise C. Arthrocentesis and injection of joints and soft tissues. In: Harris, Edward D Jr, Budd RC, et al., eds. Kelley's Textbook of Rheumatology. 7th ed. Philadelphia: W.B. Saunders, 2005:692–709.
8. Zuckerman JD, Meislin RJ, Rothberg M. Injections for joint and soft tissue disorders: when and how to use them. Geriatrics 1990; 45:45–52, 55.
9. Hollander JL. Intra-articular hydrocortisone in the treatment of arthritis. Ann Intern Med 1953; 39:735–746.
10. Hollander JL, Brown EM Jr, Jessar RA, Brown CY. Hydrocortisone and cortisone injected into arthritic joints; comparative effects of and use of hydrocortisone as a local antiarthritic agent. J Am Med Assoc 1951; 147:1629–1635.
11. Kirwan JR, Rankin E. Intra-articular therapy in osteoarthritis. Baillieres Clin Rheumatol 1997; 11:769–794.

12. Tanaka N, Sakahashi H, Sato E, Hirose K, Ishima T, Ishii S. Intra-articular injection of high molecular weight hyaluronan after arthrocentesis as treatment for rheumatoid knees with joint effusion. Rheumatol Int 2002; 22:151–154.
13. Weitoft T, Uddenfeldt P. Importance of synovial fluid aspiration when injecting intra-articular corticosteroids. Ann Rheum Dis 2000; 59:233–235.
14. Jaffer AM, Schmid FR. Hemarthrosis associated with sodium warfarin. J Rheumatol 1977; 4:215–217.
15. Parrillo SJ, Fisher J. Arthrocentesis. In: Roberts JR, Hedges JR, eds. Clinical Procedures in Emergency Medicine. 4th ed. Philadelphia: W.B. Saunders, 2005:1042–1057.
16. Wild JH, Zvaifler NJ. Hemarthrosis associated with sodium warfarin therapy. Arthritis Rheum 1976; 19:98–102.
17. Thumboo J, O'Duffy JD. A prospective study of the safety of joint and soft tissue aspiration and injections in patients taking warfarin sodium. Arthritis Rheum 1998; 41:736.
18. Nelson KH, Briner W Jr, Cummins J. Corticosteroid injection therapy for overuse injuries. Am Fam Physician 1995; 52:1811–1816.
19. Foley B, Christopher TA. Injection therapy of bursitis and tendinitis. In: Roberts JR, Hedges JR, eds. Clinical Procedures in Emergency Medicine. 4th ed. Philadelphia: W.B. Saunders, 2004:1020–1041.
20. McGee D. Local and topical anesthesia. In: Roberts JR, Hedges JR, eds. Clinical Procedures in Emergency Medicine. 4th ed. Philadelphia: W.B. Saunders, 2004: 532–551.
21. Pfenninger JL. Joint and soft tissue aspiration and injection (arthrocentesis). In: Pfenninger JL, Fowler GC, eds. Pfenninger and Fowler's Procedures for Primary Care. 2nd ed. St. Louis: Mosby, 2003:1479–1500.
22. Cardone DA, Tallia AF. Joint and soft tissue injection. Am Fam Physician 2002; 66:283–288.
23. Creamer P. Intra-articular corticosteroid injections in osteoarthritis: do they work and if so, how? Ann Rheum Dis 1997; 56:634–636.
24. Kerlan RK, Glousman RE. Injections and techniques in athletic medicine. Clin Sports Med 1989; 8:541–560.
25. Pelletier JP, Cloutier JM, Martel-Pelletier J. In vitro effects of NSAIDs and corticosteroids on the synthesis and secretion of interleukin 1 by human osteoarthritic synovial membranes. Agents Actions Suppl 1993; 39:181–193.
26. Snibbe JC, Gambardella RA. Use of injections for osteoarthritis in joints and sports activity. Clin Sports Med 2005; 24:83–91.
27. De Ceulaer K, Balint G, El-Ghobarey A, Dick WC. Effects of corticosteroids and local anaesthetics applied directly to the synovial vascular bed. Ann Rheum Dis 1979; 38:440–442.
28. Eymontt MJ, Gordon GV, Schumacher HR, Hansell JR. The effects on synovial permeability and synovial fluid leukocyte counts in symptomatic osteoarthritis after intraarticular corticosteroid administration. J Rheumatol 1982; 9:198–203.
29. Fauci AS. Glucocorticoid effects on circulating human mononuclear cells. J Reticuloendothel Soc 1979; 26:727–738.
30. Fauci AS, Dale DC, Balow JE. Glucocorticosteroid therapy: mechanisms of action and clinical considerations. Ann Intern Med 1976; 84:304–315.
31. Jones AK, al-Janabi MA, Solanki K, et al. In vivo leukocyte migration in arthritis. Arthritis Rheum 1991; 34:270–275.
32. Youssef PP, Cormack J, Evill CA, et al. Neutrophil trafficking into inflamed joints in patients with rheumatoid arthritis, and the effects of methylprednisolone. Arthritis Rheum 1996; 39:216–225.
33. Genovese MC. Joint and soft-tissue injection. A useful adjuvant to systemic and local treatment. Postgrad Med 1998; 103:125–134.
34. Speed CA. Fortnightly review: corticosteroid injections in tendon lesions. BMJ 2001; 323:382–386.
35. Fernandez C, Noguera R, Gonzalez JA, Pascual E. Treatment of acute attacks of gout with a small dose of intraarticular triamcinolone acetonide. J Rheumatol 1999; 26:2285–2286.

36. McCarty DJ, Harman JG, Grassanovich JL, Qian C. Treatment of rheumatoid joint inflammation with intrasynovial triamcinolone hexacetonide. J Rheumatol 1995; 22:1631–1635.
37. Neidel J, Boehnke M, Kuster RM. The efficacy and safety of intraarticular corticosteroid therapy for coxitis in juvenile rheumatoid arthritis. Arthritis Rheum 2002; 46: 1620–1628.
38. Padeh S, Passwell JH. Intraarticular corticosteroid injection in the management of children with chronic arthritis. Arthritis Rheum 1998; 41:1210–1214.
39. Pelletier JP, Martel-Pelletier J. Protective effects of corticosteroids on cartilage lesions and osteophyte formation in the pond-nuki dog model of osteoarthritis. Arthritis Rheum 1989; 32:181–193.
40. Pelletier JP, Mineau F, Raynauld JP, Woessner JF Jr, Gunja-Smith Z, Martel-Pelletier J. Intraarticular injections with methylprednisolone acetate reduce osteoarthritic lesions in parallel with chondrocyte stromelysin synthesis in experimental osteoarthritis. Arthritis Rheum 1994; 37:414–423.
41. Assendelft WJ, Hay EM, Adshead R, Bouter LM. Corticosteroid injections for lateral epicondylitis: a systematic overview. Br J Gen Pract 1996; 46:209–216.
42. Pando JA, Klippel JH. Arthrocentesis and corticosteroid injection: an illustrated guide to technique. Cons 1996; 36:2137–2148.
43. Green M, Marzo-Ortega H, Wakefield RJ, et al. Predictors of outcome in patients with oligoarthritis: results of a protocol of intraarticular corticosteroids to all clinically active joints. Arthritis Rheum 2001; 44:1177–1183.
44. Louis DS, Hankin FM, Eckenrode JF. Cutaneous atrophy after corticosteroid injection. Am Fam Physician 1986; 33:183–186.
45. Mens JM, Nico de Wolf A, Berkhout BJ, Stam HJ. Disturbance of the menstrual pattern after local injection with triamcinolone acetonide. Ann Rheum Dis 1998; 57:700.
46. Fitzgerald RH Jr, Intrasynovial injection of steroids uses and abuses. Mayo Clin Proc 1976; 51:655–659.
47. Gray RG, Tenenbaum J, Gottlieb NL. Local corticosteroid injection treatment in rheumatic disorders. Semin Arthritis Rheum 1981; 10:231–254.
48. Hollander JL, Jessar RA, Brown EM Jr, Intra-synovial corticosteroid therapy: a decade of use. Bull Rheum Dis 1961; 11:239–240.
49. Anderson KJ, LeCocq JF. Rupture of the triceps tendon. J Bone Joint Surg Am 1957; 39-A:444–446.
50. Anderson RL. Traumatic rupture of the triceps tendon. J Trauma 1979; 19:134.
51. Bach BR Jr, Warren RF, Wickiewicz TL. Triceps rupture. A case report and literature review. Am J Sports Med 1987; 15:285–289.
52. Ismail AM, Balakrishnan R, Rajakumar MK, Lumpur K. Rupture of patellar ligament after steroid infiltration: report of a case. J Bone Joint Surg Br 1969; 51:503–505.
53. Halpern AA, Horowitz BG, Nagel DA. Tendon ruptures associated with corticosteroid therapy. West J Med 1977; 127:378–382.
54. Karpman RR, McComb JE, Volz RG. Tendon rupture following local steroid injection: report of four cases. Postgrad Med 1980; 68:169–174.
55. Kleinman M, Gross AE. Achilles tendon rupture following steroid injection: report of three cases. J Bone Joint Surg Am 1983; 65:1345–1347.
56. Mankin HJ, Conger KA. The acute effects of intra-articular hydrocortisone on articular cartilage in rabbits. J Bone Joint Surg Am 1966; 48:1383–1388.
57. Melmed EP. Spontaneous bilateral rupture of the calcaneal tendon during steroid therapy. J Bone Joint Surg Br 1965; 47:104–105.
58. Read MT, Motto SG. Tendo achillis pain: steroids and outcome. Br J Sports Med 1992; 26:15–21.
59. Stannard JP, Bucknell AL. Rupture of the triceps tendon associated with steroid injections. Am J Sports Med 1993; 21:482–485.
60. Alarcon-Segovia D, Ward LE. Marked destructive changes occurring in osteoarthric finger joints after intra-articular injection of corticosteroids. Arthritis Rheum 1966; 9:443–463.

61. Behrens F, Shepard N, Mitchell N. Alterations of rabbit articular cartilage by intra-articular injections of glucocorticoids. J Bone Joint Surg Am 1975; 57:70–76.
62. Bentley G, Goodfellow JW. Disorganisation of the knees following intra-articular hydrocortisone injections. J Bone Joint Surg Br 1969; 51:498–502.
63. Chandler GN, Jones DT, Wright V, Hartfall SJ. Charcot's arthropathy following intra-articular hydrocortisone. Br Med J 1959; 46:952–953.
64. Chandler GN, Wright V. Deleterious effect of intra-articular hydrocortisone. Lancet 1958; 2:661–663.
65. Oikarinen AI, Vuorio EI, Zaragoza EJ, Palotie A, Chu ML, Uitto J. Modulation of collagen metabolism by glucocorticoids. Receptor-mediated effects of dexamethasone on collagen biosynthesis in chick embryo fibroblasts and chondrocytes. Biochem Pharmacol 1988; 37:1451–1462.
66. Oxlund H, Manthorpe R, Viidik A. The biochemical properties of connective tissue in rabbits as influenced by short-term glucocorticoid treatment. J Biomech 1981; 14: 129–133.
67. Steinberg CL, Duthie RB, Piva AE. Charcot-like arthropathy following intra-articular hydrocortisone. JAMA 1962; 181:851–854.
68. Sweetnam DR, Mason RM, Murray RO. Steroid arthropathy of the hip. Br Med J 1960; 5183:1392–1394.
69. Bellamy N, Campbell J, Robinson V, Gee T, Bourne R, Wells G. Viscosupplementation for the treatment of osteoarthritis of the knee. Cochrane Database Syst Rev 2005; 2:CD005321.
70. Glaser DL, Schildhorn JC, Bartolozzi AR. Do you really know what is on the tip of your needle? The inadvertent introduction of skin into the joint (abstract). Arthritis Rheum 2000; 43:497.
71. Cawley PJ, Morris IM. A study to compare the efficacy of two methods of skin preparation prior to joint injection. Br J Rheumatol 1992; 31:847–848.
72. Abeles M, Garjian P. Do spray coolant anesthetics contaminate an aseptic field? Arthritis Rheum 1986; 29:576.
73. Chatham W, Williams G, Moreland L, et al. Intraarticular corticosteroid injections: should we rest the joints? Arthritis Care Res 1989; 2:70–74.
74. Moore GF. Arthrocentesis technique and intraarticular therapy. In: Koopman WJ, ed. Arthritis and Allied Conditions. 14th ed. Philadelphia: Lippincott Williams & Wilkins, 2001:848–859.
75. McCarty DJ. Basic guide to arthrocentesis. Hosp Med 1968; 4:77–97.
76. Leversee JH. Aspiration of joints and soft tissue injections. Prim Care 1986; 13:579–599.
77. Larson HM, O'Connor FG, Nirschl RP. Shoulder pain: the role of diagnostic injections. Am Fam Physician 1996; 53:1637–1647.
78. Stahl S, Kaufman T. The efficacy of an injection of steroids for medial epicondylitis. A prospective study of sixty elbows. J Bone Joint Surg Am 1997; 79:1648–1652.
79. Morrey BF, Regan WD. Tendinopathies about the elbow. In: DeLee JC, Drez DJ, eds. DeLee and Drez's Orthopaedic Sports Medicine. 2nd ed. Philadelphia: W.B. Saunders, 2003:1213–1236.
80. Smith DL, McAfee JH, Lucas LM, Kumar KL, Romney DM. Septic and nonseptic olecranon bursitis. Utility of the surface temperature probe in the early differentiation of septic and nonseptic cases. Arch Intern Med 1989; 149:1581–1585.
81. Smith DL, McAfee JH, Lucas LM, Kumar KL, Romney DM. Treatment of nonseptic olecranon bursitis. A controlled, blinded prospective trial. Arch Intern Med 1989; 149:2527–2530.
82. Harvey FJ, Harvey PM, Horsley MW. De quervain's disease: surgical or nonsurgical treatment. J Hand Surg [Am] 1990; 15:83–87.
83. Neustadt DH. Local corticosteroid injection therapy in soft tissue rheumatic conditions of the hand and wrist. Arthritis Rheum 1991; 34:923–926.
84. Richie CA, 3rd, Briner WW Jr. Corticosteroid injection for treatment of de quervain's tenosynovitis: a pooled quantitative literature evaluation [Review, 8 refs]. J Am Board Fam Pract 2003; 16:102–106.
85. Grundberg AB, Reagan DS. Pathologic anatomy of the forearm: intersection syndrome. J Hand Surg [Am] 1985; 10:299–302.

86. Gelberman RH, Aronson D, Weisman MH. Carpal-tunnel syndrome. Results of a prospective trial of steroid injection and splinting. J Bone Joint Surg [Am] 1980; 62:1181–1184.

87. Pfenninger JL. Injections of joints and soft tissue: part II. Guidelines for specific joints. Am Fam Physician 1991; 44:1690–1701.

88. Lambert MA, Morton RJ, Sloan JP. Controlled study of the use of local steroid injection in the treatment of trigger finger and thumb. J Hand Surg [Br] 1992; 17:69–70.

89. Murphy D, Failla JM, Koniuch MP. Steroid versus placebo injection for trigger finger. J Hand Surg [Am] 1995; 20:628–631.

90. Rhoades CE, Gelberman RH, Manjarris JF. Stenosing tenosynovitis of the fingers and thumb. Results of a prospective trial of steroid injection and splinting. Clin Orthop Relat Res 1984; 190:236–238.

91. Oni JA. Treatment of ganglia by aspiration alone. J Hand Surg [Br] 1992; 17:660.

92. Zubowicz VN, Ishii CH. Management of ganglion cysts of the hand by simple aspiration. J Hand Surg [Am] 1987; 12:618–620.

93. Leopold SS, Battista V, Oliverio JA. Safety and efficacy of intraarticular hip injection using anatomic landmarks. Clin Orthop Relat Res 2001; 391:192–197.

94. Shbeeb MI, O'Duffy JD, Michet CJ Jr, O'Fallon WM, Matteson EL. Evaluation of glucocorticosteroid injection for the treatment of trochanteric bursitis. J Rheumatol 1996; 23:2104–2106.

95. Bellamy N, Campbell J, Robinson V, Gee T, Bourne R, Wells G. Intraarticular corticosteroid for treatment of osteoarthritis of the knee. Cochrane Database Syst Rev 2005; 2:CD005328.

96. Roberts WN, Hayes CW, Breitbach SA, Owen DS Jr. Dry taps and what to do about them: a pictorial essay on failed arthrocentesis of the knee. Am J Med 1996; 100: 461–464.

97. Jackson DW, Evans NA, Thomas BM. Accuracy of needle placement into the intraarticular space of the knee. J Bone Joint Surg Am 2002; 84-A:1522–1527.

98. Hoffman GS. Tendinitis and bursitis. Am Fam Physician 1981; 23:103–110.

99. Williams P, Gumpel M. Aspiration and injection of joints (1). Br Med J 1980; 281: 990–992.

100. Pisani G, Pisani PC, Parino E. Sinus tarsi syndrome and subtalar joint instability [Review 45 refs]. Clin Podiatr Med Surg 2005; 22:63–77.

101. Young CC, Rutherford DS, Niedfeldt MW. Treatment of plantar fasciitis. Am Fam Physician 2001; 63:467–474, 477–478.

102. Leach R, Jones R, Silva T. Rupture of the plantar fascia in athletes. J Bone Joint Surg [Am] 1978; 60:537–539.

103. Evans CH, Ghivizzani SC, Smith P, Shuler FD, Mi Z, Robbins PD. Using gene therapy to protect and restore cartilage. Clin Orthop Relat Res 2000; 379(suppl):S214–S219.

104. Evans CH. Gene therapies for osteoarthritis. Curr Rheumatol Rep 2004; 6:31–40.

105. Trippel SB, Ghivizzani SC, Nixon AJ. Gene-based approaches for the repair of articular cartilage. Gene Ther 2004; 11:351–359.

106. Ghivizzani SC, Oligino TJ, Glorioso JC, Robbins PD, Evans CH. Gene therapy approaches for treating rheumatoid arthritis. Clin Orthop Relat Res 2000; 379(suppl):S288–S299.

107. Gray RG, Gottlieb NL. Intra-articular corticosteroids. an updated assessment. Clin Orthop Relat Res 1983; 177:235–263.

108. Broy SB, Schmid FR. A comparison of medical drainage (needle aspiration) and surgical drainage (arthrotomy or arthroscopy) in the initial treatment of infected joints. Clin Rheum Dis 1986; 12:501–522.

109. Nalbant S, Martinez JA, Kitumnuaypong T, Clayburne G, Sieck M, Schumacher HR Jr. Synovial fluid features and their relations to osteoarthritis severity: new findings from sequential studies. Osteoarthritis Cartilage 2003; 11:50–54.

110. McCarthy GM, McCarty DJ. Intrasynovial corticosteroid therapy. Bull Rheum Dis 1994; 43:2–4.

111. Rostron PK, Calver RF. Subcutaneous atrophy following methylprednisolone injection in osgood-schlatter epiphysitis. J Bone Joint Surg [Am] 1979; 61:627–628.

Viscosupplementation

Luis E. Palacio
Thomas Jefferson University, Philadelphia, Pennsylvania, U.S.A.

Peter C. Vitanzo
Rothman Institute, Thomas Jefferson University, Philadelphia, Pennsylvania, U.S.A.

INTRODUCTION

Arthritis has a tremendous impact on the U.S. economy and a substantial impact on functional capacity and activities of daily living of those who are affected. In 1997 alone, arthritic conditions cost the U.S. economy an estimated $86.2 billion, or nearly 1% of the entire U.S. gross domestic product for that same year (1). An estimated 40 million Americans had some form of arthritis in 1995. By the year 2020, an estimated 59.4 million will be affected (2). Specifically, osteoarthritis (OA) of the knee affects 6.1% of persons over age 30 (3). Osteoarthritis is the most common rheumatic disease, and it is second only to cardiovascular diseases in producing chronic disability (4).

Conservative treatments of OA include use of oral medications, physical therapy, weight loss, and dietary supplements (i.e., glucosamine). When these modalities fail to relieve pain, injection therapy is often recommended. Currently, the primary injectable options for knee OA include steroids and joint fluid therapy products [i.e., intra-articular hyaluronic acid (IA HA)]. Steroid injections relieve pain for a variable amount of time, and effects may wear off prior to their recommended readministration period. In these patients, IA HA therapy may be the next appropriate step in management.

Viscosupplementation is the exogenous administration of HA for the treatment of OA. IA HA injections should be considered if conservative treatment options fail, are not tolerable, or for patients who are not good candidates for a knee replacement (5,6). Viscosupplementation is a useful tool in the armamentarium of physicians dealing with OA in their daily practice.

INTRA-ARTICULAR FLUID CHANGES IN ARTHRITIS

Synovial fluid functions as a joint lubricant, and HA is one of its major components. It also functions as a transport medium for nutrients, protein, and intra-articular degradation products (7). It is made up of repeating disaccharides of D-glucuronic acid and N-acetylglucosamine forming a large glycosaminoglycan (8,9) and is present in many tissues throughout the body including synovial fluid, aqueous humor, skin, and articular cartilage. It contributes to the gel-like consistency of the extracellular matrix and helps cartilage resist compression and shear forces (10).

In OA, the synovial fluid properties are altered. Its overall molecular weight diminishes, and the concentration of HA within the joint fluid decreases as well (11). Depolarization of HA also occurs, which may help explain some of these structural changes (12). It is unknown whether these changes are secondary to dilution of the joint fluid, degradation of the HA, or problems with its production (13,14). As a result, the synovial fluid loses its protective effects, including viscosity and elasticity, which affects its ability to absorb and transmit shock as well as lubricate the joint. These changes leave the articular cartilage more vulnerable to damage (4,11,14).

Synovial inflammation has been noted in OA and is thought to play an important role. Synovial fluid in OA also contains high levels of inflammatory mediators (15–19) and elevated levels of C-reactive protein (20,21).

HISTORY OF THE VISCOSUPPLEMENTATION CONCEPT

Viscosupplementation is the exogenous administration of HA for the treatment of OA. Balazs (9,14) proposed that exogenous administration of HA might help restore synovial fluid properties and promote its synthesis within the joint. Balazs assumed this would result in better joint function and decreased pain (14).

Meyer and Palmer gave HA its name in 1934 after isolating it in bovine vitreous humor. They derived the name from the Greek word "hylos," which means glass-like. In 1986, Balazs introduced the term "hyaluronan" (14). As a result, the terms HA, sodium hyaluronate, and hyaluronan all describe the same substance.

Hyaluronic acid has been utilized in veterinary medicine for many years. It has been used in race horses for treatment of OA through intravenous administrations (11). Its approval by the Food and Drug Administration (FDA) for use in humans occurred in 1997 (8).

The HA used for exogenous administration is obtained primarily from rooster and chicken combs. It has also been obtained from human umbilical cord and through bacterial cultures. Preparation for use includes purification and removal of inflammatory, immunogenic, and chemotactic fractions (14).

MECHANISM OF ACTION

The exact mechanism of action of administered HA is unclear. Proposed theories regarding mechanism of action include the following: (*i*) HA restores the physical and biomechanical properties (i.e., viscoelasticity) of synovial fluid, (*ii*) it acts as a nocioceptor analgesic, (*iii*) it stimulates endogenous HA production by synoviocytes, (*iv*) it acts as an anti-inflammatory, and/or (*v*) stimulates chondrocyte growth and collagen biosynthesis and decreases chondrocyte apoptosis.

In vitro studies utilizing human synoviocytes have demonstrated that the addition of exogenous HA stimulates de novo HA production within the synoviocyte. It also diminishes the concentration of arachidonic acid and prostaglandin E_2 in the human synoviocyte. It also has many direct effects on the leukocyte. It influences leukocyte adherence, proliferation, migration capacity, and phagocytic function (22), all of which protect against cellular damage (4).

Studies have demonstrated that IA HA reduces proinflammatory cytokines, prostaglandin E_2 levels, and cyclic adenosine monophosphate (AMP) in the synovial fluid of OA patients (7,14,23,24). This may play a large role in its efficacy.

Once administered, IA HA usually clears from the synovial fluid compartment within 24 to 48 hours, on average (11). For this reason, it has been suggested that higher molecular weight formulations may be more effective in keeping the HA within the joint for a longer period of time. Higher molecular weight formulations have been utilized, but these have been shown to last only 17 hours to one-and-a-half days, which is not much longer than the lower molecular weight predecessors (24).

EMPIRICAL EVIDENCE
Animal Studies
Hyaluronic acid has been used to enhance performance in animals since the early 1970s (25). It was first used in track horses for traumatic arthritis, and its proven success sparked its wide use in veterinary medicine. Cartilage preservation has been demonstrated following HA administration in these animal studies (7,13,14,26). The evidence of the effects of HA primarily comes from animal testing. These animal studies, as well as some human studies, suggest that HA may have a protective effect on cartilage. It certainly has a direct effect on the inflammatory process (14). It is also thought to reduce pain by acting directly on cell receptors.

Human Study
Listrat et al. (27) reported that patients who received a series of three IA HA injections at an interval of three months showed a statistically significant difference for two of three structural parameters in favor of HA when compared with controls who received conventional treatment without IA HA injection. Deterioration was less in the IA HA group in overall assessment by a blinded arthroscopy reviewer utilizing a Visual Analog Scale (VAS) (VAS scores 5.1 ± 12.7 vs. 16.7 ± 18.3, $P = 0.016$, $n = 36$). The Société Française d'Arthroscopie (SFA) scoring system also demonstrated less deterioration in favor of the IA HA group (SFA scores $= 3.7 \pm 7.3$ versus $+9.0 \pm 11.5$, $P = 0.05$) (27). Quality of life was improved in the IA HA group using the Arthritis Impact Measurement Scale (AIMS$_2$) (AIMS$_2$ scores $= -0.42 \pm 0.67$ versus $+0.18 \pm 0.88$, $P < 0.05$). Bellamy et al. (28), writing for the Cochrane group, reanalyzed Listrat's data and detected no statistical significance with these findings. Listrat's study (27) has also been criticized because of its small sample size and the possible treatment effect of joint lavage during the arthroscopic procedure. Furthermore, arthroscopy was used to assess the degree of OA, and cartilage thickness is not directly measured during this procedure (14).

Mixed Trial Results
The efficacy of viscosupplementation is still under scrutiny. There seems to be some disparity among study results regarding its value (Table 1). There is, however, substantial evidence that IA HA is at least as effective as treatment with nonsteroidal anti-inflammatory medications, but without the significant side effects associated with these. Altman et al. (4) conducted a double blind, multicenter trial with three treatment groups comparing IA HA, IA placebo (saline), and naproxen ($n = 495$). Altman reported that gastrointestinal problems resulted in discontinuation of 14 patients (8%) from the naproxen group versus four (2%) from the HA and placebo groups ($P < 0.0001$, Fisher exact test). One meta-analysis of HA trials (5) by Modawal et al. suggested HA treatment is moderately effective at 5 to 12 weeks (change in VAS at 5–7 weeks $= 17.6$, 95% CI $= 7.5$–28; change in VAS at 8 to 12 weeks $= 18.1$, 95% CI $= 6.3$–29.9); but not at 15 to 22 weeks (change in VAS $= 4.4$, 95% CI $= 15.3$–24.1, $P > 0.05$) (5). Other studies suggest

TABLE 1 Comparison of Viscosupplementation Studies

Study	HA treatment regimen	Treatments compared	Pain measurement method	Follow-up length	Mean age	Results of HA	Note
Altman et al. (4)	Five weekly injections of Hyalgan® (Sanofi-Aventis, Bridgewater, New Jersey, U.S.A.)	HA vs. placebo injection or naproxen	50-feet walk test 10 cm VAS WOMAC	26 wks	62	At least as effective as naproxen with less side effects	Acetaminophen allowed for escape analgesia
Carborn et al. (7)	Three weekly injections of Synvisc® (Genzyme Biosurgery, Cambridge, Massachusetts, U.S.A.)	Hylan G-F 20 vs. IA triamcinolone	10 cm VAS WOMAC	26 wks	63	Longer duration of effect over IA steroid	HA had a later onset of effect
Huskisson et al. (33)	Five weekly injections Hyalgan®	HA vs. placebo injection (2-cc saline)	10 cm VAS (pain on walking)	6 mos	66	Superior to placebo with effects lasting 6 mos.	Placebo did have some benefit
Jubb et al. (34)	Three weekly injections of Hyalgan®, repeated every 4 months 3 times	HA vs. placebo injection (2-cc saline)	10 cm VAS LFI S-F36[a]	1 yr	64	No symptom benefit over placebo, but less progression of joint space narrowing	Radiographs used to assess joint space loss at beginning and end; concomitant analgesia and NSAID were allowed

Study	Regimen	Comparison	Outcome measures	Duration	Age	Result	Comment
Karlsson et al. (32)	Three weekly injections of Artzal® (AstraZeneca US, Wilmington, Delaware, U.S.A.) or Synvisc®	Hyaluronan vs. hylan G-F 20 vs. placebo injection (3-cc saline)	WOMAC LFI SF-36[a]	1 yr	70–72	Hyaluronan had a significantly longer duration of benefit	Older patient group; hyaluronan-treated groups were pooled
Leopold et al. (57)	Three weekly injections of Synvisc®	HA vs. IA betamethasone	10 cm VAS WOMAC	6 mos	66	HA was equally effective as betamethasone	One betamethasone injection was given; 48% of patients requested second dose
Wobig et al. (25)	Three weekly injections of Synvisc® or LMW HA[b]	Hylan G-F 20 vs. LMW HA[b]	10 cm VAS WOMAC	12 wks	60	Hylan G-F 20 had greater efficacy over LMW HA[b]	Youngest age group; outcomes were much better than in other trials

[a]SF-36 health survey questionnaire.
[b]Low-molecular weight hyaluronic acid (unspecified).
Abbreviations: HA, hyaluronic acid; IA, intra-articluar; LFI, Lequesne functional index; NSAID, nonsteroidal anti-inflammatory drug; VAS, Visual Analog Scale; WOMAC, Western Ontario and McMaster Universities Osteoarthritis Index.

that maximum therapeutic effects are achieved at 8 to 12 weeks and last nearly six months (7,29). For patients who perceive improvement, relief may not be fully experienced until five to seven weeks after the last injection (5).

Some studies have also compared HA treatment with intra-articular steroid injections. These studies have shown various outcomes. Some report that there is no difference between the two (30–32), while others have suggested that HA treatment is superior (4,8,33,34). The consensus seems to be that corticosteroids show improvement more rapidly than HA treatment, but HA treatment seems to have a longer lasting effect (up to six months). Huskisson (33) demonstrated the prolonged effects of IA HA by measuring VAS at six months after final injection of HA (Hyalgan®, Sanofi-Aventis, Bridgewater, New Jersey, U.S.A.) versus a control arm [receiving IA placebo (saline); age matched with the HA group] and showed better VAS scores in the HA-treated group than the control group [VAS score (lower numbers represent less pain) for HA vs. control = 39.4 ± 27.8 vs. 53.7 ± 29.9, respectively, $P = 0.012$, $n = 80$] (33).

Hyaluronic acid treatment seems to be more effective in relieving symptoms when used in earlier stages of OA. Patients with advanced arthritis, on average, receive minimal benefit from IA HA injections. Studies suggesting that IA HA injections delay OA progression have used evolution of radiographic findings as a surrogate endpoint (27,34). Luissier (35) reported that radiographic grade of OA (grading scale used was not specified) influenced response to IA HA. More of the early and intermediate stage subjects reported better or much better results than those with late stage OA (per unvalidated five-point ordinal scale, chi-squared analysis, $P < 0.05$) (35). These findings suggest that early intervention with these injections may be more beneficial for OA patients (36,37).

Synergistic Effects
Patients with joint effusion experience symptomatic pain relief with arthrocentesis. There has also been a noted relief in control groups receiving placebo injections (i.e., saline). Kirwan (38) suggested that benefits obtained by IA HA may be secondary to a knee arthrocentesis placebo effect.

An analysis by Lo et al. (8) suggests that the efficacy of IA HA is controversial. A total of 22 trials were compared (HA vs. placebo). It was noted that HA patients did marginally better than patients treated with placebo (pooled effect = 0.32, 95% CI = 0.17–0.47, $P < 0.001$). As a frame of reference, a large effect is generally 1.0 or more, and a total knee replacement effect size is between 1.0 and 1.8 (8,39). It has also been noted that outcomes in various studies vary significantly.

Most studies have demonstrated that viscosupplementation is effective in about 70% of treated patients for varying periods of time (13). Treatments repeated every six months have provided relief for about two years, but its effects may be even longer (33).

Low- vs. High-Molecular Weight Formulations
Intra-articular hyaluronic acid therapy is not classified as a drug. Its approval was obtained through consideration as a medical device. There are many that believe that its mechanism of action involves more than just mechanical effects. This raises the question of whether or not its molecular weight truly plays an important role (21,40).

TABLE 2 Viscosupplementation Agents Available in the United States

Trade name	Component	Number of Injections	Molecular Weight (Daltons)
Euflexxa® (Bio-Technology General (Israel), Kiryat Malachi, Israel)	Sodium hyaluronate	3 weekly	2.4–3.6 million
Hyalgan® (Sanofi-Aventis, Bridgewater, New Jersey, U.S.A.)	Sodium hyaluronate	3–5 weekly	0.50–0.73 million
Orthovisc® (DePuy Mitek, Inc., Raynham, Massachusetts, U.S.A.)	High-molecular weight hyaluronan	3–4 weekly	1.0–2.9 million
Supartz® (Orthopedics Smith & Nephew, Inc., Memphis, Tennesse, U.S.A.)	Sodium hyaluronate	5 weekly	0.62–1.17 million
Synvisc® (Genzyme Biosurgery, Cambridge, Massachusetts, U.S.A.)	Hylan G-F 20	3 weekly	6.0 million

Because IA HA usually dissipates from the joint space within 24 to 48 hours after administration, some believe that utilizing a higher molecular weight IA HA might allow it to remain in the joint longer. Theoretically, this may produce a superior effect. Studies have been performed to help validate this theory. However, variability in their results has made it difficult to reach a conclusion.

Currently, there are five FDA-approved IA HA products available in the United States (Table 2). Hylan G-F 20 (Synvisc®, Genzyme Biosurgery, Cambridge, Massachusetts, U.S.A.) is an example of a high-molecular weight formulation. It was noted to have statistically significantly greater efficacy and duration of action compared with low-molecular weight HA. Wobig et al. (25) compared Hylan G-F 20 with low-molecular weight HA and used VAS to measure pain. There was reported improvement in overall symptoms by study subjects at week 12 [38 mm (high-molecular weight preparation) vs. 25 mm (low-molecular weight preparation), $P < 0.05$, $n = 73$] (25). The authors directly attributed pain relief to the elastoviscosity of the material used in the product (14,25,41).

INDICATIONS AND USAGE

The economic cost of gastrointestinal adverse effects secondary to nonsteroidal anti-inflammatory use has been estimated to be greater than $500 million annually (42). The American College of Rheumatology recommends the use of IA HA for OA treatment in patients who have not responded to nonpharmacologic therapy, or patients who have a contraindication to nonsteroidal anti-inflammatories or COX-2 inhibitors (Fig. 1) (6).

Patients who require multiple corticosteroid injections are also good candidates, as excessive corticosteroid may accelerate OA and joint damage (7). Corticosteroid arthropathy has been demonstrated in rabbit studies (43,44), but this has not been reproducible in primates (45), and has not been noted to affect outcomes such as a need for earlier knee replacement (46). The authors agree that steroid injections should not exceed three to four per year. Young and middle-aged patients with premature knee OA that need to delay joint replacement may also be good candidates for IA HA (47).

As with all IA HA injections, any suggestion of infection within the joint or in the overlying skin at the injection sight is a contraindication for their use. These products should also be avoided in patients with overlying skin conditions such

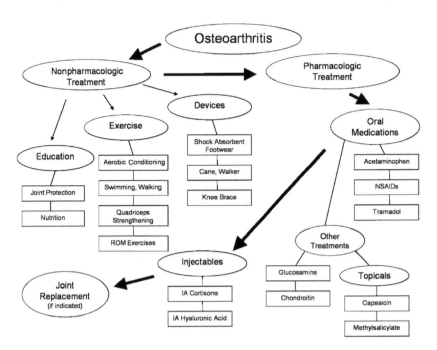

FIGURE 1 Algorithm demonstrating treatment options for patients with osteoarthritis *Abbreviations:* ROM, range of motion; IA, intra-articular; NSAIDs, nonsteroidal anti-inflammatory drugs. *Source:* Adapted from American College of Rheumatology Subcommittee on Osteoarthritis Guidelines.

as psoriasis. Additionally, IA HA should not be used in patients with known hypersensitivity (allergy) to sodium hyaluronate preparations or avian proteins, feathers, and egg products.

Intra-articular hyaluronic acid is not indicated for inflammatory-type arthritis (i.e., rheumatoid arthritis or gout). In theory, its anti-inflammatory effect may be beneficial for these patients but data is lacking (13).

Some concerns about these injections include their high cost and the inconvenience of three to five weekly injections (5). Additionally, these multiple injections and missed work for office visits can cause patient anxiety. However, the author's (Vitanzo PC) own extensive clinical experience with these injections has shown this to be a relatively infrequent occurrence.

ADMINISTRATION
Technique
Any significant effusion should be aspirated prior to administering the IA HA. This will minimize any potential dilution of the IA HA product (13). It should be administered in the appropriate intra-articular compartment. This is more challenging in obese patients and those without an effusion. While various knee joint injection sites can be utilized (i.e., anterolateral, anteromedial, and the lateral mid-patellar approach), Jackson et al. (48) demonstrated that the lateral mid-patellar approach had the highest accuracy rate for administration (Fig. 2).

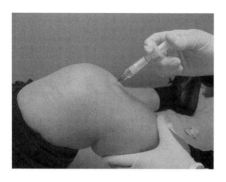

FIGURE 2 Intraarticular injection demonstrating the anterolateral approach.

Adverse Reactions

Overall, HA products are extremely safe. Trials with up to one year follow up have not demonstrated any systemic adverse effects (14). Local flares, including pain and swelling at the injection site, occur in 1% to 3% of patients and tend to be self-limited, resolving within one to three days (35,42). Hylan G-F 20 (Synvisc®) has been known to cause a greater amount of reactions than lower molecular weight HA (i.e., Supartz®, Hyalgan®). Hylan G-F 20 undergoes a process utilizing formaldehyde and vinylsulfone during its development. This process involves covalent cross-linking (Hylan A and Hylan B) to increase its molecular weight (12). This may help explain why it produces more adverse reactions than its counterparts, but this theory has yet to be proven. These reactions have been termed severe acute inflammatory reactions (SAIRs), and they seem to differ from typical allergic type reactions. Marino et al. (49) suggest reactions related to Hylan G-F 20 are a type IV (cell-mediated) hypersensitivity reaction. Clinical characteristics of a typical SAIR include severe inflammation with an effusion and pain in the joint usually within 24 to 72 hours of injection. Generally, such a reaction requires exposure to more than one IA HA injection in a series (50). These reactions can resemble a septic knee but joint fluid analyses in these patients are negative for crystals and organisms both on gram stain and culture. Therefore, they have also been labeled "pseudoseptic reactions" (12).

Local Reactions

Some common local reactions include mild to moderate pain and swelling near the injection site in up to 20% of patients (42). Therefore, it is very important to counsel patients on these possible adverse effects. Many theories have been proposed on these side effects, such as an immune-mediated response, stimulation of inflammatory mediators, and induction of pyrophosphate dehydrate (51).

Granulomatous Reactions

A few cases of local granulomatous reactions have been reported following IA HA injection (42). All have been in patients who received Hylan G-F 20 (Synvisc®). Some have been severe enough to require surgical intervention. Chronic synovitis and foreign body giant cell reaction was observed in these patients. These patients developed symptoms within two days of the last injection, and gradually resolved within one to two weeks after the last injection. Chen et al. (42) believe that the highly cross-linked molecular structure is directly responsible for its higher reaction rate, but also felt that contaminants during its preparation may play a role. These reactions do not seem to be related to crystal deposition (50).

Treatment
Reactions are uncommon and may be treated with standard treatments such as nonsteroidal anti-inflammatory drugs (NSAIDs), corticosteroid injections, arthrocentesis, or arthroscopic intervention (rarely) (13).

Acute Care
Pressure, rest, ice, compression, and elevation (PRICE) in addition to NSAIDs are first-line treatment options. If a patient is nonresponsive to these measures and a septic joint is suspected, joint aspirate should be sent for gram stain/cultures, and antibiotics should be started until culture results are available (12). A septic joint is extremely rare following IA injection, but patients should not receive corticosteroid injection as a method of treatment unless septic joint has been ruled out (52).

Chronic Care
Many clinicians continue to treat these patients with IA HA despite prior reactions. However, labeling lists prior adverse reactions as a contraindication. Chen et al. (42) report that these patients may be at an increased risk for forming local granulomas.

ADDITIONAL RESEARCH
Study Design Issues
Some difficulties with research involve the use of placebo, as there is improvement with placebo injections as well. Blinding is also an issue, because many of these substances are much thicker than the placebo substance that is used, making it easy for the clinician to differentiate the two simply by feeling during the injection. Many of the trials also allow the use of rescue medications such as acetaminophen and NSAIDs, which may also alter results.

Use in Other Joints
Intra-articular hyaluronic acid is currently FDA-approved only for knee OA, but there are various clinical studies in progress evaluating the use of IA HA in other OA joints including the hip (53), shoulder, elbow, ankle (54), foot, and first carpometacarpal joint of the thumb. Preliminary outcomes in the shoulders and hips seem to demonstrate similarities to knee studies. Future IA HA use may include these other joint indications (13,14,40).

Long-Term Studies
More long-term studies are required to assess IA HA. Currently, the Measurement of Outcomes from Viscosupplementation Effectiveness (MOVE) Study is measuring the outcome of 1301 patients compared with 559 control subjects. It is a multicenter, prospective study comparing Hylan G-F 20 with IA corticosteroid. It is the longest trial thus far measuring outcomes for a total of four years and results are not available at the time of publication.

The Future of Viscosupplementation

In the near future, IA HA therapy will likely receive FDA approval for other joints, given its similar performance in recent trials. Further data is required to determine whether or not these treatments should be given much earlier than currently indicated. The findings in animal studies, and a few human studies suggest that there may be a delay in progression of disease with these agents. If this is the case, IA HA may, ultimately, be indicated repeatedly in patients at six-month intervals, regardless of whether they are symptomatic or not.

Grecomoro et al. (55) discovered a possible synergistic effect by co-administration of low-dose corticosteroids along with HA. It may be worth investigating the possibility of administering these agents along with a low-dose corticosteroid in patients who are resistant to IA HA treatment alone. This may decrease the amount of damage that higher-dose steroids may inflict on the joint. Also, Tytherleigh-Strong et al. (56) administered IA HA shortly after osteochondral grafting surgery in sheep, and reported that IA HA may help improve articular cartilage flow at the graft edge when compared with a control group (IA buffer solution). Although this was a small trial ($n = 12$), these findings illustrate the importance of further investigation into other important uses for IA HA.

CONCLUSION

Intra-articular hyaluronic acid injections are a safe and effective treatment option for patients with knee OA. They should definitely be considered after acetaminophen and nonpharmacologic approaches have failed. It is at least as effective as treatment with NSAIDs with a much better safety profile, and it may even help diminish OA disease progression. It is a great option for patients who are not candidates for joint replacement. It is still unclear whether higher- versus lower-molecular weight formulas impact their efficacy, but they all seem to add some clinical benefit to patients with knee OA.

REFERENCES

1. Yelin E, Cisternas MG, Pasta DJ, Trupin L, Murphy L, Helmick CG. Medical care expenditures and earnings losses of persons with arthritis and other rheumatic conditions in the United States in 1997: total and incremental estimates. Arthritis Rheum 2004; 50:2317–2326.
2. Lawrence RC, Helmick CG, Arnett FC, et al. Estimates of the prevalence of arthritis and selected musculoskeletal disorders in the United States. Arthritis Rheum 1998; 41:778–799.
3. Felson DT, Zhang Y. An update on the epidemiology of knee and hip osteoarthritis with a view to prevention. Arthritis Rheum 1998; 41:1343–1355.
4. Altman RD, Moskowitz R. Intraarticular sodium hyaluronate (hyalgan) in the treatment of patients with osteoarthritis of the knee: a randomized clinical trial. Hyalgan Study Group. J Rheumatol 1998; 25:2203–2212.
5. Modawal A, Ferrer M, Choi HK, Castle JA. Hyaluronic acid injections relieve knee pain. J Fam Pract 2005; 54:758–767.
6. American College of Rheumatology Subcommittee on Osteoarthritis Guidelines. Recommendations for the medical management of osteoarthritis of the hip and knee: 2000 update. Arthritis Rheum 2000; 43:1905–1915. Available from: http://www.rheumatology.org/publications/guidelines/oa-mgmt/oa-mgmt.asp.
7. Caborn D, Rush J, Lanzer W, Parenti D, Murray C, Synvisc 901 Study Group. A randomized, single-blind comparison of the efficacy and tolerability of hylan G-F 20 and

triamcinolone hexacetonide in patients with osteoarthritis of the knee. J Rheumatol 2004; 31:333–343.

8. Lo GH, LaValley M, McAlindon T, Felson DT. Intra-articular hyaluronic acid in treatment of knee osteoarthritis: a meta-analysis. JAMA 2003; 290:3115–3121.

9. Balazs EA, Denlinger JL. Viscosupplementation: a new concept in the treatment of osteoarthritis. J Rheumatol Suppl 1993; 39:3–9.

10. Kelley WN, Harris ED Jr., Ruddy S, Sledge CB, Walsh DA, Blak DR, eds. Textbook of Rheumatology. 5th ed. Philadelphia, PA: WB Saunders Co, 1997.

11. Felson DT, Anderson JJ. Hyaluronate sodium injections for osteoarthritis: hope, hype, and hard truths. Arch Intern Med 2002; 162:245–247.

12. Goldberg VM, Coutts RD. Pseudoseptic reactions to hylan viscosupplementation: diagnosis and treatment. Clin Orthop Relat Res 2004; 419:130–137.

13. Marshall KW. Viscosupplementation for osteoarthritis: current status, unresolved issues, and future directions. J Rheumatol 1998; 25:2056–2058.

14. George E. Intra-articular hyaluronan treatment for osteoarthritis. Ann Rheum Dis 1998; 57:637–640.

15. Houssiau FA, Devogelaer JP, Van Damme J, de Deuxchaisnes CN, Van Snick J. Interleukin-6 in synovial fluid and serum of patients with rheumatoid arthritis and other inflammatory arthritides. Arthritis Rheum 1988; 31:784–788.

16. Brozik M, Rosztoczy I, Meretey K, et al. Interleukin 6 levels in synovial fluids of patients with different arthritides: correlation with local IgM rheumatoid factor and systemic acute phase protein production. J Rheumatol 1992; 19:63–68.

17. Kuryliszyn-Moskal A. Comparison of blood and synovial fluid lymphocyte subsets in rheumatoid arthritis and osteoarthritis. Clin Rheumatol 1995; 14:43–50.

18. Hrycaj P, Stratz T, Kovac C, Mennet P, Muller W. Microheterogeneity of acute phase proteins in patients with clinically active and clinically nonactive osteoarthritis. Clin Rheumatol 1995; 14:434–440.

19. Schlaak JF, Pfers I, Meyer Zum Buschenfelde KH, Marker-Hermann E. Different cytokine profiles in the synovial fluid of patients with osteoarthritis, rheumatoid arthritis and seronegative spondylarthropathies. Clin Exp Rheumatol 1996; 14:155–162.

20. Spector TD, Hart DJ, Nandra D, et al. Low-level increases in serum C-reactive protein are present in early osteoarthritis of the knee and predict progressive disease. Arthritis Rheum 1997; 40:723–727.

21. Ghosh P, Guidolin D. Potential mechanism of action of intra-articular hyaluronan therapy in osteoarthritis: are the effects of molecular weight dependent? Semin Arthritis Rheum 2002; 32:10–37.

22. Ghosh P. The role of hyaluronic acid (hyaluronan) in health and disease: interactions with cells, cartilage and components of synovial fluid. Clin Exp Rheumatol 1994; 12:75–82.

23. Pasquali Ronchetti I, Guerra D, Taparelli F, et al. Morphological analysis of knee synovial membrane biopsies from a randomized controlled clinical study comparing the effects of sodium hyaluronate (hyalgan) and methylprednisolone acetate (depomedrol) in osteoarthritis. Rheumatology (Oxford) 2001; 40:158–169.

24. Brandt KD, Smith GN, Jr., Simon LS. Intraarticular injection of hyaluronan as treatment for knee osteoarthritis: what is the evidence? Arthritis Rheum 2000; 43:1192–1203.

25. Wobig M, Bach G, Beks P, et al. The role of elastoviscosity in the efficacy of viscosupplementation for osteoarthritis of the knee: a comparison of hylan G-F 20 and a lower-molecular-weight hyaluronan. Clin Ther 1999; 21:1549–1562.

26. Gomis A, Pawlak M, Balazs EA, Schmidt RF, Belmonte C. Effects of different molecular weight elastoviscous hyaluronan solutions on articular nociceptive afferents. Arthritis Rheum 2004; 50:314–326.

27. Listrat V, Ayral X, Paternello F, et al. Arthroscopic evaluation of potential structure modifying activity of hyaluronan (hyalgan) in osteoarthritis of the knee. Osteoarthritis Cartilage 1997; 5:153–160.

28. Bellamy N, Campbell J, Robinson V, Gee T, Bourne R, Wells G. Viscosupplementation for the treatment of osteoarthritis of the knee. Cochrane Database Syst Rev 2005; (2):CD005321.

29. Waddell DD. The tolerability of viscosupplementation: low incidence and clinical management of local adverse events. Curr Med Res Opin 2003; 19:575–580.
30. Creamer P, Sharif M, George E, et al. Intra-articular hyaluronic acid in osteoarthritis of the knee: an investigation into mechanisms of action. Osteoarthritis Cartilage 1994; 2:133–140.
31. Brandt KD, Block JA, Michalski JP, Moreland LW, Caldwell JR, Lavin PT. Efficacy and safety of intraarticular sodium hyaluronate in knee osteoarthritis. ORTHOVISC study group. Clin Orthop Relat Res 2001; 385:130–143.
32. Karlsson J, Sjogren LS, Lohmander LS. Comparison of two hyaluronan drugs and placebo in patients with knee osteoarthritis. A controlled, randomized, double-blind, parallel-design multicentre study. Rheumatology (Oxford) 2002; 41:1240–1248.
33. Huskisson EC, Donnelly S. Hyaluronic acid in the treatment of osteoarthritis of the knee. Rheumatology (Oxford) 1999; 38:602–607.
34. Jubb RW, Piva S, Beinat L, Dacre J, Gishen P. A one-year, randomized, placebo (saline) controlled clinical trial of 500–730 kDa sodium hyaluronate (hyalgan) on the radiological change in osteoarthritis of the knee. Int J Clin Pract 2003; 57:467–474.
35. Lussier A, Cividino AA, McFarlane CA, Olszynski WP, Potashner WJ, De Medicis R. Viscosupplementation with hylan for the treatment of osteoarthritis: findings from clinical practice in Canada. J Rheumatol 1996; 23:1579–1585.
36. Kemper F, Gebhardt U, Meng T, Murray C. Tolerability and short-term effectiveness of hylan G-F 20 in 4253 patients with osteoarthritis of the knee in clinical practice. Curr Med Res Opin 2005; 21:1261–1269.
37. Wang CT, Lin J, Chang CJ, Lin YT, Hou SM. Therapeutic effects of hyaluronic acid on osteoarthritis of the knee. A meta-analysis of randomized controlled trials. J Bone Joint Surg Am 2004; 86-A:538–545.
38. Kirwan J. Is there a place for intra-articular hyaluronate in osteoarthritis of the knee? Knee 2001; 8:93–101.
39. Liang MH, Larson MG, Cullen KE, Schwartz JA. Comparative measurement efficiency and sensitivity of five health status instruments for arthritis research. Arthritis Rheum 1985; 28:542–547.
40. Conrozier T, Bertin P, Mathieu P, et al. Intra-articular injections of hylan G-F 20 in patients with symptomatic hip osteoarthritis: an open-label, multicentre, pilot study. Clin Exp Rheumatol 2003; 21:605–610.
41. Vitanzo PC, Jr., Sennett BJ. Hyaluronans: is clinical effectiveness dependent on molecular weight? Am J Orthop 2006; 35(9):421–428.
42. Chen AL, Desai P, Adler EM, DiCesare PE. Granulomatous inflammation after hylan G-F 20 viscosupplementation of the knee: a report of six cases. J Bone Joint Surg [Am] 2002; 84-A:1142–1147.
43. Mankin HJ, Conger KA. The acute effects of intra-articular hydrocortisone on articular cartilage in rabbits. J Bone Joint Surg [Am] 1966; 48:1383–1388.
44. Moskowitz RW, Davis W, Sammarco J, Mast W, Chase SW. Experimentally induced corticosteroid arthropathy. Arthritis Rheum 1970; 13:236–243.
45. Schumacher HR, Chen LX. Injectable corticosteroids in treatment of arthritis of the knee. Am J Med 2005; 118:1208–1214.
46. Roberts WN, Babcock EA, Breitbach SA, Owen DS, Irby WR. Corticosteroid injection in rheumatoid arthritis does not increase rate of total joint arthroplasty. J Rheumatol 1996; 23:1001–1004.
47. Cefalu CA, Waddell DS. Viscosupplementation: treatment alternative for osteoarthritis of the knee. Geriatrics 1999; 54:51–54, 57.
48. Jackson DW, Evans NA, Thomas BM. Accuracy of needle placement into the intra-articular space of the knee. J Bone Joint Surg [Am] 2002; 84-A:1522–1527.
49. Marino AA, Waddell DD, Kolomytkin OV, Pruett S, Sadasivan KK, Albright JA. Assessment of immunologic mechanisms for flare reactions to synvisc(r). Clin Orthop Relat Res 2006; 442:187–194.
50. Pullman-Mooar S, Mooar P, Sieck M, Clayburne G, Schumacher HR. Are there distinctive inflammatory flares after hylan g-f 20 intraarticular injections? J Rheumatol 2002; 29:2611–2614.

51. Leopold SS, Warme WJ, Pettis PD, Shott S. Increased frequency of acute local reaction to intra-articular hylan GF-20 (synvisc) in patients receiving more than one course of treatment. J Bone Joint Surg [Am] 2002; 84-A:1619–1623.
52. Puttick MP, Wade JP, Chalmers A, Connell DG, Rangno KK. Acute local reactions after intraarticular hylan for osteoarthritis of the knee. J Rheumatol 1995; 22:1311–1314.
53. Migliore A, Tormenta S, Martin Martin LS, et al. The symptomatic effects of intra-articular administration of hylan G-F 20 on osteoarthritis of the hip: clinical data of 6 months follow-up. Clin Rheumatol 2005; 25:1–5.
54. Salk R, Chang T, D'Costa W, Soomekh D, Grogan K. Viscosupplementation (hyaluronans) in the treatment of ankle osteoarthritis. Clin Podiatr Med Surg North Am 2005; 22:585–597, vii.
55. Grecomoro G, Piccione F, Letizia G. Therapeutic synergism between hyaluronic acid and dexamethasone in the intra-articular treatment of osteoarthritis of the knee: a preliminary open study. Curr Med Res Opin 1992; 13:49–55.
56. Tytherleigh-Strong G, Hurtig M, Miniaci A. Intra-articular hyaluronan following autogenous osteochondral grafting of the knee. Arthroscopy 2005; 21:999–1005.
57. Leopold SS, Redd BB, Warme WJ, Wehrle PA, Pettis PD, Shott S. Corticosteroid compared with hyaluronic acid injections for the treatment of osteoarthritis of the knee. A prospective, randomized trial. J Bone Joint Surg [Am] 2003; 85-A:1197–1203.

4   Treatment of Trigger Points in Myofascial Pain Syndrome

Mendel Kupfer
Thomas Jefferson University Hospital, Philadelphia, Pennsylvania, U.S.A.

E. Anthony Overton
Rothman Institute, Thomas Jefferson University Hospital, Philadelphia, Pennsylvania, U.S.A.

INTRODUCTION

Trigger points are tender, irritable areas found in muscle, which can be active or latent and can cause local or referred pain. They are the key feature of myofascial pain syndrome. This pain syndrome is encountered in clinical practice in 30% (1) to 85% (2) of patients. This chapter will discuss the treatment of trigger points with the emphasis on interventional options.

CLINICAL PRESENTATION

Myofascial pain syndrome and trigger points are often confused with fibromyalgia and tender points. The diagnosis of fibromyalgia is based on a history of widespread pain, defined as pain present bilaterally, in the upper and lower body, as well as the axial skeleton, and the presence of excessive tenderness on applying pressure to 11 of 18 specific tender point sites (3,4). These tender points by definition become painful at 4 kg of pressure and are not all over the muscle (4). Myofascial pain is characterized by the presence of trigger points. It is in a regional distribution, owing to muscle only, and refers to specific patterns. Fibromyalgia is more frequently accompanied by sleep disorders and emotional distress.

    Myofascial trigger points are defined as hyperirritable areas in skeletal muscle that are associated with hypersensitive palpable nodules in a taut band, a rope-like component of affected muscles. When a taut band is found, the examiner palpates along the taut band parallel to the fiber direction (5). The trigger point is a firm nodular density about 2 to 5 mm in diameter (6). In an active trigger point, this palpation will elicit the patient's pain complaint, including pain in the muscle's referral pattern, and may yield a "jump sign" (7). An active trigger point is further confirmed by a "local twitch response," a transient contraction of the muscle fibers associated with the trigger point. The local twitch response is triggered by manipulation of the trigger point either manually or with a needle. Latent trigger points may have the characteristics of active trigger points except that they are painful only when palpated (5).

    The diagnosis of myofascial pain is determined by the examination of trigger points (Table 1).Gerwin et al. (8) reported a failure to establish a high degree of

TABLE 1 Palpation Techniques

Palpation type	Method	Muscle type	Examples
Flat palpation	Examiner uses the fingertip to slide over muscle tissue	Superficial muscles that have only one surface available	Extensor digitorum communis
Pincer palpation	Examiner rolls muscle between the thumb and index finger	Easily accessible muscles	Upper trapezius, biceps brachii
Deep palpation	Examiner exerts finger pressure over the motor point and attachment areas trying to evoke tenderness that is specific to a direction of pressure	Muscles that are relatively inaccessible	Quadratus lumborum

Source: From Ref. 5.

agreement among novice examiners for any of the features of the myofascial trigger points. In Phase II of the study, examiners received training where definitions of the features of the trigger points were reviewed. After completion of this training, examiners established a high degree of agreement (74%) for identification of the presence of trigger points.

DIAGNOSTIC TESTING

At present, there are no universally accepted tests that are diagnostic for the identification of a trigger point. Several studies have investigated the use of electromyography as a diagnostic test but the results remain controversial. Weeks and Travell (9), as well as Hubbard and Berkoff (10) identified high-frequency potentials in trigger points while the remainder of the muscle was electrically silent. Simons and Hong (11) identified high-amplitude endplate spike potentials in addition to low-voltage endplate potentials after increasing the amplification fivefold and the sweep speed 10-fold (11). Electromyographers often identify these same findings as normal endplate potentials or endplate noise.

Ultrasound is an evolving imaging modality in musculoskeletal medicine. Ultrasound, though, has not been proven useful in locating trigger points (12). One method to confirm and monitor trigger point location is by using algometry (13–16). An algometer is used to measure the amount of pressure needed to elicit pain. The area over trigger points will be more sensitive to pressure than normal tissue. One can also objectively monitor treatment progress using this tool.

PATHOPHYSIOLOGY

The etiology of trigger points is unclear. Travell and Simons proposed the "Integrated trigger point hypothesis," which was updated in 2004 (17). It postulates that in injured muscle, there is facilitation of acetylcholine (ACh) release at the neuromuscular junction, decreased ACh break down, and upregulation of ACh receptors. This leads to persistent muscle contraction, a trigger point. In the process, there is muscle ischemia and damage from the prolonged contraction causing release of inflammatory and nociceptive mediators. An additional area of interest is how peripheral nociception, such as pain from a trigger point, might cause central nervous system upregulation of pain sensitivity (17).

PERPETUATING FACTORS

The clinical importance of perpetuating factors is often neglected in the evaluation and treatment of patients with trigger points. Perpetuating factors can be classified as mechanical (structural asymmetry, posture, ergonomics, and the like), nutritional, metabolic (hypothyroidism, hypoglycemia, and the like), psychologic, or infectious. These factors must be addressed to have an optimal outcome from the treatment.

TREATMENT
Physical Interventions
The mainstay of treatment for myofascial pain syndrome and trigger points centers around physical interventions. The first goal is to restore normal motion to muscles and then to strengthen them while retraining maladaptive postural habits that precipitated the whole process. Restoring normal kinetics to a muscle is accomplished by two complementary approaches, stretching and inactivating trigger points. Initiating a strengthening program too early can overload muscles and exacerbate trigger points.

"Spray and stretch" entails spraying a stream of vapo-coolant in the direction of the muscle fibers as it is placed in a prolonged stretch (Table 2). It is an efficient and minimally painful technique to treat a single muscle or muscle group trigger point and re-establish normal muscle length. The coolant spray minimizes pain and reflex spasm and thereby facilitates a maximal stretch. Common vapo-coolant spray options include ethyl chloride and flouri methane. Ethyl chloride is cooler than flouri methane but is also potentially toxic, flammable, and explosive. Flouri methane is not toxic or flammable but older preparations contained ozone-depleting pollutants. Ozone-safe products are now available. Ice can also be used, but it may be more cumbersome. The ice can be wrapped in plastic to avoid dripping as the wetness will diffuse the cooling effect (5,13).

Spray and stretch can be coupled with injection therapy or combined with "postisometric relaxation," a stretch technique described by Lewit and Simons (18). In this technique, the muscle is passively brought to its end point, gently activated isometrically for about five seconds, and then passively stretched to the new end point. This cycle is repeated three to five times.

TABLE 2 Spray and Stretch Technique

1. The patient is placed in a comfortable position with limbs and back supported.
2. Vapo-coolant spray is held about 45 cm away from the target body area. The stream is applied in long, slow (10 cm/sec) sweeps in a single direction over the entire muscle, moving parallel to the muscle fibers. The stream is most effective if it contacts the skin at an angle of about 30°.
3. After several sweeps of the spray, the muscle is stretched by placing steady tension, avoiding force strong enough to cause pain; jerky, rapid movements should be avoided.
4. The stretch is enhanced by having the patient take slow deep breaths while looking upward and exhaling fully while gazing downward.
5. Following the spray and stretch, the muscle should be warmed with heating pads and then moved through a full active range of motion.

Source: From Refs. 5,13.

Stretching is contraindicated in hypermobile joints. Alternative techniques should be utilized. Coolant treatments should be avoided in patients where the skin is already cold, there is a history of sensitivity to the cold, the patient has a history of allergy to the substances being used, or Raynaud's syndrome (5).

"Ischemic compression" is another means of inactivating a trigger point. It is effective and noninvasive, the major drawback is that it is painful for the patient and may be tiring for the clinician. Pressure is applied with one's thumb to a trigger point causing a tolerable but moderate amount of pain. The pressure is increased to keep the pain at a constant level. When the trigger point is pain-free, 15 seconds to one minute later, the pressure is relieved. A more gentle variation is "trigger point pressure release" where the clinician gently palpates the trigger point while stretching the muscle. Only mild pressure is placed on the trigger point, causing mild discomfort as the muscle is passively lengthened (5).

There are many additional physical techniques than can be used to treat trigger points, from osteopathic muscle energy strategies to Shiatsu massage. They all revolve around the premise of stretching the muscle and restoring normal mobility (5).

Modalities can also be employed in the treatment of myofascial pain. Ultrasound, transcutaneous electrical nerve stimulation, hot packs, and cold packs have all been used to treat myofascial pain syndrome with varying successes (19,20). Physical therapy is prescribed to teach proper stretching and postural techniques as well as to teach the patient a home exercise program. Proper posture and good body mechanics is a lifetime endeavor and must be an ongoing process.

Medication

Medication is best used as an adjuvant therapy for myofascial pain syndrome to treat comorbid or complicating conditions (sleep disorders, depression, and so on) and as a temporizing measure while the other, more active therapies are instituted. Research-validating specific medications in myofascial pain are wanted.

Nonsteroidal anti-inflammatory drugs (NSAIDs) combined with other medications for the treatment of fibromyalgia, have only shown a small contribution to symptom relief (21,22). Tramadol has been shown to be efficacious in fibromyalgia (23), osteoarthritis (24), and low back pain (25), although it has not been studied directly in myofascial pain. It has also shown efficacy when used in combination with acetaminophen (26).

The antidepressants commonly used in treatment of pain are the tricyclic antidepressants (TCA), the selective serotonin reuptake inhibitors (SSRI), and the selective serotonin norepinephrine reuptake inhibitors (SSNRI). TCA medications have been shown to be effective in nociceptive and neuropathic pain (27–29) and fibromyalgia (28). These agents are associated with significant anticholinergic and cardiac side effects, which limit their use. SSRIs have shown to be of some benefit in fibromyalgia, but the literature is mixed as to their efficacy (30,31). SSNRIs are a newer class of medication that have demonstrated some utility in treating neuropathic pain (31) and in fibromyalgia (32).

Membrane stabilizers (antiepileptics), particularly gabapentin, have shown usefulness in the management of neuropathic pain (30,33). Only one retrospective study found gabapentin to be useful in the treatment of myofascial pain (34).

Muscle spasmolytics or "relaxants" are commonly prescribed for musculoskeletal pain complaints. This broad category of medication includes barbiturates, benzodiazepines, baclofen, cyclobenzaprine, carisoprodolol, methocarbamol, chlorzoxazone, and metaxalone. There is no data documenting the efficacy of these medications in myofascial pain syndrome and their use is discouraged by Travell and Simons (5).

Opiate analgesia may increase the ability of a patient to participate in physical and psychological therapies (35–37) and as such, may have a role in the management of myofascial pain. Opiates do not address the underlying pain generators and should only be used as part of a comprehensive rehabilitation program. This should be discussed with the patient, who would then be required to sign an opiate contract that outlines the responsibilities of both the clinician and patient (27).

Injection Therapy

Injection treatments are used in myofascial pain syndromes when more conservative treatments fail, or when it is decided that aggressive treatment is needed because of the severity of the pain. "Trigger point injections" can be performed safely in an office setting, using aseptic technique, provided that the clinician has a thorough understanding of the anatomy and is able to recognize and treat potential complications. These injections should be used as a component of a broader treatment plan and are often maximally effective when immediately followed by stretching exercises.

Contraindications to injection therapy include the presence of systemic infection or a local infection in the area of the contemplated injection. Injections should be avoided in patients who are pregnant or appear to be ill. Caution must be exercised in injecting patients who are taking anticoagulants or have coagulopathies (13). Injection pain can be minimized by using a vapo-coolant spray and by inserting the needle with a quick motion of the wrist. The patient should be warned that there may be pain involved, especially with dry needling, and that muscle twitches may be elicited. The pain can last for several days before resolving.

Needle selection is determined by the body habitus of the patient, the anatomical areas to be injected, and which, if any, medication is to be injected. Larger diameter needles (i.e., 22 gauge) are less likely to bend and provide more tactile feedback. Smaller bore needles (i.e., 27 gauge) cause less pain and ecchymosis but may be difficult to use in dense tissue. The needle should be long enough to reach the trigger point without being inserted to the hub, the most common breaking point of a needle (5). An 1.5-inch 25 to 27-gauge needle is sufficient for most patients (38).

There are a variety of medications and injection options. Sterile water, isotonic saline, local long- and short-acting anesthetics, diclofenac, steroids, or botulinum toxin (BTX) can be injected into trigger points. "Dry needling" is the most basic form of "trigger point injection." A small bore needle or acupuncture needle is used to mechanically break up the trigger point without injecting anything into the site. There is no agent that has been proven to be more efficacious than any other option or consistently better than dry needling (5,39,40). Performing the injection with a local anesthetic does decrease the postinjection soreness (40,41). Epinephrine should be avoided as it can increase the myotoxicity and postinjection pain. Another strategy to manage postinjection pain is to prescribe NSAIDs or acetaminophen prospectively or following the injection. Corticosteroids are widely used in trigger point injections but there is no consistent data that supports this practice (5,19,20).

Cummings and White (39) demonstrated that the efficacy of the trigger point injection is not dependent on the individual technique. However, a local twitch response with injection has been associated with a better outcome (41). Techniques for the injection of specific muscles are reviewed at length elsewhere and are beyond the scope of this chapter (5,42).

A common method of injection is:

1. Prepare the patient and equipment using usual aseptic technique.
2. Palpate a trigger point within a taut band and trap it between two fingers.
3. Insert a needle at 30°, between the two fingers, directed toward the trigger point.
4. Pierce the trigger point, which should feel like mobile dense fibrotic tissue, reproducing the patient's pain and eliciting a local twitch response.
5. Once the trigger point is reached, about 1 mL of lidocaine is injected, depending on the muscle size and amount of trigger points to be injected. (Pull the syringe plunger out before injecting to minimize the risk of intravascular injection.)
6. The needle is withdrawn to the subcutaneous level and redirected so that the trigger point is injected in a fan-like distribution, with about 1 mL being injected in each quadrant until the "local twitch response" ceases and the taut band softens. Ten milliliter of 1% lidocaine is a typical amount of injectate (5,13,43,44).

Variations of injection techniques include Hong's "fast in-fast out," preinjection blocks, solid needle, or hollow, beveled needle (18). Hong's fast in-fast out simply refers to the innovation of trying to spear the trigger point with rapid movements to try to elicit local twitch responses. A "drop" of local anesthetic is injected after each twitch response (5,41). Preinjection block refers to the method developed by Andrew Fischer where local anesthetic is deposited along the trigger point and taut band in the area of innervation. The anesthetized trigger point is then vigorously needled. The purpose of this technique is to minimize the pain associated with needling (45). Acupuncture needles have a solid rounded tip, which causes less tissue damage. A hollow needle is typically beveled and is used to inject pharmacologic agents (19).

Postinjection care allows activity but strenuous exercise should be avoided for three to four days (44). Stretching after injection is encouraged and at a minimum, the muscle which is injected should be slowly moved through its full range of motion three times. Multiple trigger points may be injected at one visit depending on the severity of trigger point involvement and patient tolerance. Injections can be repeated once the postinjection soreness resolves in three to four days. Trigger points may require multiple injections. If three injections have not helped relieve the pain, then re-evaluation of the diagnosis is warranted (5).

Botulinum toxin is being used more frequently for the treatment of trigger points and myofascial pain. It is used to treat spasticity; it prevents ACh release from the presynaptic terminal. It is injected in the symptomatic muscle and it diffuses throughout the muscle. The injection should be performed under electromyographic guidance to ensure proper placement. BTX is found in multiple serotypes: BTX-A and BTX-B are commercially available at present. These serotypes are dosed differently and guidelines for dosing are different. These injections can be given every three months to avoid the formation of antibodies. There is some evidence that BTX has a pain-modulating effect and may provide prolonged relief from trigger point pain (43,46). The best technique for BTX administration has yet to be ascertained, but it would stand to reason that the BTX should be injected into the motor endplate and not into the trigger point itself (5). There is experimental evidence that is consistent with this conclusion. BTX can be injected in a grid pattern in a muscle to provide relief (47) whereas BTX injected into trigger points was not better than lidocaine, dry needling (40), or placebo, though the placebo was not inert (saline injections) (48).

Acupuncture is often successfully used in the treatment of pain (49). Interestingly, it has been found that 71% of trigger points share location and pain distribution patterns with acupuncture points (50). The role of acupuncture in myofascial pain treatment must still be determined (19).

Resuscitation equipment and drugs should be available. The most common complication of trigger point injection is vasovagal syncope. One must be aware of the cardiac complications of vasovagal episodes. Anxious patients or patients with a tendency to be come vasovagal should lay down for the injection. Pneumothorax can occur during cervical or thoracic injections. The presentation can be subtle, so the patient and the clinician should take any respiratory complaints seriously. Coughing or chest pain may signal pleural irritation. Bubbling during needle aspiration may indicate that the needle is in the lung space. A chest X-ray should be obtained if there is any suspicion of a pneumothorax. Intravascular complications are generally avoided by aspirating prior to injection and by injecting low volumes and concentrations. Local anesthetics are myotoxic, proarrythmogenic, and can rarely precipitate seizures. The shorter-acting local anesthetics such as procaine, an ester anesthetic, tend to be less myotoxic than the longer-acting medications (5), but also tend to cause more anaphylaxis then amide anesthetics, such as lidocaine (43). Lidocaine toxicity can cause ringing in the ears and tingling in the face and mouth. More severe symptoms are seizures and cardiac arrhythmias. Hematomas can also develop secondary to puncture of a vein or artery. Direct pressure should be placed on the area if bleeding is suspected. Care should be taken that a hematoma does not compress other structures or cause a compartment syndrome. Abdominal injections can injure the kidney when injecting the quadratus lumborum or the liver during an intercostal injection. Neurologic injuries can occur if peripheral nerves are injured either by the needle or by a toxic reaction to the injected medication. If any paresthesia is reported during needle placement, the needle should be repositioned prior to the injection. Trigger point infiltration can cause a benign paresthesia sensation. However, this will not usually occur in a specific nerve distribution. Other complications include infection, allergic reaction, and anaphylaxis. Patients should report any skin changes, warmth, or swelling. An allergy history should be obtained prior to injection and dry needling can be used if there is any question of allergy to the injectable medication (13,43).

Long-term outcome studies of trigger point injection are scarce and do not isolate the efficacy of the injection itself (19). The success of trigger point injection is dependent on many factors including postinjection physical therapy and comorbidities. In the short term, trigger point injection improves pain, function, and range of motion in up to 100% of patients (51). A review of needling therapies concluded that any effect of the needling intervention is secondary to the needle or placebo as opposed to the substance, which is injected. It is not clear as to whether or not these procedures provide any special beneficial effect (39). Treatment failure may be because of inadequate treatment of perpetuating factors, misdiagnosis of the underlying pain generator, or undertreatment of the trigger points owing to technical issues such as nonpenetration of the trigger point with the needle. If treatment fails, it would be reasonable to repeat the interventions while re-evaluating the perpetuating factors and diagnosis.

Myofascial pain syndrome is a common and important cause of pain. The treatment modalities used are physical interventions, trigger point injections, and medication. The treatment plan must be individualized to the patient and must revolve around the successful management of perpetuating factors. Patient compliance is important in successful treatment and the patient should be engaged as a part of the treating team (5).

REFERENCES

1. Skootsky SA, Jeager B, Oye RK. Prevalence of myofascial pain in general internal medicine practice. West J Med 1989; 151:157–160.
2. Fishbain DA, Goldberg M, Meagher BR, et al. Male and female chronic pain patients categorized by DSM-III psychiatric diagnostic criteria. Pain 1986; 26:181–197.
3. Goldenberg DL, Burckhardt C, Crofford L. Management of fibromyalgia syndrome. JAMA 2004; 292(19):2388–2395.
4. Wolfe F, Smythe HA, Yunus MB, et al. The American College of Rheumatology 1990 criteria for the classification of fibromyalgia: report of the Multicenter Criteria Committee. Arthritis Rheum 1990; 33:160–172.
5. Travell J, Simons DG. Apropos of all muscles. In: Travell J, Simons DG, eds. Myofascial Pain and Dysfunction. Vol. 1. 2nd ed. Baltimore: Williams & Wilkins, 1999:94–177.
6. Fricton JR. Clinical care for myofascial pain. Dent Clin North Am 1991; 35(1):1–28.
7. Kraft GH, Johnson EW, LaBan MM. The fibrositis syndrome. Arch Phys Med Rehabil 1968; 49(30):155–162.
8. Gerwin RD, Shannon S, Hong CZ, et al. Inter-rater reliability in myofascial trigger point examination. Pain 1997; 69:65–73.
9. Weeks VD, Travell J. How to give painless injections. In: AMA Scientific Exhibits. New York: Grune & Stratton, 1957:318–322.
10. Hubbard DR, Berkoff GM. Myofascial trigger points show spontaneous needle EMG activity. Spine 1993; 18:1803–1807.
11. Simons DG, Hong C-Z, Simons LS. Spontaneous electrical activity of trigger points. J Musculoskeletal Pain 1995; 3(suppl 1):124.
12. Lewis J, Tehan P. A blinded pilot study investigating the use of diagnostic ultrasound for detecting active myofascial trigger points. Pain 1999; 79:39–44.
13. Rachlin ES, Rachlin IS. Trigger Point management. In: Rachlin ES, Rachlin IS, eds. Myofascial Pain and Fibromyalgia: Trigger Point Management. 2nd ed. St. Louis: Mosby, 2002:231–258.
14. Delaney GA, McKee AC. Inter- and intra-rater reliability of the pressure threshold meter in measurement of myofascial trigger point sensitivity. Am J Phys Med Rehabil 1993; 72(3):136–139.
15. Fischer AA. Introduction: pressure algometry in quantification of diagnosis and treatment outcomes. J Musculoskeletal Pain 1998; 6(1):1–29.
16. Fischer AA. Tissue compliance meter for objective, quantitative documentation of soft tissue consistency and pathology. Arch Phys Med Rehabil 1987; 68:122–124.
17. Gerwin RD, Dommerholt J, Shah JP. An expansion of Simons' integrated hypothesis of trigger point formation. Curr Pain Headache Rep 2004; 8:468–475.
18. Lewit K, Simons DG. Myofascial pain: relief by post-isometric relaxation. Arch Phys Med Rehabil 1984; 65:45.
19. Borg-Stein J. Simons DG. Focused review: myofascial pain. Arch Phys Med Rehabil 2002; 83(3 suppl 1):S40–S47.
20. Rudin NJ. Evaluation of treatments for myofascial pain syndrome and fibromyalgia. Curr Pain Headache Rep 2003; 7(6):433–442.
21. Wolfe F, Szaho S, Lane N. Preferences for nonsteroidal anti-inflammatory drugs over acetaminophen by rheumatic disease patients: a survey of 1799 patients with osteoarthritis, rheumatoid arthritis and fibromyalgia. Arthritis Rheum 1999; 42(suppl):S296.

22. Goldenberg DL, Felson DT, Dinerman H. A randomized, controlled trial of amitriptyline and naproxen in the treatment of patients with fibromyalgia syndrome. Arthritis Rheum 1986; 29:1371–1377.
23. Russell IJ, Kamin M, Bennett RM, et al. Efficacy of tramadol in treatment of pain in fibromyalgia. J Clin Rheumatol 2000; 6:250–257.
24. Katz WA. Pharmacology and clinical experience with tramadol in osteoarthritis. Drugs 1996; 52(3):39–47.
25. Schnitzer TJ, Gray WL, Paster RZ, et al. Efficacy of tramadol in treatment of chronic low back pain. J Rheumatol 2000; 27(3):772–778.
26. Bennett RM, Kamin M, Karin R, Rosenthal N. Tramadol and acetaminophen combination tablets in the treatment of fibromyalgia pain: a double-blind, randomized, placebo-controlled study. Am J Med 2003; 114:537–545.
27. Wheeler AH. Myofascial pain disorders: theory to therapy. Drugs 2004; 64(1):45–62.
28. O'Malley PG, Balden E, Tomkins G, et al. Treatment of fibromyalgia with antidepressants. J Gen Intern Med 2000; 15(9):659–666.
29. Goldenberg DL, Mayskiy M, Mossey CJ, et al. A randomized, double-blind crossover trial of fluoxetine and amitriptyline in the treatment of fibromyalgia. Arthritis Rheum 1996; 39:1852–1859.
30. Sindrup S. Efficacy of pharmacological treatments of neuropathic pain: an update and effect related to mechanism of drug action. Pain 83(3):389–400.
31. Irving GA. Contemporary assessment and management of neuropathic pain. Neurology 2005; 64(12 suppl 3):S21.
32. Goldenberg DL. Burckhardt C. Crofford L. Management of fibromyalgia syndrome. JAMA 2004; 292(19):2388–2395.
33. Gorson K, Schott C, Hermen R, et al. Gabapentin in the treatment of painful diabetic neuropathy: a placebo controlled, double blind, crossover trial. J Neurol Neurosurg Psychiatry 1999; 66:251–252.
34. Rosenberg JM, Harrell C, Ristic H, et al. The effect of gabapentin on neuropathic pain. Clin J Pain 1997; 13(3):251–255.
35. Wheeler AH, Hanley EN, Jr. Nonoperative treatment for low back pain. Rest to restoration. Spine 1995; 20(3):375–378.
36. Argoff CA, Wheeler AH. Spinal and radicular pain disorders. Neurol Clin 1998; 23:1662–1667.
37. Rashiq S, Koller M, Haykowsky M, Jamieson K. The effect of opioid analgesia on exercise test performance in chronic low back pain. Pain 2003; 106(1–2):119–125.
38. Borg-Stien J, Stein J. Trigger points and tender points. Rheum Dis Clin N Am 1996; 22(2):305–322.
39. Cummings MT, Adrian R. White AR. Needling therapies in the management of myofascial trigger point pain: a systematic review. Arch Phys Med Rehabil 2001; 82:986–992.
40. Kamanli A, Kaya O, Ozgocmen S, et al. Comparison of lidocaine injection, botulinum toxin injection, and dry needling to trigger points in myofascial pain syndrome. Rheumatol Int 2005; 25:604–611.
41. Hong CZ. Lidocaine injection versus dry needling to myofascial trigger point. The importance of the local twitch response. Am J Phys Med Rehabil 1994; 73:256–263.
42. Rachlin ES. Injection of specific trigger points. In: Rachlin ES, Rachlin IS, eds. Myofascial Pain and Fibromyalgia: Trigger Point Management. 2nd ed. St. Louis: Mosby, 2002: 259–402.
43. Criscuolo CM. Interventional approaches to the management of myofascial pain syndrome. Curr Pain Headache Rep 2001; 5(5):407–411.
44. Alverez DJ, Rockwell PG. Trigger points: diagnosis and management. Am Fam Physician 2002; 65(4):653–660.
45. Fischer A. New injection techniques for treatment of musculoskeletal pain. In: Rachlin ES, Rachlin IS, eds. Myofascial Pain and Fibromyalgia: Trigger Point Management. 2nd ed. St. Louis: Mosby, 2002:403–419.
46. Lang AM. Botulinum toxin type A therapy in chronic pain disorders. Arch Phys Med Rehabil 2003; 84(3 suppl 1):S69–S73, quiz S74–S75.

47. Lang AM. A pilot study of Botulinum toxin type A administered using a novel injection technique for the treatment of myofascial pain. Am J Pain Manage 2000; 10: 108–112.

48. Ferrente FM, Bearn L, Rothrock R, et al. Evidence against trigger point injection technique for the treatment of cervicothoracic myofascial pain with Botulinum toxin type A. Anesthesiology 2005; 103:377–383.

49. Acupuncture. NIH Consensus statement 1997; 15(5):1–34.

50. Melzack R, Stillwell DM, Fox EJ. Trigger points and acupuncture points for pain; correlations and implications. Pain 1977; 3:3–23.

51. Hong CZ, Hsueh TC. Difference in pain relief after trigger point injections in myofascial pain patients with and without fibromyalgia. Arch Phys Med Rehabil 1996; 77: 1161–1166.

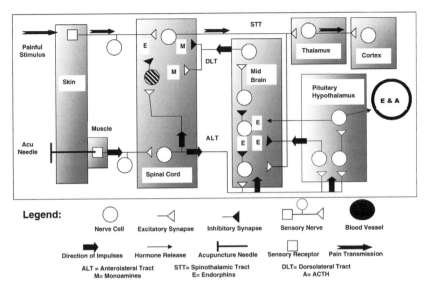

FIGURE 1 Acupuncture analgesia. *Abbreviations*: A, adrenocorticotrophic hormone; ALT, anterolateral tract; DLT, dorsolateral tract; E, endorphins; M, monoamines; STT, spinothalamic tract. *Source*: Adapted from Ref. 85.

Numerous studies have shown that the use of low (2–8 Hz) and high (50–200 Hz) frequencies achieves two different types of analgesia (21–23). Low-frequency electrical stimulation generates an endorphin-mediated analgesia through activation of all three centers. This endorphinergic analgesia is supra-segmental; relieving pain not only in the territory of the nerve being stimulated but also providing pain relief to the entire body. It is slow in onset (initiated after approximately 20–30 minutes of electrical stimulation), long-lasting, and the effects of repeated treatments are cumulative (repeated placebo treatments typically see a diminution of therapeutic effect). The analgesia of high-frequency stimulation bypasses the endorphin system activating primarily the neural pathway illustrated by the cross-hatched nerve cell in Figure 1, and to a lesser degree through the midbrain. This pathway is monoamine-dependent and segmental, relieving pain only in the distribution of the spinal segment of the stimulated peripheral nerve. The onset of pain relief is rapid, of short duration, and the effects of repeated treatments are not cumulative. Stimulation with high-frequency currents is considered to be similar to conventional transcutaneous electrical nerve stimulation (TENS).

Persistent Inflammatory Pain

Much of the wealth of information learned about AA over the past 30 years is derived from animal models with acute and transient laboratory-induced pain. Pain models in rats have been developed recently, which create a persistent inflammatory condition, through the injection of inflammatory agents under the skin. This produces inflammation that can last months, and gives researchers pain models that more closely approximate to clinically relevant disorders such as rheumatoid arthritis and other inflammatory conditions. These pain models also allow more time to evaluate posttreatment effects of EA and the dose response effect of multiple EA treatments.

The effect of different EA frequencies on chronic inflammatory pain seems to be consistent with results seen in acute transient pain, namely that lower frequency currents provide analgesia of slow onset and long duration, while the analgesia of higher frequency stimulation is of more rapid onset and shorter duration (24). In addition to increasing pain thresholds, EA at low-frequency stimulation has also been demonstrated to decrease edema in rats' paws when compared with placebo controls (25). The persistent inflammatory pain model has also been used to assess the efficacy of EA and drugs used in combination. It was recently demonstrated that EA at both high and low frequencies, combined with lower doses of morphine and indomethacin, produced better analgesic effects than EA or either drug alone (26,27).

Autonomic Regulatory Therapy

The endorphin hypothesis offers an explanation of how acupuncture can relieve pain, but it does not explain how it can help relieve nausea or the myriad of other problems it is used for. The ability of acupuncture to inhibit gastric acid secretion (28), stimulate intestinal motility (29), and impact blood pressure (BP) (30) and heart rate (HR) (31) in animal models all point towards the involvement of the autonomic nervous system (ANS). The western correlate to the Chinese concept of Yin and Yang is the idea of homeostasis, a process largely controlled by the sympathetic and parasympathetic nervous systems. One of the ways acupuncture seems to "re-establish balance" in the body is through manipulation of the ANS.

Peripheral nerve stimulation with acupuncture needles appears to have bidirectional "balancing" effects in some disturbances of systems controlled by the ANS. Needling the same acupuncture points can normalize disturbed physiological parameters like HR and BP, from conditions of hypo- or hyperfunctioning. For example, it has been demonstrated that strains of rats bred to be congenitally hyper- or hypotensive have their BP and HR normalized with acupuncture (32). Pharmacologic studies indicate that the pressor effects of acupuncture are mediated by central cholinergic mechanisms, while the BP-lowering effects in hypertensive rats involve release of endorphins and serotonin (33). These normalizing effects have also been noted in laboratory animals whose BPs have been acutely manipulated. Rats made hypotensive by withdrawing blood and dogs made hypertensive by intravenous infusions of epinephrine had their BP brought back near baseline with acupuncture (34,35). Studies on cardiovascular function in normal human subjects meanwhile have shown little effect on mean HR and BP, suggesting that an "imbalance" is necessary for acupuncture to have a significant effect (36).

More germane to the topic of this book is how acupuncture, by stimulation of the ANS, can impact the cardiovascular system to relieve musculoskeletal pain. There is evidence from animal models that the placement of a needle into a spastic, painful skeletal muscle causes it to relax by improving blood flow to the contracted area. The needling of a spastic muscle has been shown in an elegant series of animal experiments (37) to trigger a sympathetically mediated vasodilation with subsequent relief of spasm and pain in the involved muscle. This autonomic reflex was achieved both locally with needles directly into the spastic muscle, and at a distance with needles placed into the ipsilateral paravertebral musculature overlying the nerve roots supplying the spastic muscle. The relief of muscle spasm and myofascial pain with needling has also been independently observed in humans with the treatment of trigger points.

First described by Dr. Janet Travell (38), trigger points are hyperirritable loci in myofascial structures which when compressed can cause characteristic referred pain, tenderness, motor dysfunction, and autonomic phenomena. Travell et al. (39,40) observed that dry needling (needling without injection of drugs) produced pain relief and muscle relaxation. Several authors (41,42) have noted that a majority of acupuncture points correspond to Travell's trigger points. Melzack et al. (42) found a concordance of 71% between classical acupuncture points and trigger points. This overlap of acupuncture points and disturbed areas of muscle should not be that surprising when we recall that small-diameter muscle afferents are necessary components for pain relief with acupuncture.

Summary

There is strong basic science evidence that acupuncture is a peripheral nerve stimulation technique that achieves effects like analgesia, muscle relaxation, and improved blood flow in treated areas through a variety of neural pathways. The AA model reveals that pain relief achieved by peripheral nerve stimulation with acupuncture needles can have segmental effects through the action of endorphins and monoamines in the spinal cord and midbrain, as well as suprasegmental or systemic effects with the release of B-endorphin and ACTH into the blood and spinal fluid by the hypothalamus/pituitary complex. Acupuncture analgesia seems to work on both acute transient and persistent inflammatory pain induced in the laboratory. Finally, relief of musculoskeletal pain and improved range of motion and blood flow in areas with tight spastic muscles can be achieved with an acupuncture needle directly in the affected muscles or in distant anatomically relevant paraspinal muscles via a sympathetically mediated vasodilation. Despite the strides made in understanding some of the physiological mechanisms of acupuncture, the results of clinical research to date have been less than clear.

CLINICAL RESEARCH

The acupuncture treatments used in most research trials are not a particularly accurate reflection of what is used in daily practice. The clinical practice of acupuncture involves individualized acupuncture point selection based on patient-specific systemic imbalances determined by oriental diagnostic techniques. To adhere to generally accepted research guidelines, the majority of acupuncture trials use fixed protocol treatments (same acupuncture points and the same number and duration of treatments) to treat a problem defined by biomedical diagnostic criteria. While not ideal, this "cookbook" approach to acupuncture is currently the best solution available to begin to elucidate the clinical effects of acupuncture.

The National Institutes of Health Consensus Conference

Since the early 1970s, almost 500 randomized controlled trials (RCTs) have evaluated acupuncture's efficacy. More than half of these trials were placebo- or sham-controlled, with the remainder comparing acupuncture alone or in combination with conventional care to standard conventional care alone. The National Institutes of Health (NIH) held a consensus conference (43) in 1997 to evaluate the scientific and medical data on the uses, risks, and benefits of acupuncture for a variety of conditions. A panel of experts representing the fields of acupuncture, pain, psychology, drug abuse, psychiatry, physical medicine and rehabilitation, family medicine, internal medicine, health policy, statistics, epidemiology, physiology, and biophysics reviewed data and heard testimony from 25 experts in these same fields.

The consensus conference found clear evidence of acupuncture's efficacy in adult postoperative nausea and the nausea of chemotherapy as well as for postoperative dental pain. They also found evidence that acupuncture may be useful as an adjunct treatment, an acceptable alternative, and can be considered in a comprehensive management program for conditions such as addiction, stroke rehabilitation, headache, menstrual cramps, tennis elbow, fibromyalgia, myofascial pain, osteoarthritis (OA), low back pain, carpal tunnel syndrome, and asthma. It was their conclusion that many of the acupuncture studies to date provide equivocal or contradictory results because of design, sample size, inadequate follow-up, and other methodological issues shared by studies in other areas of medicine.

Unique Methodological Issues

In addition to the usual difficulties inherent in any clinical trial there are also problems unique to performing acupuncture RCTs. There are relatively few acupuncturists with biomedical training and even fewer that work in academic institutions. The blinding of acupuncturists to avoid performance bias is difficult, if not impossible. Blinding patients is also challenging in situations where subjects are familiar with true acupuncture treatment.

The lack of uniformity in what makes up an acupuncture treatment is a significant obstacle to consistent research. First, there are numerous styles of acupuncture which makes it possible to have a variety of treatments, using different points, for the same problem. Second, within a given style of acupuncture, there is also variability in the number, frequency, and duration of treatments, as well as the depth of puncture used. It is no surprise then, that the most consistent and reproducible evidence for acupuncture comes from trials that use a single point for a particular symptom (emesis or dental pain), even though this method bears little resemblance to clinically practiced acupuncture (44).

Problem of Placebo

Finding a matching control for an acupuncture treatment, one that is identical in appearance and sensation, practical, and physiologically inert has been a challenge for researchers. The wide variety of control techniques used in acupuncture trials over the years can be divided into two major categories: noninvasive (placebo) and invasive (sham). Placebo acupuncture creates the appearance of needle insertion without ever penetrating the skin. Past attempts at placebo techniques, such as rubbing or affixing blunted needles over the skin, were not thought to be very credible. The recent development of a validated placebo needle is a significant breakthrough in this area. The placebo needle is blunted and has a shaft that telescopes into the handle of the needle giving the appearance that it has been shortened and inserted into the skin. In several randomized trials, patients with these needles were unable to discern whether they had received true or placebo acupuncture (45,46).

The most commonly used control treatment in acupuncture trials has been sham needling or the needling of sites irrelevant to the condition being treated. Sham needling was initially thought to be ineffective and the ideal placebo until researchers noted that needling of these nonacupuncture points had a much higher rate of response than expected for an inert placebo. In 1983, Lewith and Machin (47) made the observation that in some trials sham acupuncture appeared to have an analgesic effect in

40% to 50% of patients compared with a 60% response rate with real acupuncture. Further investigation of this phenomenon has indeed revealed that the needling of nonacupuncture points can produce some analgesia through anatomically distinct brain pathways and the use of different neurotransmitters than those used by true acupuncture points (48,49).

This finding puts into question much of the earlier research using sham needling as a control. The potential physiological effects of sham needling may produce treatment outcomes that are intermediate between those of true acupuncture and no treatment making statistical significance of results more difficult to achieve. Many real versus sham acupuncture trials then, may only offer information about the most effective sites of needling, not about the specific effects of acupuncture.

The act of needling alone then appears to have some physiological effects, but does it really matter where the needles are placed? In the treatment of acute pain, the answer appears to be yes. Numerous animal studies (50,51) demonstrate that stimulation of true acupuncture points works better than sham needling in acute laboratory-induced pain. Several experimenters have also shown for acute lab-induced pain in humans, the needling of true acupuncture points provided marked analgesia while stimulation of sham points had only weak effects (52–54). While the specificity of acupuncture points has been well documented in acute pain studies in humans it has yet to be studied properly in patients with chronic pain.

Studies suggest that sham points seem to be more effective than placebo in relieving chronic pain working 33% to 50% of the time, while true acupuncture points are effective in 55% to 85% of patients in chronic pain. To detect differences in response rates on this order of magnitude requires over 120 subjects per study, and until recently there were no clinical acupuncture trials of this size (47). It appears then that until larger clinical trials are completed, analyzing pooled data from acupuncture RCTs may be the best way to evaluate acupuncture's efficacy for chronic conditions.

Systematic Reviews

The past 30 years have seen significant advances in the understanding of the neurophysiology of acupuncture, with the majority of information coming from animal studies. Clinical efficacy, however, requires the demonstration in humans of a favorable treatment effect as compared with placebo or another treatment using a rigorous methodological design. The gold standard for assessing clinical efficacy is a large, well-designed, RCT; however, most acupuncture trials to date have been small studies with few meeting the description of a large RCT. As a result, the best measure of acupuncture efficacy currently is a systematic review (SR).

The Cochrane collaboration was formed in 1993 with the sole purpose of conducting, maintaining, and disseminating SRs relevant to all areas of healthcare. In the future, it should be one of the most important sources of comprehensive summaries on the clinical effectiveness of acupuncture (55). In the area of musculoskeletal medicine we will look briefly at recent SRs examining the effects of acupuncture on chronic pain, low back and neck pain, OA, lateral epicondylar pain, and fibromyalgia.

Chronic Pain

The most recent SR assessing the efficacy of acupuncture for chronic pain (defined as pain present for longer than three months) looked at 51 RCTs published in

TABLE 2 Best Evidence Synthesis Method

Strong evidence: multiple, relevant, high-quality RCTs with generally consistent outcomes
Moderate evidence: one relevant high quality RCT and one or more relevant low-quality RCTs with generally consistent outcomes
Limited evidence: one relevant, high-quality RCT or multiple relevant, low-quality RCTs with generally consistent outcomes
Inconclusive evidence: only one relevant low-quality RCT, no relevant RCTs or RCTs with inconsistent outcomes

---

Abbreviation: RCT, randomized control trial.
Source: Adapted from Ref. 56.

English (56). Study quality was assessed using the validated Jadad Scale (57). Three-fourths of the studies received a low-quality score and low-quality scores were significantly associated with favorable results. The substantial clinical heterogeneity of conditions, treatments, control groups, and outcome measures did not allow meta-analysis or statistical pooling. The best evidence synthesis method (58) (Table 2), which takes into account both the quality and outcome of studies, was used instead. The authors found limited evidence that acupuncture was better than no treatment (waiting list) and inconclusive evidence that acupuncture was better than sham/placebo acupuncture or standard of care. An interesting secondary finding was observed related to the number of treatments needed for a good clinical effect. Six or more acupuncture treatments were significantly associated with favorable outcomes ($P = 0.03$) even after adjusting for study quality.

Low Back Pain

Prior to 1999, evidence supporting acupuncture's efficacy in low back pain was inconclusive owing to low quality, small size, and heterogeneity of the existing trials (59). Since 1999, there have been a number of larger, methodologically rigorous trials completed that have been incorporated into a recent meta-analysis and SR. Both of these publications suggested that acupuncture effectively relieved chronic low back pain.

The meta-analysis by Manheimer et al. (60) evaluated 33 RCTs, and used the standardized mean difference (SMD) as the principal measure of effect size as the trials assessed the same outcome but measured it in various ways. For the SMD, 1 unit of effect size corresponds with a 25-point difference on the Visual Analog Scale (VAS) and a 2-point difference on the Roland Disability Score (RDS). Using the standards established by the Cochrane Back Group Editorial Board, a minimum of a 10 mm difference on the VAS and a 2-point difference on the RDS was considered to be clinically significant. Using short-term pain relief as the primary outcome, acupuncture was more effective than sham acupuncture [SMD = 0.54, 95% confidence interval (CI) = 0.35 to 0.73, seven trials] and no additional treatment (SMD = 0.69, 95% CI = 0.40 to 0.98, eight trials) for providing short-term relief of chronic low back pain. This short-term relief seems to be sustained in the long-term, but follow-up data was limited in quality and quantity. The data also suggested enhanced functional capacity in the short-term compared with no additional treatment (SMD = 0.62, 95% CI = 0.30 to 0.95, 14 trials). The evidence comparing acupuncture with other active treatments in chronic low back pain was inconclusive, as was the evidence for its efficacy in acute low back pain.

Furlan et al. (61) evaluated 35 RCTs covering 2861 patients in their SR. They also reported pain relief and improved function in patients with chronic low back pain treated with acupuncture compared with those with no treatment or sham treatment. The pooled analysis of two lower quality RCTs ($n = 90$) comparing acupuncture treatment with no treatment found that acupuncture was more effective for short-term pain relief with an SMD of -0.73 (95% CI $= -1.19$ to -0.28) and short-term functional improvement with an effect size of 0.63 (95% CI $= 0.19$ to 1.08). There is also limited evidence (one lower quality RCT, $n = 40$) that acupuncture was also more effective at intermediate follow-up for outcomes of pain. The pooled analysis comparing acupuncture treatment with sham therapy revealed strong evidence that acupuncture was more effective for the relief of pain immediately after treatment [weighted mean difference (WMD) $= -10.21$, 95% CI $= -14.99$ to -5.44, $n = 314$] and for the three month period following treatment (WMD $= -17.70$, 95% CI $= -25.5$ to -10.07, $n = 138$).

Furlan et al. (61) further reported that while acupuncture was not more effective than other conventional and alternative treatments, when added to other conventional therapies it relieved pain and improved function better than conventional therapies alone. Four higher-quality trials ($n = 281$ subjects) assessed the additive effects of acupuncture with other therapies (exercises, nonsteroidal anti-inflammatory drugs, aspirin, nonnarcotic analgesic, mud packs, infrared heat, back care education, ergonomics, and behavioral modification) and compared them with these therapies alone. The pooled analysis shows that acupuncture used in combination with the other therapies was more effective; immediately after sessions (four higher-quality trials, SMD $= -0.76$, 95% CI $= -1.02$ to -0.5, $n = 289$), at short-term follow-up (three higher-quality trials, SMD $= -1.1$, 95% CI $= -1.62$ to -0.58, $n = 182$), and at the intermediate follow-up (two higher-quality trials, SMD $= -0.76$, 95% CI $= -1.14$ to -0.38, $n = 115$). These effects were also observed for functional outcomes immediately after sessions (three higher-quality trials, SMD $= -0.95$, 95% CI $= -1.27$ to -0.63, $n = 173$), at the short-term follow-up (SMD $= -0.95$, 95% CI $= -1.37$ to -0.54), and at the intermediate follow-up (SMD $= -0.55$, 95% CI $= -0.92$ to -0.18).

Although the conclusions found positive results with acupuncture, the magnitude of the effects was thought to be relatively small. The average pain reduction (measured on scales like VAS) in the acupuncture group with chronic low back pain was 32% (16 studies), versus 23% in the sham group (six studies) versus 6% in the no treatment group (six studies). Finally, there was again insufficient evidence to make any recommendations for acupuncture's use in acute low back pain.

Neck Pain

There have been two recent SRs of trials of acupuncture for neck pain. One found that trials were equally split between positive and negative outcomes (62). The other, using a newly developed tool to assess validity of findings of RCTs, found no convincing evidence for the analgesic efficacy of acupuncture in chronic neck and back pain (63). Both reviews noted that the methodologic quality of the trials was poor. As these reviews were published, a large ($n = 177$), methodologically rigorous RCT examining the effect of acupuncture on neck pain was performed comparing true acupuncture with massage and a sham laser treatment (64). One week after five treatments, the acupuncture group showed significantly greater improvement in motion-related pain compared with massage on a 100-point VSA (SMD $= 24.22$, 95% CI $= 16.5$ to 31.9; $P = 0.0052$), but not compared with sham laser. This finding suggests that while acupuncture may relieve neck pain its success is likely because of the placebo effect. A subsequent reanalysis of this raw data (65) using a regression analysis model rather than paired t-tests came to a different conclusion. This reanalysis adjusted for baseline score and depression and found true acupuncture reduced pain scores 11.5 points (95% CI 3.5 to 19.5 points; $P = 0.005$) more than those in the sham or massage group. When the analysis of the data was limited to just those who had received sham laser or true acupuncture, acupuncture resulted in a reduction of pain score of 9.4 points greater than sham laser (95% CI 0.9 to 18.0 points; $P = 0.031$).

Osteoarthritis
The most recent SR was published in 1997, and found highly contradictory results in the 13 OA trials evaluated (66). There were positive results found in seven trials and no significant results in the remaining six studies. Most of the studies with positive findings had a number of methodological flaws; no placebo control, no randomization, small sample size, or no formal statistical analysis. Ezzo et al. (67) identified seven trials ($n = 393$) for inclusion in an SR looking specifically at OA of the knee. A best evidence synthesis was performed to determine the strength of evidence by control group. Compared with waiting list or treatment, there was limited evidence that acupuncture was superior when using pain relief and functional status as endpoints. Compared with sham acupuncture, there was strong evidence that real acupuncture is more effective for pain relief but inconclusive evidence that it was any better in improving the function. There was also insufficient evidence for determining whether acupuncture was as efficacious as other treatments.

These SRs were completed before the largest randomized placebo-controlled acupuncture trial ever undertaken ($n = 570$) was published (68). This trial, evaluating the use of acupuncture in knee OA, involved a more intensive acupuncture regimen (23 sessions) for a longer period (26 weeks) than any other trial to date. In this three-armed study, patients either received true EA, sham treatment, or education. Patients were allowed to stay on their usual pain medicines or pursue any nonpharmacologic therapy they or their physicians wished. The primary outcome measures were changes in the validated Western Ontario and McMaster Universities Osteoarthritis Index (WOMAC) pain and function scores and a patient global assessment at 8 and 26 weeks (refer Table 3 for subjects' baseline values). At eight weeks, subjects in the true acupuncture group experienced greater improvement in WOMAC function scores (mean difference $= -2.9$, 95% CI $= -5.0$ to -0.8; $P = 0.01$), but not in WOMAC pain score or the patient global

TABLE 3 Baseline Scores

	True acupuncture ($n = 190$)	Sham acupuncture ($n = 191$)	Education control ($n = 189$)	Total ($n = 570$)
WOMAC pain score (0–20[a])	8.92 ± 3.42	8.90 ± 3.39	9.01 ± 3.70	8.94 ± 3.50
WOMAC function score (0–68[a])	31.31 ± 12.06	31.29 ± 12.00	32.48 ± 11.81	31.69 ± 11.96
Patient global assessment (1–5[a])	2.95 ± 0.97	3.08 ± 0.88	2.94 ± 0.88	2.99 ± 0.91

[a]Range.
Abbreviation: WOMAC, Western Ontario and McMaster Universities Osteoarthritis Index.
Source: Adapted from Ref. 68.

assessment. At 26 weeks, true acupuncture saw a significant decrease in WOMAC pain (mean difference = -0.87, 95% CI = -1.58 to -0.16; $P = 0.003$) and function scores compared with sham at 26 weeks (mean difference = -2.5, 95% CI = -4.7 to -0.4; $P = 0.01$). This decrease in WOMAC pain and function scores was in the order of 40% from baseline in each. There was also a significant improvement in patient global assessment at 26 weeks (mean difference = 0.26, 95% CI = 0.07 to 0.45; $P = 0.02$).

Lateral Epicondylar Pain
The only SR published in the Cochrane review series evaluating lateral epicondylar pain concluded that there was insufficient evidence to support or refute the use of acupuncture in the treatment of lateral elbow pain (69). This review did demonstrate needle acupuncture to be of short-term benefit with respect to pain, but this conclusion was based on the results of two small trials, the results of which were not able to be combined in meta-analysis because of study heterogeneity. No benefit lasting more than 24 hours post-treatment was demonstrated. Four new clinical trials meeting the inclusion criteria have been published since this Cochrane review, and a new SR evaluating the evidence in all six trials has been completed (70). All six of the studies included in this review were rated as high-quality RCTs, and five of these six indicated that acupuncture treatment was more effective than control treatments in the short-term relief of pain (Table 4). A best evidence synthesis approach was used and determined that there was strong evidence suggesting that acupuncture was effective in short-term relief of lateral epicondylar pain.

The Molsberger study (82) cited in Table 4 is a good example of suprasegmental pain relief with acupuncture. In this study, a single treatment with one needle placed below the head of the fibula reduced the pain scores by 55.8% in patients with chronic tennis elbow compared with 15% in the placebo group ($P < 0.01$, X^2-test).

Fibromyalgia
A recent SR of acupuncture for the treatment of fibromyalgia included both RCTs and cohort studies (71). Quality assessment of these studies revealed only one methodologically rigorous RCT of the three studies reviewed (72). This randomized single-blinded study involving 70 subjects, evaluated the effects of six acupuncture or sham treatments administered over a three-week period. Assessment after the final treatment found that true acupuncture was more effective than sham acupuncture in relieving pain (VAS), increasing pain thresholds (as measured by blinded assessors using algometry), improving subjective global ratings, and reducing morning stiffness (Tables 5A, 5B). The pain threshold, considered to be the primary outcome measure, improved by 70% in the EA group and 4% in the control group. The lower quality studies' results were also positive. The duration of benefit following treatment is not known.

Summary
Much of the clinical evidence for acupuncture's effectiveness is inconclusive (Table 6). There is some emerging evidence of clinical efficacy; however, there is still a great need for better quality research. Large-scale multicenter trials that address the issues of adequate placebo control, uniformity of the definition of the problem and treatment, and the use of objective outcomes are needed to further validate this technique.

TABLE 4 Studies Evaluating Acupuncture for Lateral Epicondylar Pain

Study type	Intervention	Treatment plan	Assessment scale	Outcome measures
Randomized, single-blind trial (77)	Treatment group (n = 8) Acupuncture producing De Qi (see page 94) Ultrasound group (n = 9) Pulsed ultrasound for 10 min	8 treatments 2–3X/week	Visual Analog Pain Scale before each treatment Pain-free grip strength scores	No significant difference in grip strength scores between groups
Randomized controlled double-blind trial (78)	Treatment group (n = 20) Acupuncture producing De Qi Control group (n = 22) Sham needle acupuncture Points 5 cm away from the points used above	10 treatments 2X/week	Pain assessed at rest, in motion, during exertion as well as duration and frequency on 0–5 scale. Functional impairment assessed with DASH questionnaire.	Pain: treatment group improved significantly more than control at two weeks (both groups significantly improved at all follow ups) Functional impairment: treatment group improved significantly more than control at two weeks and two months
Randomized trial (79)	Treatment group (n = 20) Acupuncture Ultrasound group (n = 20) Pulsed ultrasound therapy over central and peripheral area of lateral epicondyle for 5 min	Treatment group 10 treatments 1–2X/week for two months Ultrasound group 12 treatments Daily for 12 days	Visual Analog Scale (1–10) measuring pain Maigne functional recovery test	Pain and functional recovery significantly improved immediately after treatment and at 6 months follow-up in treatment group compared with ultrasound group
Randomized, double-blinded trial (80)	Group A: treatment (n = 44) Acupuncture producing De Qi Group B: control (n = 38) Superficial needle insertion Same points as Group A	10 treatments 2–3X/week	5-point scale describing present condition: 1 = excellent 2 = good	Pain improvement after treatment: Group A 10 days n = 44 3 months n = 43

Study design	Groups	Treatment	Outcome measures	Results
			3 = improved 4 = slightly improved 5 = unchanged/worse	

Continuation (scale results):

	10 days *n* = 38	3 months *n* = 35
1/2	22 (50%)	33 (77%)
3	17 (39%)	3 (07%)
4/5	5 (11%)	7 (16%)

Group B

	10 days *n* = 38	3 months *n* = 35
1/2	8 (21%)	22 (60%)
3	17 (45%)	9 (26%)
4/5	13 (34%)	5 (14%)

Study design	Groups	Treatment	Outcome measures	Results
Double blinded quasi-randomized trial (81)	*Treatment group* (*n* = 25) Acupuncture points *Control group* (*n* = 25) Sham needle acupuncture Points one thumb-width away from those used in treatment group	Three treatments within 10 days	Pressure pain threshold Pain-free grip strength Impairment caused by pain (1–10)	At 14 day follow-up: *Treatment group* 59% had decrease in impairment; 7 subjects had full recovery *Control group* 24% had decrease in impairment; 0 subjects had full recovery
Randomized placebo-controlled, double-blinded trial (82)	*Treatment group* (*n* = 24) Acupuncture point on ipsilateral leg *Placebo group* (*n* = 24) Stimulation with pencil-like probe to simulate needle insertion over the T3 ipsilateral paravertebral muscles	One treatment	Pain ranked numerically on a scale of (0–10)	Immediately after treatment: *Treatment group* 19 reported pain relief of ≥50%; 55.8% mean pain reduction *Placebo group* Six reported pain relief of ≥50%; 15% mean pain reduction

Source: Adapted from Ref. 70.

TABLE 5A Fibromyalgia Study: Clinical Parameters

	Before treatment		After treatment	
	Control (n = 27)	Acupuncture (n = 28)	Control (n = 27)	Acupuncture (n = 28)
Pain threshold (kg/cm^2)	1.47 (0–24) [0.97–1.98]	1.36 (0.21) [0.94–1.79]	1.54 (0.23) [1.07–2.01]	2.3 (0.32) [1.67–2.98]
Pain on Visual Analog Scale (1[a]–100 mm)	60.89 (4.07) [52.52–69.25]	56.61 (3.19) [50.06–63.15]	53.78 (4.37) [44.80–62.76]	39.89 (4.97) [29.70–50.06]
Morning stiffness (minutes)	82.04 (13.11) [55.09–108.98]	57.86 (11.80) [33.65–82.07]	83.15 (15.51) [51.26–115.03]	40.89 (10.64) [19.06–62.73]
Patient's subjective global assessment (1–10[a])	4.59 (0.26) [4.07–5.12]	4.82 (0.31) [4.18–5.46]	5.07 (0.37) [4.31–5.84]	6.46 (0.43) [5.58–7.35]
Evaluating physician's subjective global assessment (1–10[a])	4.70 (0.33) [4.03–5.38]	5.21 (0.32) [4.56–5.87]	5.04 (0.45) [4.12–5.96]	7.00 (0.41) [6.17–7.83]

Note: Mean values are expressed with (SE) and (95% confidence interval).
[a]Best value.
Source: Adapted from Ref. 72.

TABLE 5B Fibromyalgia Study: Differences in Clinical Parameters After Acupuncture

	P value for intragroup changes[a]		P value for intergroup differences[b]	
	Control	Acupuncture	Before treatment	After treatment
Pain threshold	0.6378	0.0027	0.8990	0.0303
Pain on VAS	0.0619	0.0020	0.2699	0.0246
Morning stiffness	0.8684	0.0627	0.1126	0.0321
Patient's assessment	0.2360	0.0018	0.4353	0.0111
Physician's assessment	0.4080	0.0001	0.2266	0.0034

[a]Wilcoxon-matched pairs signed rank test, two-tailed.
[b]Mann-Whitney U and Wilcoxon rank sum W test, two-tailed, corrected for ties.
Abbreviation: VAS, Visual Analog Scale.
Source: Adapted from Ref. 72.

TABLE 6 Systematic Reviews and Meta-Analyses of Randomized Controlled Trials of Acupuncture for Musculoskeletal Conditions

Condition	Trials, *n*	Subj., *n*	Findings	Conclusions
Chronic pain (55)	51	2423	21 positive and 27 negative. Acupuncture vs. placebo trials 15 positive and 17 negative	Inconclusive evidence for acupuncture vs. placebo or standard care; limited evidence better than waiting room
BP (meta-analysis) (59)	33	2416	Short-term pain relief. 25 positive 6 negative. Only three trials of acute BP	*Chronic BP:* Acupuncture superior to sham and no treatment in short-term pain relief *Acute BP:* Inconclusive
LBP (60)	35	2861	Only 14 trials of high methodological standards 24 positive and 6 negative; only three trials of acute LBP	*Chronic LBP:* Acupuncture superior to sham and no treatment for pain relief and functional improvement in short-term; useful adjunct to other therapies *Acute LBP:* Inconclusive
Chronic neck and LBP (62)	13	522	Five positive and eight negative. Most valid trials negative	No convincing evidence for efficacy
Neck pain (61)	14	724	Seven positive and seven negative. Acupuncture no better than placebo in four of five trials	Inconclusive
Osteoarthritis (64)	13	437	Seven positive and six negative. Most trials with methodological flaws. The most rigorous studies suggest acupuncture not superior to sham in reducing pain.	Inconclusive
Osteoarthritis of the knee (65)	7	393	Acupuncture compared with: wait list two positive trials, placebo two of three positive, physical therapy two negative	May play a role in treatment of OA
Lateral epicondyle pain (68)	6	282	All positive. All six studies rated as high quality.	Strong evidence for efficacy in short-term relief of pain
Fibromyalgia (69)	3	149	All positive. Only one of the three trials was methodologically rigorous.	Positive with reservations owing to small size

Abbreviations: BP, blood pressure; LBP, low back pain; OA, osteoarthritis

ADVICE FOR PATIENTS
Practitioners
Many styles of acupuncture have evolved over the millennia. China, Japan, and Korea all have their own distinct versions of acupuncture as do many western countries. There is also a wide variety of acupuncture practitioners in North America. In 1987, the American Academy of Medical Acupuncture was formed as the first national physician and surgeon organization dedicated to the advancement of acupuncture within America. Approximately 3000 physicians have undergone acupuncture training, usually completing 300 hours of formal education. A physician's approach is more often a synthesis of traditional practice combined with a western understanding of myofascial trigger points, the nervous system, and recent scientific discoveries about the potential mechanisms of acupuncture. Practitioners with a more traditional approach to acupuncture include Oriental Medical Doctors (OMDs) and Licensed Acupuncturists (LAcs). To become an OMD, a four-year training course in traditional Chinese medical therapies including herbal medicine, therapeutic massage (tuina) and exercise (Qi gong), and acupuncture must be completed. The two years of training required to become an LAc is limited to acupuncture only. Finally, chiropractic and naturopathic physicians often perform acupuncture as part of their clinical practice.

Treatment
People have different experiences with acupuncture needling, but it is not thought to be particularly painful by most. One usually feels a slight jab when the needle is inserted, and it is then manipulated briefly to achieve a brief sensation of numbness or fullness known as "de qi." "De qi" or the "arrival of qi" is associated with the activation of nerve afferents that mediate acupuncture's effects. Once the needles are in place, there should be no discomfort felt. Depending on the problem, the needles can be either left in place undisturbed, or stimulated manually, with a burning herb (moxa) or electricity.

Acupuncture needles produce much less tissue trauma than hypodermic needles. They are solid with a smooth point designed to push tissue aside as opposed to hypodermic needles, which are hollow with beveled edges that cut through the tissue. Acupuncture needles are also significantly thinner, with the average needle able to fit easily inside the lumen of a 25-gauge hypodermic needle. Anywhere from 5 to 15 needles are used in an average session and most acupuncturists now use disposable needles which minimizes the risk of infection.

Patients can expect to be seen once or twice a week initially with treatments being spaced out or stopped as clinical improvement is observed. A fair trial of treatment in most chronic musculoskeletal problems is about six visits (55) and if there is significant improvement, treatments should continue until the problem is completely resolved or symptoms plateau. In acute soft-tissue injuries, treatments can be performed as frequently as once or twice a day at the outset with the frequency of treatment decreasing with improvement.

Adverse Effects
Treatment with acupuncture, generally speaking is very safe if performed by a competent practitioner. Reports of serious side-effects like pneumothorax, infection, spinal lesions, and problems associated with organ punctures and broken needles beneath the skin have been reported in the literature but are rare. A

recent SR of prospective studies of acupuncture safety found only two cases each of pneumothorax and broken needles in a quarter of a million treatments (73). Two recent prospective surveys in the United Kingdom found no serious adverse events in over 66,000 treatments (74,75). To put this in perspective, gastropathy caused by nonsteroidal anti-inflammatory drugs, the most popular medicines in the world for musculoskeletal pain, is responsible for an estimated 100,000 hospitalizations and 10,000 deaths annually in the United States alone (76). Minor complications with acupuncture are also infrequent (in the order of 14 per 10,000 treatments) and transient, seldom lasting more than a week. The most common minor adverse events noted in these British studies were fainting, nausea, forgotten needles, and headache.

CONCLUSION

Patients with musculoskeletal pain can sometimes be faced with unappealing therapeutic options like surgery, or the long-term use of narcotics, antiseizure, or psychotropic medications. Acupuncture offers practitioners and their patients a low cost, low risk, drug-free alternative, or adjunct treatment with almost no side-effects. Extensive laboratory evidence of physiological mechanisms suggests that it can not only relieve pain and inflammation but it can also relax tight, spastic muscles by improving blood flow. Despite 3000 years of empirical evidence suggesting that acupuncture may relieve musculoskeletal pain, its clinical efficacy has yet to be firmly established largely because of methodological shortcomings of RCTs performed over the last 30 years. For the time being then, acupuncture remains a therapeutic intervention of great practical potential still in need of proper clinical validation.

REFERENCES

1. Pelletier K, Astin J. Integration and reimbursement of complementary and alternative medicine by managed care and insurance providers: 2000 update and cohort analysis. Altern Ther Health Med 2002; 8(1):38–44.
2. Diehl D, Kaplan G, Coulter I, et al. Use of acupuncture by American physicians. J Altern Comp Med 1997; 3(2):119–126.
3. Paramore L. Use of alternative therapies: estimates from the Robert Woods Johnson Foundation national access to care survey. J Pain Symptom Manag 1996; 13:83–89.
4. Mayer D, Price D, Raffii A. Antagonism of acupuncture analgesia in man by the narcotic antagonist naloxone. Brain Res 1977; 121:368–372.
5. Shen J, Wenger N, Glaspy J, et al. Electroacupuncture for control of myeloablative chemotherapy-induced emesis: a randomized controlled trial. JAMA 2000; 284:2755–2761.
6. Dorfer L, Moser M, Bahr I, et al. A medical report from the Stone Age? Lancet 1999; 354:1023–1025.
7. Helms J. Acupuncture Energetics: A Clinical Approach for Physicians. Berkeley: Medical Acupuncture Publishers, 1995:3–17.
8. Osler W. The Principles and Practice of Medicine. New York: D. Appleton and Company, 1892:280, 820.
9. Reston J. Now about my operation in Peking. NY Times 1971, July 26:1, 6.
10. Taylor H. The uncharted wilderness of acupuncture. Presented at National Conference on Physicians, Schools, and Communities. October 1973, http://www.acuwatch. org/hx/taylor.shtml.
11. Helms J. Acupuncture Energetics: A Clinical Approach for Physicians. Berkeley: Medical Acupuncture Publishers, 1995.

12. Pomeranz B. Electroacupuncture and transcutaneous electrical nerve stimulation. In: Stux G, Pomeranz B, Berman B, eds. Basics of Acupuncture. 5th ed. Berlin: Springer-Verlag, 2003:315–316.
13. Dung H. Anatomical features contributing to the formation of acupuncture points. Am J Acupunct 1984; 12:139–143.
14. Pomeranz B, Chiu D. Naloxone blocks acupuncture analgesia and causes hyperalgesia: endorphin is implicated. Life Sci 1976; 19:1757–1762.
15. Pomeranz B, Berman B. The scientific basis of acupuncture. In: Stux G, Pomeranz B, Berman B, eds. Basics of Acupuncture. 5th ed. Berlin: Springer-Verlag, 2003:17.
16. Pomeranz B, Berman B. The scientific basis of acupuncture. In: Stux G, Pomeranz B, Berman B, eds. Basics of Acupuncture. 5th ed. Berlin: Springer-Verlag, 2003:18–19.
17. Peets J, Pomeranz B. CXBX mice deficient in opiate receptors show poor electroacupuncture analgesia. Nature 1978; 273:675–676.
18. Kishioka S, Miyamoto Y, et al. Effects of a mixture of peptidase inhibitors on met-enkephalin, beta-endorphin, dynorphin (1-13) and electroacupuncture induced antinociception in rats. Jpn J Pharm 1994; 66:337–345.
19. Lung C, Sun A, Tsao C, et al. An observation of the humoral factor in acupuncture analgesia in rats. Am J Chin Med 1978; 2:203–205.
20. Pomeranz B, Berman B. The scientific basis of acupuncture. In: Stux G, Pomeranz B, Berman B, eds. Basics of Acupuncture. 5th ed. Berlin: Springer-Verlag, 2003:9–24.
21. Pomeranz B, Berman B. The scientific basis of acupuncture. In: Stux G, Pomeranz B, Berman B, eds. Basics of Acupuncture. 5th ed. Berlin: Springer-Verlag, 2003:14–16.
22. Anderson S. Pain control by sensory stimulation. In: Bonica J, ed. Vol. 3. Advances in Pain Research and Therapy. New York: Raven, 1979:561–585.
23. Han J, Chen X, Sun S, et al. Effect of low- and high-frequency TENS on met-enkephalin-arg-phe and dynorphin A immunoreactivity in human lumbar CSF. Pain 1991; 47:295–298.
24. Pomeranz B, Berman B. The scientific basis of acupuncture. In: Stux G, Pomeranz B, Berman B, eds. Basics of Acupuncture. 5th ed. Berlin: Springer-Verlag, 2003:24–27.
25. Zhang R, Lao L, Wang X, et al. Electroacupuncture attenuates inflammation in a rat model. J Altern Comp Med 2005; 11:135–142.
26. Zhang R, Lao L, Wang X, et al. Electroacupuncture combined with indomethacin enhances antihyperalgesia in inflammatory rats. Pharmacol, Biochem Behav 2004; 78:793–797.
27. Zhang R, Lao L, Wang X, et al. Involvement of opiod receptors in electroacupuncture-produced anti-hyperalgesia in rats with peripheral inflammation. Brain Res 2004; 1020:12–17.
28. Jin H, Zhou L, Lee K, et al. Inhibition of acid secretion by electrical acupuncture is mediated by endorphin and somatostatin. Am J Physiol 1996; 271:524–530.
29. Iwa M, Matsushima M, Nakade Y, et al. Electroacupuncture at ST-36 accelerates colonic motility and transit in freely moving conscious rats. Am J Physiol Gastrointest Liver Physiol 2005; 290:G285–G292.
30. Hoffman P, Thoren P. Long lasting cardiovascular depression induced by acupuncture like stimulation of the sciatic nerve in unanesthetized rats. Effects of arousal and type of hypertension. Acta Physiologica Scandanavica 1986; 127:119–126.
31. Clifford D, Lee M, Lee D. Cardiovascular effects of atropine on acupuncture, needling with electrostimulation at Tsu San Li (St36) in dogs. Am J Vet Res 1977; 38:845–849.
32. Yao T. Acupuncture and somatic nerve stimulation: mechanism underlying effects on cardiovascular and renal activities. Scand J Rehab Med Suppl 1993; 29:7–18.
33. Yao T, Andersson S, Thoren T. Long lasting cardiovascular depressor response following sciatic stimulation in SHR. Evidence for the involvement of central endorphin and serotonin systems. Brain Res 1982; 244:295–303.
34. Sun X, Yu J, Yao T. Pressor effect produced by stimulation of somatic nerve on hemorrhagic hypotension in conscious rats. Acta Physiol Sin 1983; 35:264–270.
35. Li P, Sun F, Zhang A. The effect of acupuncture on blood pressure: the interrelation of sympathetic activity and endogenous opiod peptides. Acupunct Electrother Res 1983; 8:45–56.
36. Nishijo K, Mori H, Yosikawa K, et al. Decreased heart rate by acupuncture stimulation in humans via facilitation of cardiac vagal activity and suppression of cardiac sympathetic nerve. Neurosci Lett 1997; 227:165–168.

37. Takeshige C. Mechanism of relief of muscle pain by needle insertion into acupoints. Acupunct Sci Int J 1990; 1:7–12.
38. Travell J, Simons D. Myofascial Pain and Dysfunction: The Trigger Point Manual. Baltimore: Williams and Wilkins, 1998.
39. Gunn G. The Gunn Approach to the Treatment of Chronic Pain: Intramuscular stimulation for Myofascial Pain of Radiculopathic Origin. London: Churchill Livingstone, 1996.
40. Lewit K, The needle effect in the relief of myofascial pain. Pain 1979; 6:83–90.
41. Gunn G, Milbrandt W, et al. Dry needling of muscle motor points for chronic low back pain. Spine 1980; 5:279–291.
42. Melzack R, Stillwell DM, Fox EJ, Trigger points and acupuncture points for pain: correlations and implications. Pain 1977; 3:3–23.
43. NIH Consensus Conference, Acupuncture. JAMA 1998; 280:1518–1524.
44. Kaptchuk T, Acupuncture: theory, efficacy and practice. Ann Int Med 2002; 5:374–383.
45. Streitberger K, Kleinhenz J. Introducing a placebo needle into acupuncture research. Lancet 1998; 352:364–365.
46. Park J, White A, Stevinson C, et al. Validating a new non-penetrating sham acupuncture device: two randomized controlled trials. Acupunct Med 2002; 20:168–174.
47. Lewith G, Machin D. On the evaluation of the clinical effects of acupuncture. Pain 1983; 16:111–127.
48. Takashige C. Differentiation between acupuncture and non-acupuncture points by association with an analgesia inhibitory system. Acupunct Electrother Res 1985; 10:195–203.
49. LeBars D, Villanueva L, Willers J. Diffuse noxious inhibitory controls (DNIC) in animals and man. Acupunct Med 1991; 9:47–56.
50. Pomeranz B, Chiu D, Naloxone blocks acupuncture analagesia and causes hyper algesia: endorphin is implicated. Life Science 1976; 19:1757–1762.
51. Cheng R, Pomeranz B, et al. Electroacupuncture elevates blood cortisol levels in naive horses: sham treatment has no effect. Int J Neurosci 1980; 10:95–97.
52. Stacher G, Wancura I, et al. Effective acupuncture on pain threshold and pain tolerance determined by electrical stimulation of the skin: a controlled study. Am J Chin Med 1975; 3:143–146.
53. Chapman C, Chen A, Bonica J. Effects of intrasegmental electrical acupuncture on dental pain: evaluation by threshold estimation and sensory decision theory. Pain 1977; 3: 213–227.
54. Brockhaus A, Elger C. Hypalgesic efficacy of acupuncture on experimental pain in man. Comparison of laser acupuncture and needle acupuncture. Pain 1990; 43(2):181–185.
55. Ezzo J, Lao L, Berman B. Assessing clinical efficacy of acupuncture: what has been learned from systematic reviews of acupuncture? In: Stux, Pomeranz, Berman, eds. Clinical Acupuncture: Scientific Basis. Berlin: Springer-Verlag, 2001:113–130.
56. Ezzo J, Berman B, Hadhazy V, et al. Is acupuncture effective for the treatment of chronic pain? A systematic review. Pain 2000; 86:217–225.
57. Jadad A, Moore R, Carroll D, et al. Assessing the quality of randomized clinical trials: is blinding necessary? Controlled Clin Trials 1996; 17:1–12.
58. Slavin R. Best evidence synthesis-an intelligent alternative to meta-analysis. J Clin Epidemiol 1995; 48:9–18.
59. Van Tulder M, Cherkin D, Berman B, et al. The effectiveness of acupuncture in the management of acute and chronic low back pain. A systematic review within the framework of the Cochrane Collaboration Back Review group. Spine 1999; 24:1113–1123.
60. Manheimer E, White A, Berman B. Meta-analysis: acupuncture for low back pain. Ann Intern Med 2005; 142(8):651–663.
61. Furlan A, van Tulder M, Cherkin D, et al. Acupuncture and dry needling for low back pain. Cochrane Database Sys Rev 2004; (4).
62. White A, Ernst E. A systematic review of randomized controlled trials of acupuncture for neck pain. Rheumatology (Oxford) 1999; 38:143–147.
63. Smith L, Oldman A, McQuay H, et al. Teasing apart quality and validity in systematic reviews: an example from acupuncture trials in chronic neck and back pain. Pain 2000; 86:119–132.

64. Irnich D, Behrens N, Molzen H, et al. Randomized trial of acupuncture compared with conventional massage and "sham" laser acupuncture for treatment of chronic neck pain. BMJ 2001; 322:1–6.
65. Vickers A. Acupuncture for treatment for chronic neck pain. Reanalysis of data suggests that effect is not a placebo effect. BMJ 2001; 323(7324):1306–1307.
66. Ernst E. Acupuncture as a symptomatic treatment of osteoarthritis. A systematic review. Scand J Rheumatol 1997; 26:444–447.
67. Ezzo J, Hadhazy V, Birch S, et al. Acupuncture for osteoarthritis of the knee: a systematic review. Arthritis Rheum 2001; 44:819–825.
68. Berman B, Lao L, Langenberg P, et al. Effectiveness of acupuncture as adjunctive therapy in osteoarthritis of the knee. Ann Intern Med 2004; 141:901–910.
69. Green S, Buchbinder R, Hall S, et al. Acupuncture for lateral elbow pain in adults. Cochrane Database Sys Rev 2001; CD003527.
70. Trihn K, Phillips S, Ho E, et al. Acupuncture for the alleviation of lateral epicondylar pain: a systematic review. Rheumatology 2004; 43(9):1085–1090.
71. Berman B, Ezzo J, Hadhazy V, et al. Is acupuncture an effective treatment for fibromyalgia? A clinical review. J Fam Pract 1999; 48:213–218.
72. Deluze C, Bosia L, Zirbs A, et al. Electroacupuncture in fibromyalgia: results of a controlled trial. BMJ 1992; 305:1249–1252.
73. Ernst E, White A. Prospective studies of the safety of acupuncture: a systematic review. Am J Med 2001; 110:481–485.
74. White A, Hayhoe S, Hart A, et al. Adverse events following acupuncture: prospective survey of 32000 consultations with doctors and physiotherapists. BMJ 2001; 323:485–486.
75. MacPherson H, Thomas K, Walters S, et al. The York acupuncture safety study: prospective survey of 34000 treatments by traditional acupuncturists. BMJ 2001; 323:486–487.
76. Fries J. NSAID gastropathy: the second most deadly rheumatic disease? Epidemiology and risk appraisal. J Rheumatol 1991; 18(suppl 28):6–10.
77. Davidson J, Vandervoort A, Lessard L, et al. The effect of acupuncture versus ultrasound on pain level, grip strength, and disability in individuals with lateral epicondylitis: a pilot study. Physiotherapy Can 2001; 53:195–202.
78. Fink M, Wolkenstein E, Luennmann M, et al. Chronic epicondylitis: effects of real and sham acupuncture treatment: a randomized controlled patient- and examiner-blinded long-term trial. Forsh Komplementarmed Klass Naturheilkd 2002; 9:210–215.
79. Grua D, Mattioda A, Quirico P, et al. Acupuncture in the treatment of lateral epicondylitis: evaluation of the effectiveness and comparison with ultrasound therapy. G Ital Riflessot Agopunt 1999; 11:63–69.
80. Haker E, Lundeberg T. Acupuncture in the treatment of epicondylagia: a comparative study of two acupuncture techniques. Clin J Pain 1990; 6:221–226.
81. Irnich D, Karg H, Behrens N, et al. Controlled trial on point specificity for acupuncture in the treatment of lateral epicondylitis (tennis elbow). Phys Med Rehab Kurortmed 2003; 13:215–219.
82. Molsberger A, Hille E. The analgesic effect of acupuncture in chronic tennis elbow pain. Br J Rheumatol 1994; 33:1162–1165.
83. Irnich D, Kurg H, Behrens N, et al. Controlled trial on point specificity for acupuncture in the treatment of lateral epicondylitis (tennis elbow). Phys Med Rehab Kurortmed 2003; 13:215–219.
84. Molsberger A, Hille E. The analgesic effect of acupuncture in chronic tennis elbow pain. Br J Rheumatol 1994; 33:1164–1165.
85. Pomeranz B, Berman B. The scientific basis of acupuncture. In: Stux G, Pomeranz B, Berman B, eds. Basics of Acupuncture. 5th ed. Berlin: Springer-Verlag, 2003:11.

6 Botulinum Toxin in Pain, Spasticity, and Dystonia

M. Dholakia and Guy W. Fried
Thomas Jefferson University Hospital, Philadelphia, Pennsylvania, U.S.A.

INTRODUCTION

Botulinum toxin (BTX) is an exotoxin produced by the anerobic bacterium *Clostridium botulinum* that has effects on motor, sensory, and autonomic nerves. Botulinum toxin has been used clinically for over a decade in the management of various disorders, including spasticity, dystonia, achalasia, benign prostatic hypertrophy, blepharospasm, dysphonia, dystonia, hyperhidrosis, kyphoscoliosis, low back pain, migraine, and tension-type headache, myofascial pain, nystagmus, pancreatitis, pelvic floor disorders, rectal fissures, sialorrhea, TMJ syndrome, tremor, and urinary sphincter dysfunction (1,2).

There are seven serotypically different strains of BTX (types A, B, C1, D, E, F, and G), all of which cause motor paralysis and autonomic dysfunction via inhibition of acetylcholine (ACh) release from presynaptic nerve terminals. Only BTX type A (BTX-A) and BTX type B (BTX-B) are available for commercial use. BTX-A is the most potent, widely used, and extensively studied strain of BTX.

BTX-A is available in the United States as the product Botox® (Allergan Inc., Irvine, California, U.S.A.) and in Europe as Dysport® (Ipsen Ltd., UK). Botulinum toxin type B is available in the United States as Myobloc® (Solstice Neurosciences Inc., Malvern, Pennsylvania, U.S.A.) and in Europe as NeuroBloc® (Solstice Neurosciences, Malvern, Pennsylvania, U.S.A.).

HISTORY

In 1817, the German physician Justinus Kerner first described foodborne botulism, a disease characterized by symmetric descending paralysis with intact sensation, abdominal pain, nausea, vomiting, dizziness, blurred vision, dry mouth, ptosis, decreased pupillary and deep tendon reflexes, diplopia, dysphagia, dysarthria, dysphonia, constipation, and urinary retention. *C. botulinum* was identified in 1897 by Emile van Ermangen as the organism responsible for this disease. Edward Schantz isolated BTX in 1920. In 1949, it was shown that BTX-A blocked transmission at the neuromuscular junction. In 1989, the United States Federal Drug Administration (USFDA) approved Botox for the treatment of strabismus, blepharospasm, and hemifacial spasm. In 2000, Botox and Myobloc were both approved for use in treating cervical dystonia and pain related to cervical dystonia. Botox cosmetic was approved in 2002 for treatment to reduce the appearance of glabellar frown lines. Most recently, in 2004, Botox was approved for use in the management of hyperhidrosis.

MECHANISM OF ACTION

The BTX molecule is a 150-kDa dichain consisting of a 100-kDa heavy chain and a 50-kDa light chain, linked by a disulfide bond. In its native state, the toxin is complexed to one or more nontoxic molecules that serve to stabilize it and protect it from denaturation. Within hours of ingestion or injection, the carboxyl terminal of the heavy chain binds irreversibly to a specific receptor on the membrane of the presynaptic nerve. The toxin is then endocytosed into a vesicle. The light chain portion of the toxin molecule is subsequently released into the cytosol of the nerve terminal where it cleaves one or more of a group of proteins, collectively termed the SNARE proteins, which facilitate the binding of ACh-containing vesicles to the presynaptic nerve membrane. The specific protein disrupted varies based on the serotype of the toxin; BTX-A cleaves the protein SNAP-25 (synaptosomal protein of 25 kDa), and BTX-B cleaves the protein synaptobrevin. By interfering with the exocytosis of ACh, BTX prevents the release of ACh into the synaptic cleft, thereby preventing neuromuscular junction (NMJ) transmission and muscle contraction. The onset of action occurs within a few days to two weeks. Peak effect is generally seen at approximately six weeks. The duration of action averages three months in skeletal muscle, seven to nine months in the autonomic nervous system, and up to one year in smooth muscle (e.g., detrusor).

The motor end plates that have been affected by the toxin may take up to one year to regain normal function (3). However, the recovery of neuromuscular function occurs sooner, via axonal sprouting. This circumvents the deactivated motor end plates and establishes new neuromuscular junctions.

When injected intramuscularly with the appropriate dose and localization, BTX causes a localized, partial, temporary chemical denervation that weakens the force of involuntary contraction without paralyzing the muscle. Muscle histology reveals atrophy of muscle fibers and increased variation in fiber size during the peak effect of the toxin. These effects appear to be temporary; muscle fiber size (and theoretically, neuromuscular function) returns to normal, even after repeated cycles of injection and recovery (1,4,5).

In addition to blocking the release of ACh at the NMJ of extrafusal muscle fibers, BTX reduces spasticity by decreasing intrafusal fiber contraction within the muscle spindle via inhibition of ACh release from the presynaptic terminal of the gamma motor neuron. This reduces afferent input to the spinal cord, dampening the tonic stretch reflex (i.e., decreasing activation of the alpha motor neuron) and resulting in decreased spasticity (5).

IMMUNOLOGY

In some cases, after repeated treatments, the patient may develop immunologic resistance to BTX. Blocking antibodies directed against the binding portion of the heavy chain prevent the toxin molecule from being internalized into the presynaptic nerve terminal. Clinically, the practitioner may note decreased paralytic or antiautonomic effect compared with prior treatments. The development of blocking antibodies seems to be associated with a higher dose and greater frequency of injection, in addition to a larger protein load of the toxin complex.

The heavy chain-binding portion of each BTX serotype is unique; hence, blocking antibodies directed against one serotype will not interfere with the activity of another serotype. For a patient who develops resistance to BTX-A, for example, the activity of BTX-B should not be affected. However, cross-reactivity, although rare, is possible.

COMMERCIAL PREPARATIONS

Botox is BTX-A, which is purified from bacterial cultures to create a complex of the toxin and several accessory proteins. This complex is dissolved in a solution of sodium chloride and human albumin and then vacuum dried. Each vial of Botox contains 100 units of the toxin/protein complex, 0.5 mg of albumin, and 0.9 mg of sodium chloride. Botox should be stored in a freezer ($<-5°C$), and should be used within four hours of opening the vial, to reduce the risk of protein denaturation or contamination. The product should be reconstituted with preservative-free normal saline, prior to use.

Myobloc, BTX-B, is available in 2500, 5000, or 10,000 U per vial. Unlike Botox, which is a powder that must be reconstituted prior to use, Myobloc is a liquid solution of 5000 units/mL. Myobloc can be stored at room temperature for nine months, or in refrigeration ($2-8°C$) for 30 months. Like Botox, Myobloc should be used within four hours of opening the vial (Table 1).

Although only approved in the United States for the treatment of cervical dystonia and pain caused by cervical dystonia, Myobloc appears in most cases to have a similar efficacy, duration of action, and side-effect profile when compared with Botox (3). Data directly comparing the two products is scant. Botulinum toxin type B has been noted to cause more dry mouth than BTX-A, especially when injected into the head and neck musculature. This side-effect is thought to be the result of a greater affinity of BTX-B for sympathetic nerves (3).

Although the manufacturers of both Botox and Myobloc recommend that only preservative-free normal saline be used to dilute their products, the use of preservative-free local anesthetic has not been shown to cause protein denaturation, and may reduce injection-site pain (1,3).

BTX is dosed in units, one unit being the amount of toxin that would kill 50% of a standardized mouse model (LD50) when injected intraperitoneally. It is important to note that although there are suggested conversions between the different brands of BTX (30–50:1 for Myobloc to Botox, 3–5:1 for Dysport to Botox), these are guidelines only. Owing to differences in chemical composition, manufacturing, and biological activity of the types of BTX, there is no simple conversion between units of one brand of BTX and units of another. In other words, 100 units of Botox and 5000 units of Myobloc should not be expected to produce identical clinical responses in the same patient. Thus, care must be taken when the clinician wishes to substitute one product for another.

TABLE 1 Comparison of Commercially Available (in the United States) Botulinum Toxins

	Serotype	Target protein	Form	Storage	Units per vial	Approved uses
Botox	A	SNAP-25	Vacuum-dried	$<-5°C$	100	Strabismus, blepharospasm, hemifacial spasm, cervical dystonia
Myobloc	B	Synapto brevin	Solution	$2-8°C$	2500/5000/ 10,000	Cervical dystonia

TABLE 2 Potential Adverse Reactions to Botulinum Toxin Injection

Adverse reaction	Reference
Focal weakness	(8,24)
Generalized weakness	(7)
Dysphagia	(1,2,25)
Dry mouth[a]	(3,1)
Dyspepsia	(3,1)
Flu-like syndrome	(8,39)
Injection site pain	(3,35)

[a]More common with botulinum toxin (BTX) type B than with BTX-A injection.

ADVERSE REACTIONS AND CONTRAINDICATIONS

The presence of motor neuron disease or any condition that affects the neuromuscular junction (e.g., myasthenia gravis, Eaton–Lambert syndrome, use of aminoglycoside antibiotics, etc.) is a contraindication to the injection of BTX. In addition, BTX should not be used in patients who are pregnant or breastfeeding or in those with progressive myopathy or systemic illness.

The adverse events associated with BTX (Table 2) are generally dose dependent and transient. The most common adverse event after BTX injection is excessive weakness in the target muscle or local spread of the toxin causing weakness in adjacent muscles. Injection into the muscles of the head and neck carries the risk of local spread of toxin to the salivary glands causing dry mouth and/or spread to the muscles of the pharynx and larynx, causing dysphagia. A flu-like syndrome (muscle soreness, fever, chills) can also occur after BTX injection, and is thought to be caused by the nontoxin portion of the injected molecule. Systemic spread of BTX-A can also occur, as evidenced by the finding of increased jitter on single-fiber electromyography (EMG) in muscles remote from the injection site (4,6). One author has reported three cases of local BTX-A injection causing generalized paresis (7). This systemic spread of BTX is thought to be via a hematogenous or lymphatic route. It is not yet clear whether or not BTX-B carries the same risk of systemic spread. Botulinum toxin does not enter the central nervous system to any significant degree; thus, central nervous system side-effects (e.g., sedation) are rare.

DOSING

The estimated lethal dose of Botox for the average patient is 3000 units (8). In order to decrease the risk of formation of blocking antibodies, the current recommendation for Botox is a maximum of 400 to 600 units, no more frequently than once every three months (9,10). However, doses as high as 800 units every three months have been used clinically without an apparent increase in adverse effects or more frequent development of immunologic resistance. The maximum recommended dose of Myobloc is no more than 10,000 to 15,000 units every three months (9,11), although, like Botox, higher doses have been used clinically. In children, a recent literature review suggests a maximum of 20 to 23 units/kg of Botox no more often than every three months with less than 10 units/kg in a single large muscle, divided into single injection sites of 50 units or less (12).

The selection of a dose of BTX for hypertonia should be based on several factors, including the severity of the condition, the number of muscles involved, the length of time that hypertonia has existed in a certain muscle, patient age, body mass, response to previous injections of BTX, concurrent use of other medications to control hypertonia, use of adjunctive modalities or therapies after injection, and cost. Severe hypertonia and greater patient body mass may warrant a higher dose of toxin. Use of other medications (e.g., oral or intrathecal Baclofen) to control hypertonia and/or the use of adjunctive modalities (e.g., electrical stimulation of antagonist muscles) may potentiate the effects of BTX, decreasing the amount of BTX that is necessary. More chronic hypertonia increases the likelihood that some muscle fibrosis has occurred. The presence of muscle fibrosis makes the injection of BTX less effective. The practitioner should let the clinical response to previous injections guide the selection of the appropriate dose of BTX. Dosage guidelines are outlined in Table 3.

DILUTION

Animal studies have demonstrated that dilution of injected BTX increases the degree of resultant muscle paralysis (9,13,14). On muscle histology, muscles that received a less concentrated solution of BTX showed more atrophy. The mechanism by which this effect occurs is unclear but may involve greater diffusion of BTX throughout the muscle when a larger volume of injectate is used, allowing the toxin to affect a greater number of neuromuscular junctions (9). The advantage of dilution is not only the potentially increased efficacy of the injection, but also a decrease in the amount of toxin necessary and the possibility of treating more muscle sites in a single session without exceeding the maximum suggested total dose of toxin. The disadvantages of dilution include an increased potential for spread of toxin from the target muscle to adjacent muscles, and the possibility of increased injection site pain owing to the larger volume of injectate (9). In general, no more than 0.5 cc should be injected per muscle site (10,11).

BOTULINUM TOXIN IN SPASTICITY

Spasticity is defined as a velocity-dependent increase in muscle tone. Spasticity is caused by the loss of central descending inhibitory pathways causing disinhibition of local spinal cord excitatory neurons. Spasticity can cause pain and inhibit function, in addition to predisposing the patient to the development of joint contractures and pressure ulcers. Botulinum toxin has been shown to decrease spasticity in a variety of central nervous system disorders, including stroke (15–17), spinal cord injury (SCI) (18), cerebral palsy (CP) (19,20), traumatic brain injury (TBI) (21), and multiple sclerosis (MS) (22). As explained earlier, BTX reduces spasticity through its dual effects on the alpha motor-innervated extrafusal muscle fibers and the gamma motor-innervated intrafusal muscle fibers of the muscle spindle.

Care must be taken in selecting the spastic muscles that are to be treated with BTX. In some patients, especially those with SCI and CP, spasticity may be necessary to enhance certain volitional movements. For example, some patients with SCI might utilize spasticity in the triceps muscles to aid with transfers; injecting BTX into these muscles might result in a loss of function. A diagnostic anesthetic block using a local anesthetic should be considered before BTX injection in such cases to determine the potential effect on function.

In treating spasticity, it is recommended that 10 to 50 units of Botox be injected per muscle site, depending on the variables previously mentioned. In large

TABLE 3 Suggested Dose Ranges for Botox and Myobloc in Spasticity and Dystonia

Position	Muscle	Spasticity (units per visit)		Dystonia (units per visit)		Approx. no. of injection sites
		Botox	Myobloc	Botox	Myobloc	
Adducted/internally rotated shoulder	Pectoralis complex	50–200	2500–5000	75–160	NA	2–5
	Latissimus dorsi	50–200	2500–5000	65–125	NA	2–5
	Teres major	25–100	1000–3000	50–100	NA	1–3
	Subscapularis	50–100	1000–3000	NA	NA	1–2
Flexed elbow	Brachioradialis	25–100	1000–3000	25–90	NA	2–3
	Biceps	50–200	2500–5000	25–175	NA	2–4
	Brachialis	40–150	1000–3000	25–75	NA	2
Pronated forearm	Pronator quadratus	10–50	1000–2500	10–35	500–1500	1
	Pronator teres	25–75	1000–2500	10–35	500–1500	1–2
Flexed wrist	Flexor carpi radialis	10–100	1000–3000	15–50	500–2500	1–2
	Flexor carpi ulnaris	10–100	1000–3000	15–50	500–2500	1–2
Clenched fist	Flexor dig. superficialis (per fascicle)	20–60	1000–3000	15–40	250–1500	1–2
	Flexor dig. profundus (per fascicle)	20–60	1000–3000	15–40	250–1500	1–2
Thumb-in-palm	Flexor pollicis longus	10–50	1000–2500	5–25	1000–2500	1–2
	Adductor pollicis	5–30	500–2500	5–25	500–1500	1
	Opponens pollicis	5–30	500–1500	5–25	125–250	1–2
Flexed hip	Iliopsoas	50–200	3000–7500	NA	NA	2
	Rectus femoris	50–200	2500–5000	NA	NA	2

Pattern	Muscle					
Flexed knee	Medial hamstrings	50–200	2500–7500	NA	NA	3
	Lateral hamstrings	75–200	2500–7500	NA	NA	3
	Gastrocnemius	50–150	3000–7500	NA	NA	3
Extended knee	Quadriceps	50–300	5000–7500	NA	NA	2–6
Equino-varus foot	Gastrocnemius	50–250	3000–7500	NA	NA	2–4
	Soleus	50–200	2500–5000	NA	NA	1–3
	Tibialis posterior	50–150	3000–7500	50–200	2500–7500	1–3
	Tibialis anterior	50–150	2500–5000	50–200	2500–5000	1–3
	Flexor dig. longus	50–100	2500–5000	50–100	2500–5000	1–2
	Flexor dig. brevis	20–40	2500–5000	30–80	2500–5000	1–2
	Flexor hallucis longus	25–75	1500–3500	20–100	NA	1–2
	Extensor hallucis longus	50–100	NA	20–100	2000–4000	1–2
Adducted thigh	Hip adductor group	75–400	5000–10,000	NA	NA	2–6
Extended/rotated neck	Levator scapulae	NA	NA	25–100	1000–4000	1–4
	Semispinalis capitis	NA	NA	50–150	1000–3000	1–4
	Sternocleidomastoid	NA	NA	15–75	1000–3000	1–4
	Splenius capitis	NA	NA	50–100	1000–5000	2–6
	Trapezius	NA	NA	50–150	1000–5000	2–4
	Longissimus capitis	NA	NA	50–150	1000–5000	1–4
Flexed neck	Sternocleidomastoid	NA	NA	15–75	1000–3000	1–4
	Scalenus complex	NA	NA	15–50	1000–3000	1–4

Abbreviation: NA, data unavailable.
Source: Adapted from Refs. 3, 9, 10, 11, 25, 26.

muscles, especially those in which the motor end plates are concentrated in multiple regions (e.g., gastrocnemius), multiple injection sites may produce better results than a single injection site.

BTX injection into the detrusor has been shown to be effective in SCI patients in treating refractory detrusor hyperreflexia, resulting in increased bladder capacity, increased postvoid residual volume with decreased voiding pressure, bladder compliance, and urge incontinence (23). In addition, transperineal injection of BTX into the external urethral sphincter has been used to treat detrusor-external sphincter dyssynergia, resulting in decreased maximum urethral pressure and postvoid residual volume (23).

In treating large muscle groups, the practitioner is limited by the amount of BTX that may be used at a given treatment session. In some muscles, especially the bulky muscles of the lower limb, the spasticity may be too great to be treated with BTX injection alone, even when maximal doses of toxin are used. In these cases, it may be possible to use injections of phenol, an inexpensive neurolytic agent, to block the alpha motor neuron and reduce spasticity in larger muscles, reserving BTX for treatment of smaller muscles. In addition, the effects of BTX may be enhanced by the use of physical modalities, such as splinting of the spastic muscle or electrical stimulation of antagonist muscles, after injection.

In terms of pain management, it is estimated that 75% of patients with painful spasticity will obtain some pain relief as a result of BTX injection (1). Joint or muscle pain after treatment of weight-bearing limbs may occur, and is probably a consequence of changes in the biomechanics of gait or posture. This pain should resolve with ice, rest, stretching, and the use of nonsteriodal anti-inflammatory medications (24). Another potential, though rare, complication of BTX injection for spasticity is the development of urinary retention after injection of the bilateral hip adductor muscles (24).

BOTULINUM TOXIN IN DYSTONIA

Unlike spasticity, dystonia is abnormally increased muscle tone that is not dependent on velocity. The sustained muscle contraction of dystonic muscles causes irregular, involuntary, and often painful twisting movements of the trunk, neck, and/or limbs that result in abnormal fixed or shifting body positions. The pathogenesis of dystonia is unknown, but is thought to be associated with impaired output from the basal ganglia and/or thalamus. Dystonia can occur idiopathically, as an inherited disorder, or in association with trauma, structural brain or spinal cord lesions, infection, Wilson's disease, neuroleptic medications, metaclopramide, or complex regional pain syndrome (CRPS). Typically, dystonic movements worsen during volitional motor activity or periods of emotional stress and improve with relaxation or sleep.

Dystonia is characterized as focal (involving one body part, e.g., cervical dystonia), segmental (involving two contiguous body parts, e.g., craniocervical dystonia), multifocal (involves noncontiguous body parts), or generalized (characterized by segmental lower limb dystonia and involvement of at least one other body part). The two most common focal dystonias are cervical dystonia and writer's cramp. Focal dystonias generally remain stable over time, rarely spreading to involve other body areas.

Cervical dystonia involves abnormal tone in the sternocleidomastoid, trapezius, scalenus complex, semispinalis capitis, splenius capitis, and other neck muscles. Most patients are females between the ages of 30 and 50. In the majority of cases, there is a gradual onset and progression of symptoms. The most common form of cervical dystonia is isolated rotation of the head to one side, or torticollis. Other common forms include forward neck flexion (antecollis), neck extension (retrocollis), lateral neck flexion (laterocollis), or any combination of these movements. On EMG evaluation, motor unit activity is seen in most of the muscles that are agonists in the direction of movement with relative relaxation in antagonist muscles.

Controlled clinical trials indicate that treatment with BTX is very effective in improving both the limitation in movement and pain associated with this condition. The usual starting dose is 100 to 200 units of Botox (25) or 5000 to 10,000 units of Myobloc (26), total for the muscles involved in cervical dystonia (Table 3). Smaller doses should be used when treating the anterior neck muscles, especially the bilateral sternocleidomastoid muscles, to decrease the risk of dysphagia owing to local spread of toxin to the muscles of the pharynx.

Another possible adverse effect of BTX use in cervical dystonia is weakness of the neck musculature, resulting in difficulty maintaining head posture. This complication can be managed by wearing a soft cervical collar until the effects of the toxin abate. It should also be noted that the muscles of the neck overlap in multiple layers, sometimes with agonist and antagonist muscles overlying each other. For this reason, awareness of the depth of needle insertion is critical for the treatment of cervical dystonia. Furthermore, the localization of muscles based on anatomical landmarks can be less accurate when the head is held in an abnormal position (25). Electromyographic evaluation can be useful to determine which muscles should be injected. Other potential complications of BTX injection, though rare, are pneumothorax, vascular injury, or neurologic injury (owing to the proximity of the cervical muscles to the lung apices, carotid arteries, jugular veins, and cervical nerve roots).

Writer's cramp, a form of occupational dystonia, has been described in musicians and other individuals whose activities necessitate repetitive movements of the hands. The condition typically begins with a sensation of clumsiness of the hands during fine motor activity, and progresses to slowing of movement and tightness of the grip. Involuntary muscle tone can cause abnormal posturing of the hand. In general, hyperextension or hyperflexion of the wrist and fingers occurs, associated with activity. Once the activity is ceased, the muscle contraction subsides and the symptoms should resolve. Writer's cramp can be associated with tremor, torticollis, and pain in the hand extending to the forearm or shoulder. It responds poorly to treatment with oral medications or physical therapy. BTX is the treatment of choice, and has been found to be effective in alleviating both the abnormal muscle contraction and the pain associated with this focal dystonia (27–29).

BOTULINUM TOXIN EFFECT ON NOCICEPTION

An emerging use of BTX is as an analgesic agent. In clinical use, especially in the treatment of cervical dystonia, a dissociation between muscle relaxation and pain relief has been noted. That is, the patient may experience pain relief before any muscle relaxation effects are seen, and pain relief may persist after the muscle relaxation effect has dissipated (30). This observation suggests that BTX modulates pain via a mechanism that is distinct from its mechanism of reducing muscle contraction.

Animal models support the theory that BTX has direct effects on nociception. In culture, BTX has been shown to inhibit the release of substance P—a neuropeptide involved in nociception and the neurogenic inflammatory response—from the dorsal root ganglion of embryonic rat sensory neurons (31). In this study, all subtypes of BTX tested (types A, B, C, and F) were found to decrease substance P release. However, BTX-A had the most pronounced effect. Botulinum toxin type B had the least significant effect. The inhibition of substance P release occurred as early as four hours after exposure to BTX-A, and was sustained for 15 days. In a rat model, Cui et al. (32) demonstrated that Botox reduces neurogenic inflammation and inflammation-induced pain (known as the delayed, or phase II, pain response), although it does not reduce pain caused by direct stimulation of chemical or thermal nociceptors. Current theories postulate that BTX inhibits the release of certain neuropeptides, which are important in inducing neurogenic inflammation, such as substance P, CGRP, or calcitonin gene-related peptide, from the peripheral nerve terminals of sensory neurons. The target proteins responsible for facilitating the fusion of ACh-containing vesicles with the motor neuron presynaptic membrane are thought to also facilitate the fusion of neuropeptide-containing vesicles with the peripheral sensory nerve terminal membrane. Thus, by cleaving the same target protein, BTX reduces muscle contraction, and may also reduce nociception. Furthermore, the neuropeptides that mediate neurogenic inflammation are thought to sensitize the afferent neuron, resulting in spinal cord hyperexcitability—also known as central sensitization—which may enhance the perception of pain. By blocking the release of these neuropeptides, BTX may prevent or decrease the development of central sensitization, thereby reducing the perception of pain (32,33).

BOTULINUM TOXIN IN MYOFASCIAL PAIN SYNDROME

Myofascial pain syndrome (MPS) is a regional pain disorder diagnosed by the palpation of one or more trigger points. A trigger point is a palpable, hyperirritable band of muscle which, when compressed, causes pain in a characteristic referral pattern. Dry-needling or lidocaine injection of trigger points are currently accepted treatments for MPS. However, BTX injection has become a treatment option in cases in which these measures have failed to provide adequate pain relief. BTX-A and B appear to have similar efficacy in MPS in case reports and in retrospective analyses (3). Patient selection, injection techniques, and BTX dose can all affect the success of treatment.

BOTULINUM TOXIN IN MIGRAINE HEADACHE

Several placebo-controlled trials have shown reduction in the frequency and severity of migraine headaches and a decrease in the use of rescue medications, after injection of BTX-A into muscles of the head and neck (frontalis, temporalis, procerus, corrugator, and/or trapezius) (34,35). Most of the studies used a total of 100 units of Botox or less, and the duration of effect was approximately three months. Transient brow ptosis, blepharoptosis, diplopia, and injection site pain and/or ecchymosis are potential complications of BTX injection for the treatment of migraine headaches. In the treatment of chronic tension-type headache, BTX-A has not been found more efficacious than placebo (35).

At this time, BTX cannot be considered a first-line treatment for any of the aforementioned pain disorders. Rather, its use should be reserved for those cases in which more conservative treatments have failed. A small number of reported cases describe the use of BTX in treating residual limb pain in amputees (36) and zone of injury allodynia in patients with spinal cord injuries (37). However, further studies are required to establish the efficacy of BTX in treating these disorders. Ongoing clinical trials are examining the effect of intra-articular BTX injection on joint pain owing to osteoarthritis, and the use of BTX for the treatment of painful interstitial cystitis. It seems likely that the role of BTX in pain management will continue to expand in the coming years.

INJECTION LOCALIZATION TECHNIQUES

Muscles to be injected can be grossly identified on the basis of anatomic landmarks, by using surface or needle electrical stimulation to elicit a twitch response, or with the use of EMG. Once the target muscle has been identified, the practitioner must then decide the location in the muscle to inject BTX. It has been shown in a canine model that localizing BTX-A injections at or near the neuromuscular junction maximizes the paralytic effect of the toxin (38). In most striated muscles, the greatest concentration of neuromuscular junctions (i.e., the motor end plate zone) is at the midpoint of the muscle. In these muscles, anatomic localization may suffice to identify the motor end plate zone.

In some muscles, such as those originating from the abdominal wall or those located deep in other structures, the midpoint of the muscle may not be easily discernable by palpation. In muscles with multiple sites of origin (e.g., gastrocnemius) or with fibers of varying lengths (e.g., sartorius, gracilis) the motor end plates may not be located at the anatomic midpoint of the muscle, but may, instead, be scattered throughout the muscle (38). In such cases, EMG may be used to locate the end plate region or electrical stimulation to identify the motor point. The motor point is defined as the area where a small motor nerve enters the muscle. The motor point should not be confused with the motor end plate, where the neuromuscular junction is located and ACh is released. In most muscles, the location of the motor point and the motor end plate zone are the same. However, in some muscles, such as the gastrocnemius and peroneus longus, this is not the case (38). Needle EMG is the most accurate method to identify the neuromuscular junction, allowing the smallest needed dose of BTX to be deposited closest to its site of action. Electromyography also helps to identify viable muscle, especially in patients with chronic spasticity or dystonia, in whom the muscles may have undergone fibrotic change. In patients with active spasticity or dystonia, the presence of constant motor unit activity may make identification of the end plate with EMG impossible. In these cases, the areas of the muscle with the greatest amount of motor unit activity are injected.

REFERENCES

1. Raj PP. Botulinum toxin therapy in pain management. Anes Clin North Am 2003; 21(4).
2. Jankovic J. Botulinum toxin in clinical practice. J Neurol Neurosurg Psychiatry 2004; 75:951–957.
3. Royal MA. Botulinum toxins in pain management. Phys Med Rehabil Clin N Am 2003; 14:805–820.

4. Klein AW. Complications and adverse reactions with the use of botulinum toxin. Disease Month 2002; 48:5.
5. Rosales R, et al. Extrafusal and intrafusal muscle effects in experimental botulinum toxin-A injection. Muscle Nerve 1996; 19:488–496.
6. Olney RK, Aminoff MJ, Gelb DJ, et al. Neuromuscular effects distant from the site of botulinum neurotoxin injection. Neurology 1988; 38:1780–1783.
7. Bhatia KP, Munchau A, Thompson PD, et al. Generalised muscular weakness after botulinum toxin injections for dystonia: a report of three cases. J Neurol Neurosurg Psychiatry 1999; 67:90–93.
8. Childers MK, Aoki KR. Pharmacology in pain relief. In: Childers MK, ed. The Use of Botulinum Toxin Type A in Pain Management, 2nd ed. Columbia: Academic Information Systems, 2002:35.
9. Francisco GE. Botulinum toxin: dosing and dilution. Am J Phys Med Rehabil 2004; 83:S30–S37.
10. http://www.mdvu.org/library/dosingtables/btxa_adg.html (We Move: Management of spasticity with Botulinum Toxin Type A).
11. http://www.mdvu.org/library/dosingtables/btxb_adg.html (We Move: Botulinum Toxin Type B Adult Dosing Guidelines).
12. Kinnett DK. Botulinum toxin A injections in children: technique and dosing issues. Am J Phys Med Rehabil 2004; 83:S59–S64.
13. Shaari C, Sanders I. Quantifying how location and dose of botulinum toxin injections affect muscle paralysis. Muscle Nerve 1993; 16:964–969.
14. Kim HS, Hwang JH, Jeong ST, et al. Effect of muscle activity and botulinum toxin dilution volume on muscle paralysis. Dev Med Child Neurol 2003; 45:200–206.
15. Childers MK, Brashear A, Jozefczyk P, et al. Dose-dependent response to intramuscular botulinum toxin type A for upper-limb spasticity in patients after a stroke. Arch Phys Med Rehabil 2004; 85:1063–1069.
16. Brashear A, Gordon MF, Elovic E, et al. Intramuscular injection of botulinum toxin for the treatment of wrist and finger spasticity after a stroke. N Engl J Med 2002; 347:395–400.
17. Gordon MF, Brashear A, Elovic E, et al. Repeated dosing of botulinum toxin type A for upper limb spasticity following stroke. Neurology 2004; 63:
18. Fried GW, Fried KM. Spinal cord injury and use of botulinum toxin in reducing spasticity. Phys Med Rehabil Clin N Am 2003; 14:901–910.
19. Koman LA, Mooney JF III, Smith BP, et al. Management of spasticity in cerebral palsy with botulinum A toxin: report of a preliminary, randomized, double-blind trial. J Pediatr Orthop 1994; 14:299–303.
20. Gaebler-Spira D, Revivo G. The use of botulinum toxin in pediatric disorders. Phys Med Rehabil Clin N Am 2003; 14:703–725.
21. Yablon SA, et al. Botulinum toxin in severe upper extremity spasticity among patients with traumatic brain injury: an open-labeled trial. Neurology 1996; 47:939–944.
22. Hyman N, et al. Botulinum toxin (Dysport) treatment of hip adductor spasticity in multiple sclerosis: a prospective, randomized, double-blind, placebo controlled, dose ranging study. J Neurol Neurosurg Psychiatry 2000; 68:707–712.
23. Frenkl TL, Rackley RR. Injectable neuromodulatory agents: botulinum toxin therapy. Uro Clinics N Am 2005;
24. Bell KR, Williams F. Use of botulinum toxin type A and type B for spasticity in upper and lower limbs. Phys Med Rehabil Clin N Am 2003; 14:821–835.
25. Walker FO. Botulinum toxin therapy for cervical dystonia. Phys Med Rehabil Clin N Am 2003; 14:749–766.
26. http://www.mdvu.org/library/dosingtables/btxa_adg_dys.html (We Move: Management of dystonia with Botulinum Toxin Type A).
27. Wissel J, et al. Botulinum toxin in writer's cramp: objective response evaluation in 31 patients. J Neurol Neurosurg Psychiatry 1996; 61:172–175.
28. Tsui JKC, Bhatt M, Calne S, Calne DB. Botulinum toxin in the treatment of writer's cramp: a double-blind study. Neurology 1993; 43:183–185.
29. Cole R, Hallett M, Cohen LG. Double-blind trial of botulinum toxin for treatment of focal hand dystonia. Mov Disord 1995; 4:466–471.

30. Freund B. Temporal relationship of muscle weakness and pain reduction in subjects treated with botulinum toxin A. J Pain 2003; 4:159–165.
31. Welch MJ, Purkiss JR, Foster KA. Sensitivity of embryonic rat dorsal root ganglia neurons to *Clostridium botulinum* neurotoxins. Toxicon 2000; 38:245–258.
32. Cui M, Khanijou S, Rubino J, Aoki RK. Subcutaneous administration of botulinum toxin A reduces formalin-induced pain. Pain 2004; 107:125–133.
33. Silberstein S. Botulinum neurotoxins: origins and basic mechanisms of action. Pain Pract 2004(suppl); 4:S19–S26.
34. Silberstein S, et al. Botulinum toxin type A as a migraine preventive treatment. Headache 2000; 40:445–450.
35. Winner P. Botulinum toxins in the treatment of migraine and tension-type headaches. Phys Med Rehabil Clin N Am 2003; 14:885–899.
36. Kern U, et al. Effects of botulinum toxin type B on stump pain and involuntary movements of the stump. Am J Phys Med Rehabil 2004; 83:396–399.
37. Jabbari B. Botulinum toxin A improved burning pain and allodynia in two patients with spinal cord pathology. Pain Med 2003; 4:206–210.
38. Childers MK. The importance of electromyographic guidance and electrical stimulation for injection of botulinum toxin. Phys Med Rehabil Clin N Am 2003; 14:781–792.
39. Jankovic J, Brin MF. Therapeutic use of botulinum toxin. N Engl J Med 1991; 324: 1186–1194.

7 Arthrography and Joint Injection/Aspiration: Principles and Techniques

Eoin Kavanagh
Department of Musculoskeletal Radiology, University of Pittsburgh Medical Center, Pittsburgh, Pennsylvania, U.S.A.

William B. Morrison
Thomas Jefferson University Hospital, Philadelphia, Pennsylvania, U.S.A.

INTRODUCTION

For physicians interested in diagnosis and treatment of joint disease, it is important to study the methods for needle access. Once a reliable joint access is achieved, one can inject therapeutic substances, such as lidocaine or steroid; aspirate joints suspected of harboring infection; and perform diagnostic arthrograms. Image guidance is the basis for reliable articular procedures, as definitive placement can be documented. This chapter will discuss the techniques and approaches for image-guided needle placement into the major and minor joints.

GENERAL TECHNIQUES
Conventional Arthrography

Conventional arthrography involves the percutaneous injection of contrast material into a joint followed by a series of radiographs, with specific views depending on the joint being imaged. As a diagnostic technique, conventional arthrography has been replaced by other imaging modalities in nearly all cases. Conventional arthrography is rarely performed today; however, it is essential for the practicing musculoskeletal radiologist to be familiar with the techniques used, as the injection methods employed can be applied to any advanced form of arthrographic imaging. In patients with severe claustrophobia and in centers without computed tomography (CT) or magnetic resonance imaging (MRI) technology, it may be necessary to employ the use of conventional arthrography. Many textbooks have addressed the finer nuances of the art of arthrography, and these provide a useful reference guide should one of these procedures need to be performed. The techniques used in conventional arthrography can also be applied to joint aspiration. For joint aspiration, fluoroscopy, ultrasound, or CT guidance can be used. Fluoroscopy is the most common technique to use owing to its versatility, relatively low cost, and ease of use.

For aspiration of suspected septic arthritis, an 18-gauge or larger needle is recommended for joint access, as infected joint fluid usually has a higher viscosity compared with regular joint fluid. When performing a joint aspiration, it is essential to inject a small volume of iodinated contrast material to verify the intra-articular location of the needle tip and to assess any potential abnormal communications of the joint space. If aspiration of a suspected septic joint yields no fluid, it may be useful to instill sterile saline into the joint followed by aspiration, thereafter sending any aspirated material for culture. When infection is suspected, it is best to avoid the initial intra-articular administration of iodinated contrast material which has bacteriostatic properties.

Computed Tomographic Arthrography

Computed tomographic arthrography (CTA) is useful for the demonstration of cartilaginous and osseous intra-articular bodies, cartilage defects, fracture fragments, synovial abnormalities, and ligamentous disruption (Fig. 1). It is usually reserved for patients with contraindications to MRI. The most common contraindications to MRI include patients with claustrophobia—those with implanted pacemaker/ defibrillator devices, and patients with any other internal metallic objects that specifically exclude the possibility of MRI owing to their composition or location. CTA involves the intra-articular injection of iodinated contrast material typically followed by axial CT scanning. Using multidetector CT technology, very thin sections allow for acquisition of volumetric data, therefore allowing reconstructions to be performed in any plane without loss of resolution. The newer generation multidetector CT scanners generate a higher proton flux decreasing the streak artifact that often limited CTA on older scanners. Therefore, 300-mg I/ml nonionic iodinated contrast should be used without the need for intra-articular air injection when a multidetector scanner is used, and excellent quality images can be acquired. With older generation CT scanners, it is prudent to dilute contrast with sterile saline or to use a less concentrated iodinated contrast preparation to avoid streak artifact. Many authors in the past have advocated injection of variable amounts of air as a negative contrast agent. This is useful to distend the joint without creating significant artifact, and the air can be moved about the joint by putting the patient in different positions. Some authors "coat" the synovium with only a few cubic centimeters of contrast, filling the rest of the joint with air. These techniques have fallen by the wayside with the advent of multidetector CT technology.

The techniques used for accessing the joint are exactly the same as for conventional arthrography and MR arthrography (MRA). Contraindications to CTA include patients with a history of severe contrast allergy and pregnant patients

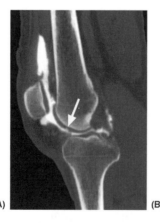 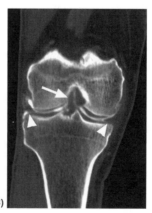

(A)   (B)

FIGURE 1 Computed tomographic arthrography. (**A**) Sagittal reformatted image shows contrast distending the joint. Cartilage is visualized at high resolution; note small cartilage defect at the trochlea (*arrow*). (**B**) Coronal reformatted image shows contrast outlining the intact anterior cruciate ligament (*arrow*) and menisci (*arrowheads*).

(owing to the teratogenic effects of radiation). As the spatial resolution achieved with CTA is greater than that of MRA, some authors feel that CTA is superior to direct MRA for the detection of subtle cartilage lesions. Computed tomographic arthrography has been studied in the evaluation of the postoperative knee, with excellent visualization of meniscal re-tears. It is also very useful in patients who have metallic orthopedic hardware in situ. Using high mAs techniques, beam-hardening artifact from implanted metal hardware can be almost completely eliminated. Such patients would typically not be candidates for MRA owing to the distortion of MR images secondary to metallic susceptibility artifact. It is likely in the near future that the use of multidetector CTA would enjoy increased use in the imaging of the postoperative joint.

Magnetic Resonance Arthrography
Direct MRA
Conventional MRI has enjoyed great success in imaging the musculoskeletal system, and has deservedly become the "gold-standard" imaging technique for suspected internal derangement of joints. There are, however, several limitations of conventional MRI examinations, including the inability to visualize small intra-articular structures, and the fact that many pathologic processes have similar signal intensity to normal anatomical structures. Postoperative findings may also be similar in signal intensity to pathological changes. Unless there is an effusion present, conventional MRI may be somewhat limited owing to nondistention of the joint.

Direct MRA involves the direct injection of dilute gadolinium, followed by MR imaging. This leads to improved intra-articular contrast owing to the T1 shortening effect of gadolinium, and also provides distention of the joint, allowing smaller intra-articular structures to be visualized (Fig. 2). The distention effect alone of saline injection has proved better than conventional MRI in some studies. The distention effect also forces intra-articular contrast through and around pathologic entities. With adequate distention, intra-articular gadolinium

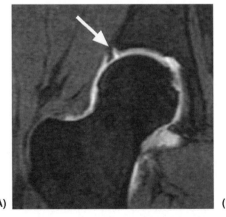
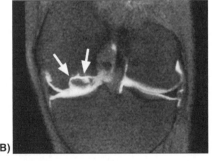

(A)   **(B)**

FIGURE 2 Direct magnetic resonance arthrography (MRA). Dilute gadolinium contrast is injected directly into the joint followed by MR imaging. (**A**) Coronal image of the hip shows bright contrast in the joint, undermining a superior labral detachment (*arrow*). (**B**) Coronal image of the knee shows an unstable osteochondral lesion of the medial femoral condyle, with high signal contrast extending under the fragment (*arrows*).

will enter any pathologic entity in communication with the joint space. Magnetic resonance arthrography provides excellent soft-tissue contrast and demonstrates many abnormalities beyond the resolution of conventional MRI. One of the main disadvantages of MRA is the artifacts seen in patients with implanted prostheses and metallic hardware.

To perform direct MRA, the gadolinium injected should be diluted to 2.5 mM. To achieve this concentration, we add 0.1 cc of gadopentetate dimeglumine to 20 cc of normal saline. This admixture is then shaken to allow for uniform dilution. The final gadolinium dilution ratio should be 1:200. It has been demonstrated that iodinated contrast reduces the T1 shortening effect of gadolinium. This effect is seen on both high and low field-strength systems. It is therefore advisable to use as little iodinated contrast as is needed when performing direct MRA examinations. For direct MRA, the quality of the examination is not affected by patient exercise. We therefore encourage patients to ambulate normally to the MRI suite postinjection, but do not routinely prescribe nor avoid exercise postinjection for direct MRA.

Current indications for direct MRA include assessment of the glenoid labrum in the shoulder and acetabular labral tears in the hip. Direct MRA is also useful for the imaging of cartilage lesions. Magnetic resonance arthrography can also be used for accurate determination of the congruity of the rotator cuff and to distinguish between rotator cuff tendonosis and a full thickness tear (when gadolinium would pathologically enter the subacromial-subdeltoid bursa). Direct MRA is useful in imaging the postoperative joint (especially the shoulder and knee). Direct MRA is also useful in assessing intraosseous ligament tears in the wrist and the ligament tears about the elbow joint. In the ankle, direct MRA can determine the patency of the anterior talo-fibular ligament in patients with ankle sprain. Direct MRA is a safe procedure with no adverse effects reported with the use of intra-articular gadolinium over a 15-year period.

Indirect MRA

Indirect MRA involves the injection of a standard dose of 0.1 mmol/kg of intravenous gadolinium, followed by delayed imaging, to create an "arthrographic effect" as the contrast diffuses into the joint (Fig. 3). As the gadolinium diffuses from the blood stream into the synovial compartment of the joint being imaged, the degree of arthrographic effect will depend on the volume of synovial fluid present within the joint and the degree of synovial vascularity. One of the main disadvantages of indirect arthrography is the lack of joint distention (unless a pre-existing effusion was present). Typically, patients with small to moderate joint effusions will achieve a better arthrographic effect using this technique. A tense effusion may prevent or delay contrast uptake owing to increased intra-articular pressure. In addition, a large effusion may cause heterogeneous or incomplete filling of the joint with gadolinium. Smaller joints, such as the wrist and ankle, and the small joints of the hands and feet achieve a more consistent arthrographic effect owing to the high synovial area/joint volume ratio. Patient exercise postinjection of intravenous gadolinium will increase diffusional flow into the joint and improve the arthrographic effect. One of the main advantages of indirect arthrography is the fact that it can be performed offsite without the need for an invasive procedure. This technique may also be more acceptable to patients as it involves an intravenous injection only.

Indirect arthrography is not optimal for the evaluation of the acetabular labrum. Heterogeneous enhancement within large joints can lead to misdiagnosis, and optimally cases should be monitored and additional delay or exercise employed if

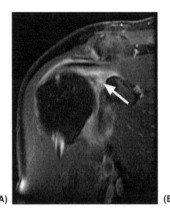 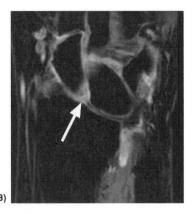

(A)   **(B)**

FIGURE 3 Indirect magnetic resonance arthrography (MRA). This technique involves the injection of a standard dose of gadolinium contrast intravenously. The contrast accumulates in the joint and MR imaging is performed after a delay, usually 30 minutes or greater. Unlike direct MR arthrography, vascular and hyperemic structures outside the joint also enhance. **(A)** Indirect MR arthrogram of the shoulder in oblique coronal plane shows enhancement of the joint fluid and pericapsular structures. Note irregular enhancement under the superior labarum (*arrow*) consistent with tear. **(B)** Coronal indirect MR arthrogram of the wrist shows contrast extending through the scapholunate ligament (*arrow*) representing a tear.

this is the case. Interpreter errors can occur with this technique owing to enhancement of normal intra-articular structures (such as the periphery of the triangular fibrocartilage complex). Indirect arthrography is also useful in the postoperative patient, but is considered less useful than direct MRA because postoperative granulation tissue can also enhance and may be confused for recurrent tear.

Complications
Complications of direct arthrography are rare and usually self-limiting. The most commonly reported complications are transient pain and restricted range of motion of the joint injected. These complications will usually resolve several hours postarthrography as the injectate is absorbed and the degree of joint distention abates.

    Infection is a potential risk of arthrography, but with appropriate sterile technique, this complication is rarely encountered in clinical practice. Hemarthrosis is another potential risk of arthrography, which is rarely encountered, except in patients on anticoagulant therapy. There is also a potential risk of iatrogenic damage to normal articular or extra-articular structures with arthrography. In general, arthrography is a safe procedure. Proper patient positioning and technique will ensure that arthrography of any joint will be a safe procedure with very few complications encountered.

Contraindications
Relative contraindications to arthrography include coagulopathy (International Normalized Ratio >1.4 or platelets $<50,000/\text{mm}^3$), systemic infection, contrast allergy and pregnancy. In patients with an increased tendency for bleeding, a smaller access needle can be used, and ultimately, the radiologist should weigh the benefits versus the risks to the patient in conjunction with the referring clinician. Smaller, compressible joints are less problematic than deep joints in this setting.

Systemic infection is only a relative contraindication, as in some cases, aspiration with arthrography may be indicated to determine an occult source of sepsis (e.g., in a patient with sepsis after total hip arthroplasty). For those patients with a history of prior allergy to iodinated contrast material, it is advisable to prescribe pretreatment with 32 mg of oral methylprednisolone at 12 and two hours prior to the procedure. Pregnancy is also a relative contraindication to arthrography owing to the potentially teratogenic effects of radiation. In pregnant patients who require arthrography, consideration should be given to ultrasound-guided joint injection.

There are very few absolute contraindications to arthrography, but they include; patient/caretaker unwilling or unable to consent to the procedure and active infection at the site of skin puncture.

General Fluoroscopic Technique (Table 1)
The procedure, its risks, alternatives, and potential complications are explained to the patient. A consent form is signed. The patient is positioned on the fluoroscopy table, and once the desired patient position is achieved, preliminary radiographs are obtained. It is essential to review the preliminary radiographs prior to commencing the arthrographic procedure. A metallic marker is placed over the expected needle entry site. Using real-time or intermittent fluoroscopy, the desired position is marked using a pen or by making a skin impression using, for example, the circular end of a needle cover. The skin over the needle entry site is prepped and draped in the usual fashion. Lidocaine is administered to the skin and subcutaneous tissues. The arthrography needle is then advanced into the joint in question using real-time or intermittent fluoroscopy. Upon entry to the joint, a small volume of iodinated contrast material can be injected via soft tubing to confirm intra-articular placement of the needle tip. If an effusion is present, it should be drained to completion. Some authors advocate the intra-articular injection of a small (1–2 cc) volume of lidocaine to provide additional diagnostic information if pain relief is achieved postarthrography. Thereafter, the injectate of choice is administered to the joint, depending on the desired arthrographic technique. Some centers advocate the addition of a small volume of epinephrine to the injectate if

TABLE 1   Equipment Needed for Fluoroscopic Guidance of Joint Injection or Aspiration

Fluoroscopy table or C-arm with facility for spot radiographs
Various sizes and shapes of cushions and bolsters for patient positioning
Metallic markers
2 × 10-cc syringes (for lidocaine and iodinated contrast—Fig. 1)
1 × 20-cc syringe (for the injectate—depending on the arthrography technique)
Insulin syringe (for gadolinium $\pm$ epinephrine)
Soft connector tubing
Sterile gloves
Sterile gauze
Sterile drapes
Various sized needles, 22, 20, and 18 gauge
Adhesive bandage
20-cc sterile saline
10-cc 1% lidocaine
10-cc iodinated contrast 300 mgI/ml.

imaging is to be performed after a delay (e.g., at an "off-site" MRI facility). The administration of intra-articular epinephrine results in synovial vasoconstriction, and delays resorption of the injectate. To add epinephrine draw 0.1 cc of 1:1000 epinephrine using an insulin syringe and add it to the injectate.

In general, low resistance is a useful sign of intra-articular position (which is why a 20-gauge needle is recommended for most joint injections), but this is limited in obese patients. If fluoroscopy shows the needle tip to lie within the joint but high resistance is encountered, then the operator should try turning the needle tip when injecting. If that is not successful, the needle should be pulled back 1 to 2 mm, as the needle tip may be embedded in cartilage. Injection should be stopped if any significant pain is encountered or when the capsule is fully distended (the operator will note a rapid increase in resistance). Injection should also be terminated when the target intra-articular injection volume has been achieved.

Ultrasound Guidance Technique

Many practicing radiologists use ultrasound-guided techniques for joint aspiration or for arthrographic joint injection (prior to CTA or MRA). The advantages of ultrasound are that it is readily available; it does not employ ionizing radiation; and it is a relatively quick and simple technique.

The procedure, its risks, alternatives, and potential complications are explained to the patient. A consent form is then signed. The patient is then placed in a comfortable position on the examination couch to allow for easy access to the joint for injection. Typically, a 5- to 12-MHz linear array transducer is used for ultrasound-guided joint access techniques. The appropriate location and window is then chosen based on known joint recesses or by targeting a specific pocket of joint fluid. Doppler evaluation is recommended to assess for vascular structures surrounding the joint for injection or along the projected potential needle approach path. Some operators find it useful to mark the chosen transducer position with indelible ink on the skin surface. The skin is then prepped and draped in the usual fashion. A sterile cover is placed over the ultrasound probe. Using a strict aseptic technique, 1% lidocaine is administered to the skin and subcutaneous tissues, and then a 20- to 22-gauge needle is inserted oblique to the skin and along the long axis of the probe in order to achieve optimal needle visualization, under direct ultrasonic guidance. The needle tip itself should be identified as a moving reflector (Fig. 4). The needle can be "jiggled" slightly, and if not immediately observed then movement of the surrounding tissues can be easily detected. The path of the needle is then adjusted under real-time ultrasonic guidance. Passage of the needle tip into a joint is generally associated with a feeling of transient capsular resistance followed by a sensation of a resistance-free space. Joint injection can then be performed under real-time sonographic observation.

Specific Fluoroscopic Joint Access Techniques
Shoulder

The most common technique used is the anterior approach with insertion of a needle at the junction of the middle and lower thirds of the glenohumeral joint. For shoulder arthrography, a 20-gauge 3.5-inch spinal needle is used for joint access.

The patient is positioned in the supine position with the arm in a position of external rotation. A sandbag is placed in the patient's upturned palm to maintain a position of external rotation. Using a metallic marker, the preferred access point is

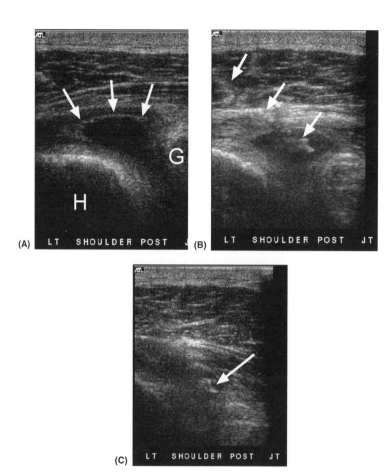

FIGURE 4 Ultrasound as guidance method. (**A**) Transverse image of the posterior aspect of the glenohumeral joint (G, glenoid; H, humeral head) shows an effusion distending the joint capsule (*arrows*). (**B**) Placement of needle creates echogenic line (*arrows*) as it is observed passing into the joint. (**C**) Aspiration with resolution of capsular distension. Note echogenic needle tip (*arrow*) remaining in posterior joint. *Source*: Images courtesy Levon Nazarian, M.D., Philadelphia, Pennsylvania, U.S.A.

marked at the lower third of the glenohumeral joint (Fig. 5). Following the administration of local anesthetic to the skin and subcutaneous tissues, the needle is placed straight down to the joint erring to the side of the humeral head to avoid abutting the glenoid labrum. This method, originally described by Schneider, is probably the most widespread technique in use today by radiologists. With this technique, the needle must traverse the subscapularis myotendinous junction and the inferior glenohumeral ligament. Therefore, there are associated potential risks of distorting or damaging anatomical structures, such as the glenoid labrum. We routinely use this approach for shoulder arthrography, and find it a safe and relatively easy technique, acceptable to patient and operator alike.

For shoulder arthrography, approximately 12 to 14 cc of injectate is instilled into the shoulder joint when assessing the glenoid labrum (depending on the

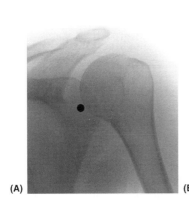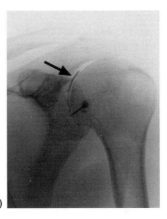

(A)   (B)

FIGURE 5 Technique for shoulder arthrography using an anterior approach. The patient is lying supine on the fluoroscopy table with the arm externally rotated. (**A**) Anteroposterior (AP) radiograph of the shoulder shows the preferred site for access at the lower third of the glenohumeral joint (*circle*). (**B**) AP radiograph of the shoulder shows needle in position and iodinated contrast in the glenohumeral joint (*arrow*).

volume of the capsule). Volumes of up to 16 cc can be used when assessing the integrity of the rotator cuff.

Some authors have advocated a modified anterior approach via the rotator interval. With this technique, the needle is directed from a position on the skin just anterior to the acromion toward the medial upper quadrant of the humeral head, entering the joint capsule via rotator interval. We have found this technique useful in obese patients in whom breast tissue overlies the shoulder in the supine position. A smaller 22- to 25-gauge needle is used for joint access using this technique. The potential difficulty with this technique of injection is that the subacromial-subdeltoid bursa overlies the superior aspect of the rotator interval, and this technique may result in inadvertent puncture of the bursa leading to difficulties with diagnostic interpretation.

A posterior approach to the joint capsule can be used, but this is most commonly used by nonradiologists without image guidance, often leading to inadvertent injection of the overlying muscle or subacromial-subdeltoid bursa. This approach has been advocated in patients with suspected anterior instability and in muscular patients. The needle tip is aimed at the upper one-third of the posterior glenohumeral joint. Positioning for fluoroscopic guidance is more challenging than for anterior approaches, as an oblique view along the glenohumeral joint must be acquired with the patient in the prone position. This position can be achieved with bolsters under the shoulder and by using a C-arm.

Conventional shoulder arthrography is still used for the detection of full thickness rotator cuff tears. For this technique, 8 cc of intra-articular contrast is administered, followed by the administration of 8 cc of intra-articular air. Both the contrast and the air can be drawn into a 20-cc syringe, and injected without disconnecting the tubing. Once the air is injected and intra-articular position is verified, the needle is withdrawn without disconnecting the syringe and tubing (otherwise air will leak out though the needle). The patient then exercises by swinging the arm. Anteroposterior views of the shoulder are obtained in internal and external rotation with and without the use of counterweights. If a full thickness rotator cuff tear is present, then contrast and air will be seen to extend from the glenohumeral joint into the subacromial-subdeltoid bursa. Sonography and MR guidance have also been used for needle positioning in shoulder arthrography.

Hip

When addressing the topic of hip arthrography, it is essential to review the anatomy of the femoral canal. The femoral canal overlies the hip joint, and is the passageway by which femoral neurovascular structures exit from the abdomen into the upper thigh. The boundaries of the femoral canal are anteriorly the inguinal ligament, medially the pubic bone and the lacunar ligament, laterally the iliopsoas muscle, and posteriorly the pubic ramus and pectineus muscle. The femoral canal is divided into two compartments by the medial border of the femoral vein. The medial compartment is termed the femoral ring. The lateral compartment contains the following structures from medial to lateral; lymphatic channels, the femoral vein, the femoral artery, and most laterally the femoral nerve. The femoral artery and vein are enclosed by the femoral sheath, an extension of the transversalis fascia. It is essential to palpate and mark the course of the femoral artery in each patient undergoing hip arthrography, to ensure that inadvertent puncture of these vessels does not occur. Reliance on anatomical landmarks is not a safe practice, as anatomical variations in this region can occur and differences in patients' body habitus can lead to misjudgment of where the femoral vessels lie.

Hip arthrography is commonly used to assess the articular cartilage for the presence of intra-articular bodies and labral tears, which may be associated with femoral-acetabular impingement. Therapeutic hip injection and diagnostic aspiration are also major indications for this technique.

Hip arthrography is most commonly performed using a direct anterior approach, with the needle inserted toward the lateral aspect of the junction of the femoral head and neck (Fig. 6). The reason for this approach is that the joint

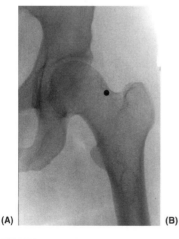 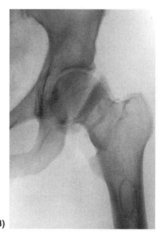

(A)   (B)

FIGURE 6   Technique for hip arthrography. (A) Anteroposterior (AP) radiograph of the hip shows the preferred site of needle access for hip arthrography at the lateral aspect of the junction of the femoral head and neck (*circle*). (B) AP radiograph of the hip shows iodinated contrast within the hip joint after needle removal.

capsule is a thick structure which is best approached at an angle. The medial joint should be avoided, as the femoral nerve and vein overlie this region. Many different techniques for hip arthrography have been reported in the radiology literature. Some authors have recommended a lateral or steep oblique supratrochanteric approach, which may be useful in obese patients with abdominal pannus. Targeting the center of the femoral neck is a commonly used technique; however, a direct approach onto the femoral neck can pinch the capsule onto the bone, resulting in high resistance or injection into the bursa. Some authors recommend caudal or cranial angulation of the needle tip during its approach. For hip arthrography, 10 to 12 cc of injectate is instilled into the hip joint, depending on the tolerated volume of the joint.

Total Hip Arthroplasty Aspiration
Aspiration of a total hip arthroplasty is a frequently requested radiological investigation. Postoperative patients with sepsis or pain may be referred for this technique. The technique of total hip aspiration is relatively straightforward, employing the use of fluoroscopic guidance.

The procedure is explained to the patient, and informed consent is obtained. Using sterile technique, the skin is prepped and draped in usual fashion. The course and position of the femoral artery is marked on the patient's skin. This is important as anatomical markers may have changed secondary to scarring of the superficial tissues in a postoperative patient. Following this, an 18-gauge needle is advanced toward the metallic femoral head or neck component of the hip prosthesis. It may be difficult to visualize the needle on the fluoroscopic images owing to the metallic nature of the total hip prosthesis. Angulation of the tube may aid visualization of the needle tip. Once the needle is felt to impress on a metallic surface, an aspiration sample is obtained. If no fluid is obtained, the needle should be "walked" around the medial and lateral aspects of the femoral neck. An alternative access method has been described, which involves advancing the aspiration needle past the lateral aspect of the shaft of the prosthesis and into the dependent portion of the joint.

If no fluid is obtained after this, then 10 cc of sterile saline should be injected through the needle and an immediate aspiration taken. The fluid obtained is then sent for culture and sensitivity, and microbiological analysis. Once the aspiration is completed, a small volume of iodinated contrast is injected to verify intra-articular position, and to evaluate for abnormal communication into any pathological entities, such as sinus tracts and abscesses, and around the prosthesis, indicating loosening. Postaspiration radiographs are then obtained.

Any fluid obtained should be placed in a sterile container and sent for Gram stain, microscopy, culture, and sensitivity. A sample of the fluid collected should also be sent for a cell count by placing a small amount of fluid within an appropriate collection tube that can be centrifuged in the microbiology laboratory.

Knee
Conventional arthrography of the knee is now rarely performed owing to the superiority of conventional MRI for the detection of internal derangement; however, injection of the knee remains common as a part of MRA or CTA. For anterolateral access to the knee joint, the patient is placed in the supine position and the knee is placed in a position of slight flexion with a roll under the popliteal fossa (Fig. 7). After the administration of subcutaneous anesthesia, the patella is then pulled

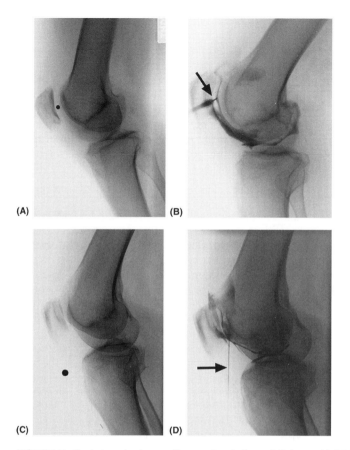

FIGURE 7 Technique for knee arthrography via the patellofemoral joint (**A, B**) and the alternative anterior approach (**C, D**). (**A**) Lateral radiograph of the knee shows the preferred site for needle access to the knee joint via the patellofemoral joint (*circle*). (**B**) Lateral radiograph of the knee with needle in position (*arrow*) and iodinated contrast in the knee joint. (**C**) Lateral radiograph of the knee shows site of access for knee arthrography via an anterior approach with the entry site medial to the patellar tendon (*circle*). (**D**) Lateral radiograph of the knee shows needle (*arrow*) in position at the trochlea and iodinated contrast within the knee joint.

medially and the puncture is made at the level of the mid-patella using a 1.5-inch 20-gauge needle (some operators find that placing the patient on their side in the "running man" position is useful for this approach). The knee joint can alternatively be accessed via a medial approach, also at the level of the mid-patella. The needle is then aimed beneath the surface of the patella. An anterior approach for knee arthrography, which mimics the route used for arthroscopy, has also been employed with success. When using this technique, the knee is imaged in the lateral plane (in the "running man" position), and following palpation of the patellar tendon, the needle is advanced medial to the tendon, in the direction of the trochlear cartilage. To perform knee arthrography via an anterior approach, a 3.5-inch 20-gauge needle is recommended.

After injection, concentric elastic bandage can be wrapped around the knee above the patella in order to prevent contrast from pooling in the suprapatellar recess. The total amount of injectate for knee arthrography is 20–30 ml.

One of the main indications for direct MRA of the knee is the assessment of the postoperative knee. Meniscal re-tears will be manifest as areas where gadolinium penetrates the substance of the meniscus. Joint distention is therefore critical when performing direct MRA of the knee, to allow for passage of gadolinium into meniscal retears.

Wrist

Wrist arthrography is typically performed for the assessment of a suspected triangular fibrocartilage complex tear or an interosseous ligament tear of either the scapholunate or lunatotriquetral ligament. Tears of these small ligaments are diagnosed by direct visualization of the tear or by extension of contrast into an adjacent compartment. There are three joint components that can be potentially evaluated in a complete wrist arthrogram—the radiocarpal joint, the midcarpal joint, and the distal radioulnar joint. Unlike arthrography of most other joints in the body, as there are multiple sites of potential communication, it is beneficial to radiographically evaluate the early flow of iodinated contrast (whether performing conventional arthrography, MRA, or CTA). Small perforations and abnormal communications can be detected on early spot radiographs. It is important to point out that these abnormalities will also be evident on later films, but the exact location of a perforation has become obscured.

The administration of subcutaneous lidocaine is optional when assessing the radiocarpal joint, as the needle used is typically a short 25-gauge needle. The patient's hand is placed with the palm facing downward (Fig. 8). When injecting the radiocarpal joint, a roll can be used to place the wrist in a small degree of flexion. The needle is then advanced into the radiocarpal joint via a dorsal approach, aiming between the distal radius and the mid scaphoid. Pitfalls of radiocarpal injection include injection into the superficial extensor tendons and targeting the osseous surface of the radial rim. A three-compartment wrist arthrogram involves initial injection of the radiocarpal joint followed by exercise. The patient is then brought back three to four hours later, and undergoes injection of the midcarpal joint, followed by injection of the distal radioulnar joint, each injection followed by exercise. The target location for injection of the midcarpal joint is at the joint space at the junction of the triquetral, capitate, hamate, and lunate bones. The location for injection of the distal radioulnar joint is at the distal aspect of the articulation between the radius and the ulna. If the distal radioulnar joint requires injection, it should be performed last, as it can be a painful procedure owing to the sensitivity of the adjacent periosteum.

Typical injection volume is 3 cc for the radiocarpal joint, 2 to 3 cc for the midcarpal joint and 1 cc for the distal radioulnar joint (the latter two joints are typically injected until resistance is felt).

Elbow

For arthrographic access to the elbow joint, the patient should be placed lying prone with the arm over their head, or sitting in a chair with their arm placed on a table with the elbow flexed to 90° (Fig. 9). The joint can be entered laterally over the radiocapitellar joint using fluoroscopic guidance or posterolaterally between the olecranon and the humerus. The advantage of the latter technique is that no major structures, including the lateral collateral ligament, need to be traversed. An 1.5-inch 20- or 22-gauge needle is used to access the radiocapitellar joint. Seven to ten cubic centimeters of the injectate is then instilled.

126 Kavanagh and Morrison

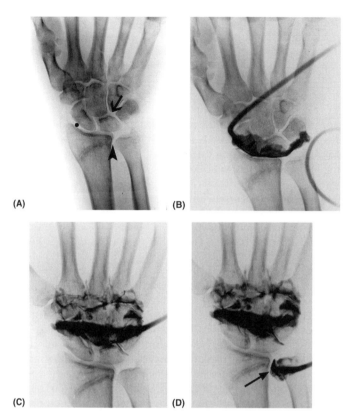

FIGURE 8 Technique for wrist arthrography (radioscaphoid, midcarpal, and distal radioulnar joints). (**A**) Anteroposterior radiograph of the wrist shows site for injection of the radioscaphoid (*circle*), the midcarpal (*arrow*), and distal radioulnar joint (*arrowhead*). (**B**) Needle within the radioscaphoid joint. Iodinated contrast is seen throughout the radiocarpal joint. (**C**) Needle within the midcarpal joint. Iodinated contrast is seen within the midcarpal joint which normally communicates with the second through fourth carpometacarpal joints. (**D**) Needle within the distal radioulnar joint (*arrow*) with iodinated contrast.

Ankle–Tibiotalar Joint

Initially, the course of the dorsalis pedis artery is palpated and marked. The artery is positioned lateral to the anterior tibialis tendon (Fig. 10). After injection of a small volume of subcutaneous lidocaine and under fluoroscopic guidance, a 1.5-inch 20-gauge needle is introduced with use of sterile medial to the anterior tibial tendon aiming for the talar dome. Approximately, 7 to 12 ml of injectate is injected into the joint. Contrast material may extend into the flexor hallucis longus tendon sheath, and may also extend into the subtalar joint (6–25% of individuals). If this occurs, then a greater volume of contrast may be required to distend the joint adequately.

Pubic Symphysis

Arthrography of the pubic symphysis is best performed under sonographic or fluoroscopic guidance. After subcutaneous injection of local anesthesia, a 22-gauge needle is targeted toward the symphyseal cleft at the upper margin of the joint, using a cranial to caudal approach (Fig. 11). Once the needle reaches the outer margin of the joint, signified by increased resistance with a firm consistency,

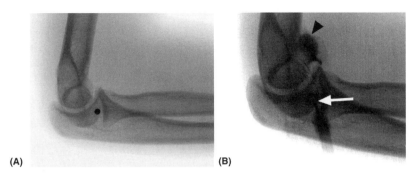

FIGURE 9 Technique for elbow arthrography. (**A**) Lateral radiograph of the 90°-flexed elbow shows site for access to the elbow joint laterally at the radiocapitellar joint (*circle*). (**B**) Needle in position (*arrow*) and iodinated contrast within the elbow joint (*arrowhead*).

the needle is advanced 1 cm farther into the cleft of the fibrocartilaginous disk. After positioning the needle, 1 cc of nonionic contrast material is injected into the symphyseal cleft to confirm the needle's position, show the morphology of the disk, and to potentially provoke symptoms. A single anteroposterior radiograph should be performed to record the appearance of the disk. Lack of imaging guidance may lead to a periarticular injection and diagnostic inaccuracy. For the treatment of osteitis pubis, an aqueous suspension composed of steroid and long-acting local analgesic can be injected into the cleft.

Acromioclavicular Joint
Arthrography of the acromioclavicular joint is typically performed under fluoroscopic guidance with a 1.5-inch 22-gauge needle introduced anterior-superiorly using cranial to caudal angulation with the patient in the supine position. A tiny volume of contrast is injected into the joint to confirm intra-articular placement of the needle tip. This procedure is usually performed for the administration of local anesthesia to the joint for documentation of symptom relief.

Metatarsophalangeal Joint
Diagnostic arthography of the metatarsophalangeal joints is rarely performed, but can be very useful for accurate evaluation of plantar plate tears and other pathological conditions affecting these joints. Using fluoroscopic guidance, an 1.5-inch

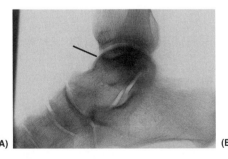
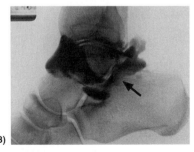

FIGURE 10 Technique for ankle arthrography. (**A**) Lateral ankle view showing location for access to the ankle joint anteriorly (*line*). The needle is placed medial to the dorsalis pedis artery and is directed toward the talar dome. (**B**) Contrast within the ankle joint. Often there is communication with the subtalar joint (*arrow*).

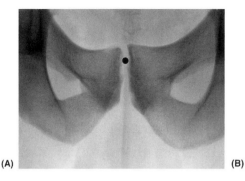 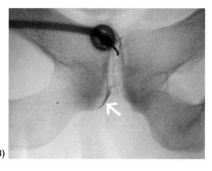

(A)   **(B)**

FIGURE 11 Technique for arthrography of the pubic symphysis. (**A**) Anteroposterior radiograph of the pelvis shows site for needle access to the pubic symphysis (*circle*). (**B**) AP radiograph of the pubic symphysis shows needle in position within the joint. Iodinated contrast is seen within the joint with a right-sided "cleft sign" (*arrow*), indicating capsular injury to the pubic symphysis.

22-gauge needle is advanced into the joint using a dorsal approach and a small volume of contrast medium injected.

SUGGESTED READING

1. Aliabadi P, Baker ND, Jaramillo D. Hip arthrography, aspiration, block, and bursography. Radiol Clin North Am 1998; 36:673–690.
2. Bergin D, Schweitzer ME. Indirect magnetic resonance arthrography. Skelet Radiol 2003; 32(10):551–558.
3. Brandser EA, El-Khoury GY, FitzRandolf RL. Modified technique for fluid aspiration from the hip in patients with prosthetic hips. Radiology 1997; 204:580–582.
4. Brenner ML, Morrison WB, Carrino JA, et al. Direct MR arthrography of the shoulder: is exercise prior to imaging beneficial or detrimental? Radiology 2000; 215(2):491–496.
5. Brown RR, Clarke DW, Daffner RH. Is a mixture of gadolinium and iodinated contrast material safe during MR arthrography? Am J Roentgenol 2000; 175:1087–1090.
6. Chung CB, Dwek JR, Feng S, Resnick D. MR arthrography of the glenohumeral joint: a tailored approach. AJR Am J Roentgenol 2001; 177(1):217–219.
7. Cicak N, Matasovic T, Barraktarvic T. Ultrasonographic guidance of needle placement for shoulder arthrography. J Ultrasound Med 1992; 11:135–137.
8. Depelteau H, Bureau NJ, Cardinal E, Aubin B, Brassard P. Arthrography of the shoulder: a simple fluoroscopically guided approach for targeting the rotator cuff interval. AJR 2004; 182:329–332.
9. Dussault RG, Kaplan PA, Anderson MW. Flouroscopy-guided sacroiliac joint injection. Radiology 2000; 214:273–277.
10. Farber JM. CT arthrography and postoperative musculoskeletal imaging with multi-channel computed tomography. Semin Musculoskelet Radiol 2004; 8(2):157–166.
11. Farmer KD, Hughes PM. MR arthrography of the shoulder: fluoroscopically guided technique using a posterior approach. AJR 2002; 178:433–434.
12. Haims A, Katz LD, Busconi B. MR orthrography of the hip. Radiol Clin North Am 1998; 36:691–702.
13. Hendrix RW, Anderson TM. Arthrographic and radiologic evaluation of prosthetic joints. Radiol Clin North Am 1981; 19:349–364.
14. Kenin A, Levine J. A technique for arthrography of the hip. Am J Roentgenol Radium Ther Nucl Med 1952; 68:107–111.
15. Kilcoyne RF, Kaplan P. The lateral approach for hip arthrography. Skelet Radiol 1992; 21:239–240.
16. Kim KS, Lachman R. In vitro effects of iodinated contrast media on the growth of staphylococci. Invest Radiol 1982; 17(3):305–309.

17. Kramer J, Recht MP. MR arthrography of the lower extremity. Radiol Clin North Am Sep 2002; 40(5):1121–1132.
18. Leopold SS, Battista V, Oliverio JA. Safety and efficacy of intraarticular hip injection using anatomic landmarks. Clin Orthop 2001; 391:192–197.
19. Masi JN, Newitt D, Sell CA, et al. Optimization of gadodiamide concentration for MR arthrography at 3 T. AJR 2005; 184:1754–1761.
20. Miller TT. MR arthrography of the shoulder and hip after fluoroscopic landmarking. Skelet Radiol 2000; 29:81–84.
21. Montgomery DD, Morrison WB, Schweitzer ME, Weishaupt D, Dougherty L. Effects of iodinated contrast and field strength on gadolinium enhancement: implications for direct MR arthrography. J Magn Reson Imaging 2002; 15(3):334–343.
22. O'Connell MJ, Powell T, McCaffrey NM, O'Connell D, Eustace SJ. Symphyseal cleft injection in the diagnosis and treatment of osteitis pubis in athletes. AJR 2002; 179(4):955–959.
23. Ozonoff MB. Controlled arthrography of the hip: a technique of fluoroscopic monitoring and recording. Clin Orthop 1973; 93:260–264.
24. Resnick D. Shoulder arthrography. Radiol Clin North Am 1981; 19:243–253.
25. Salvati EA, Freiberger RH, Wilson PD Jr Arthrography for complications of total hip replacement. A review of thirty-one arthrograms. J Bone Joint Surg [Am] 1971; 53:701–709.
26. Schneider R, Ghelman B, Kaye JJ. A simplified injection technique for shoulder arthrography. Radiology 1975; 114:738–739.
27. Schwartz AM, Goldberg MJ. The medial adductor approach to arthrography of the hip in children. Radiology 1979; 132:483.
28. Schweitzer ME, Natale P, Winalski CS, Culp R. Indirect wrist MR arthrography: the effects of passive motion versus active exercise. Skelet Radiol 2000; 29(1):10–14.
29. Steinbach LS, Palmer WE, Schweitzer ME. Special focus session. MR arthrography. Radiographics 2002; 22(5):1223–1246.
30. Straw R, Chell J, Dhar S. Adduction sign in pediatric hip arthrography. J Pediatr Orthop 2002; 22:350–351.
31. Strife JL, Towbin R, Crawford A. Hip arthrography in infants and children: the inferomedial approach. Radiology 1984; 152:536.
32. Strobel K, Pfirrmann CW, Zanetti M, Nagy L, Hodler J. MRI features of the acromioclavicular joint that predict pain relief from intraarticular injection. AJR 2003; 181(3): 755–760.
33. Trattnig S, Breitenseher M, Rand T, et al. MR imaging-guided MR arthrography of the shoulder: clinical experience on a conventional closed high-field system. AJR 1999; 172(6):157.
34. Valls R, Melloni P. Sonographic guidance of needle position for MR arthrography of the shoulder. AJR 1997; 169(3):845–847.
35. Zurlo JV, Towers JD, Golla S. Anterior approach for knee arthrography. Skelet Radiol Jun. 2001; 30(6):354–356.

8

Musculoskeletal Ultrasound Interventions

Carolyn M. Sofka and Gregory R. Saboeiro
Weill Medical College of Cornell University, Hospital for Special Surgery, New York, New York, U.S.A.

INTRODUCTION

The use of sonography to guide for interventional procedures in the musculoskeletal system has been increasing in frequency in the United States over the past few years (1–3). This may be attributed, in part, to increased familiarity of musculoskeletal radiologists with the modality and the acceptance of sonography as a diagnostic imaging tool by orthopedic surgeons and rheumatologists. The documented accuracy of sonography for diagnosing various conditions in the musculoskeletal system, and the proven reliability of sonography to guide for diagnostic and therapeutic interventions, has helped to strengthen and broaden sonography's role in musculoskeletal imaging (1–13).

This review will outline the current status of musculoskeletal sonography in performing various percutaneous interventions in the musculoskeletal system, with an emphasis on extra-articular applications, as intra-articular interventions are discussed elsewhere in this text.

This review received Institutional Review Board approval.

GENERAL CONSIDERATIONS

In general, a medium- or high-frequency linear transducer is of universal utility in performing musculoskeletal ultrasound procedures (6). The smaller structures of the hands and feet necessitate the use of a higher-frequency transducer, whereas the larger joints, such as the shoulder and hip, which are at a relatively increased depth, require a lower-frequency transducer for visualization. Depending on the patient's body habitus, a lower-frequency curved sector transducer may be employed to increase the imaging depth of penetration (9). In general, at our institution, a standoff pad is not utilized for the evaluation of superficial structures, in favor of the liberal use of ultrasound gel, although some find a standoff pad helpful.

Direct visualization of the linear echogenic needle tip entering the target of interest is the most reliable confirmation of accurate medication delivery to the area of interest. Additional confirmation of accurate needle placement can be performed with the injection of trace amounts of air mixed with saline, and observing the echogenic air bubbles within the tendon sheath, joint, or other area of interest (10,14). Test injections of local anesthetic, as well, can result in observing fluid distention of the area of interest, often with visualizing echogenic microbubbles, depending on the viscosity of the injected fluid and synovial fluid, be it fluid distending a tendon sheath or joint (1,6,14). Delivery of the therapeutic anesthetic/steroid mixture, owing to its viscosity, can result in the formation of microbubbles, yielding essentially an inherent contrast effect ("sono-arthrographic effect" in the cases of intra-articular injections), further confirming accurate needle placement (14,15).

Power Doppler is a useful adjunct in the evaluation of conditions in the musculoskeletal system. Areas of questionable inflammation can demonstrate increased power Doppler activity, thus directing therapeutic intervention to the appropriate area (16). In certain rheumatologic conditions, a quantitative and subjective change in power Doppler activity has been demonstrated in areas of inflammation status postsonographic guided steroid injections (17,18). In some rheumatological studies, the use of intravenous contrast agents [e.g., Levovist®, Berlex, Canada (99.9% galactose, 0.1% palmitic acid)] with power Doppler imaging has proven to be effective in documenting responses in synovial perfusion after intra-articular steroid injection (18). The daily clinical use of sonographic contrast agents in the musculoskeletal system, however, has not been defined.

Tendons

The majority of the tendons (tendon sheaths) throughout the musculoskeletal system can be addressed for sonographic-guided injection. The most directly approachable tendons are those that are the most superficially located, such as the ones about the wrist or ankle.

For tendon sheath injections, a preliminary scan should be performed to evaluate the presence of a tendon sheath effusion; whereas the presence of fluid in the tendon sheath enables a technically easier injection, the absence of fluid does not preclude performing an injection in the appropriate clinical setting.

Tendons are best approached in short axis (1,2) (Fig. 1). The shortest distance from the patient's skin to the tendon sheath should be determined and that route, barring any intervening neurovascular structures, should, in general, be chosen. The needle should be directed to a position circumferential to the tendon, within the tendon sheath. Ideally, if the tendon sheath of interest is directly apposed to bone, the needle should be directed deep to the tendon into the tendon sheath, directly apposed to bone, which will allow for better needle stability.

During real-time evaluation in a tendon sheath injection, the fluid being injected should flow quite readily and easily, and be visualized distending the tendon sheath. Turning the transducer along the long axis of the tendon during injection of the anesthetic steroid mixture often allows for more reliable confirmation that the tendon sheath is being distending appropriately.

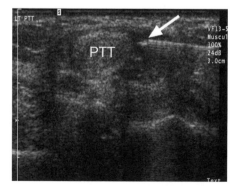

FIGURE 1 Ultrasound-guided PTT sheath injection. Short-axis sonographic image of the PTT demonstrates mild enlargement of the tendon with decreased echogenicity, consistent with tendinosis (PTT). The echogenic linear needle tip is seen within the hypoechoic tendon sheath (*arrow*). *Abbreviation*: PTT, posterior tibial tendon.

The same procedure can be used for diagnostic tendon sheath aspirations, in the setting of inflammation or potential infectious tenosynovitis. In this setting, power Doppler is often useful, usually demonstrating marked increased vascularity along the course of the tendon and tendon sheath in the setting of active inflammation or infection (16). A slightly lower gauge (larger bore) needle might be employed for diagnostic aspirations in the setting of questionable infection, as the material may be somewhat thick.

Soft-Tissue Masses

Most soft-tissue masses, and occasionally, osseous lesions, which are cortically based or those that have a significant soft-tissue component, can be addressed for sonographic guided aspiration or biopsy. Characterization of the lesion in question should be performed prior to the procedure, and correlation of the sonographic appearance of the lesion with other cross-sectional imaging studies (e.g., magnetic resonance imaging or computed tomography), should be done, as the sonographic echo characteristics may often be nonspecific (4,19).

The echotexture of the lesion; relationship to nearby neurovascular structures; and vascularity of the lesion, should all be taken into account before planning a sonographic-guided biopsy. Close communication with the referring oncologic orthopedic surgeon is vital for presurgical planning with a discussion as to the projected path of needle placement and trajectory, which generally is crucial for presurgical planning (4,19).

Large core samples, such as those obtained with standard biopsy guns, and needle aspirated for cytology can be obtained with sonographic guidance, depending on individual pathology laboratory preference.

Other soft-tissue masses that can be addressed for sonographic-guided injection include Morton's neuromas, which are not truly "tumors," but mass-like lesions in the intermetatarsal webspaces formed by chronic irritation with resultant proliferative fibrosis forming about the interdigital nerves (20) (Fig. 2). These lesions may be visualized either from the dorsal or the plantar aspect of the foot depending on the site in the webspace they are located, usually with a medium frequency linear transducer. Depending on the location where the neuroma is best visualized, the needle can be placed along the more plantar margin of the foot (usually with the patient positioned supine, with the foot dorsiflexed) or through the dorsal margin of the webspace (with the patient supine and the affected foot flat on the examining table); the latter position affords slightly greater stability of the foot with less ability of the patient to abruptly move the foot during the procedure (2).

Periarticular Conditions (Ganglia, Bursae, Calcific Tendinitis)

Various periarticular pathologies can be addressed for sonographic guided interventions. Periarticular ganglion or synovial cysts are common causes of pain, and can occasionally present clinically with an, often concerning, palpable mass. These structures are usually in close proximity to, if not directly arising from, a joint. Ganglion cysts are commonly encountered in the wrist, foot, and ankle. The ability of ultrasound to localize and define boundaries of fluid-filled structures, such as cysts has been established throughout the body, and periarticular ganglion or synovial cysts can be seen and decompressed with sonographic guidance (11).

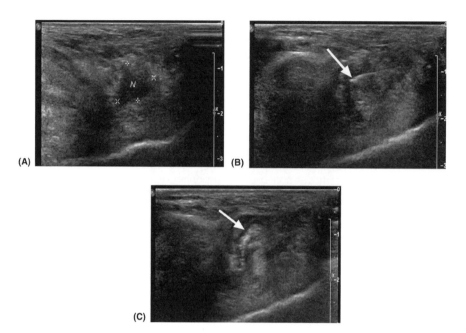

FIGURE 2   (**A**) Longitudinal ultrasound image of the third webspace of the forefoot with a medium-frequency linear transducer with color optimization demonstrates a focal hypoechoic nodule consistent with a neuroma (N). (**B**) Ultrasound-guided injection of the neuroma using a short 25-gauge needle demonstrates the needle tip (*arrow*) to be within the center of the lesion. (**C**) Injection of the neuroma with steroid/anesthetic mixture demonstrates filling of the neuroma and associated adventitial bursa with echogenic material (*arrow*) confirming accurate delivery of medication.

One of the most common periarticular cystic lesions often treated with sonographically guided injection and aspiration is a synovial cyst about the knee, located between the semimembranosis and medial head of the gastrocnemius tendons (popliteal cyst or Baker's cyst). These collections of fluid often decompress from the joint. These cysts can become quite large, and can cause mechanical symptoms, pain and often clinical concern of a more aggressive process, as a mass may be felt clinically. Cysts that are relatively simple can be readily addressed for aspiration with a short needle, as these are often localized close to the skin surface. A relatively large bore (18 gauge) needle is suggested barring other clinical contraindications, such as a bleeding diathesis, as the fluid in these cysts can be quite viscous. A spinal needle can be used for larger cysts (Fig. 3). Popliteal cysts can be internally complex, containing synovial debris, which may be calcified or ossified, occasionally limiting the applicability of sonographic-guided aspiration.

True and adventitial bursae can be injected with sonographic guidance. These can include the greater trochanteric bursa, adventitial bursae in the webspaces of the toes, often associated with intermetatarsal neuromas, and the retrocalcaneal bursa. As with other applications throughout the musculoskeletal system, directly visualizing the needle entering the fluid collection (bursa) of interest confirms accurate needle placement.

Periarticular calcification (calcium hydroxyapatite deposition) within tendons or bursae can be a cause of, occasionally fairly severe, pain and limited

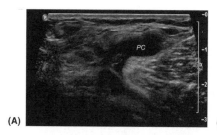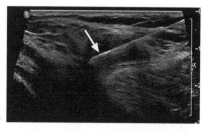

(A)   (B)

FIGURE 3 (**A**) Short axis view of the popliteal fossa with a linear transducer in a sector format demonstrates a curvilinear anechoic fluid collection in the expected distribution of a popliteal cyst (PC) coursing around the semimembranosis tendon. (**B**) Ultrasound-guided aspiration and injection of the cyst demonstrates the linear echogenic needle (*arrow*) with characteristic reverberation artifact within the cyst cavity.

range of motion (21). This most often occurs about the shoulder. Calcium deposits can be seen with sonography as areas of focal increased echogenicity, often demonstrating posterior acoustic shadowing if well mineralized and dense. Subjectively, the less well mineralized, somewhat amorphous and softer, calcifications, are most amenable to percutaneous treatment (13,22,23). Occasionally, with relatively acute onset of disease symptoms, regional flow can be seen about the calcific deposits with color or power Doppler sonography, indicating an inflammatory response (23).

Once the calcific deposit is localized with sonography, one or two needles can be inserted into the calcific deposit for injection and aspiration (Fig. 4). We recommend an 18- or a 20-gauge spinal needle. If a two-needle system is used, the needles are placed perpendicular to one another, with one needle used for injection and the other for aspiration. Ideally, mechanical lavage of the calcific deposit with 1% lidocaine results in gradual disintegration of the calcium deposit, with resultant aspiration of milky white material back into the syringe, usually with partial dispersement of the calcium into the bursa where it eventually is resorbed. Following mechanical lavage, injection of the pericalcific area with a mixture of 1% lidocaine and corticosteroid is performed. There have been several studies reporting on the excellent success of this technique, with the best results encountered when patients present relatively acutely.

Miscellaneous

Chronic heel pain owing to plantar fasciitis can be treated with sonographic-guided injections. Traditionally, blind plantar fascia injections have been performed by palpating the calcaneal tuberosity, and directing the needle into the planta fascia fibers. This has been shown to be associated with chronic dehiscence and potential tear of the plantar fascia (24). Sonography, in contrast, can be used to directly visualize the plantar fascia fibers, and thus avoid direct intrafascial injections (2,6).

Other applications of sonographic-guided interventions in the musculoskeletal system include various sclerosing therapies and sonographic guided percutaneous tenotomy. Alcohol injections of various peripheral vascular lesions, such as venous malformations, pseudoaneurysms and aneurysmal bone cysts with sonographic guidance have been demonstrated to be a reliable means of imaging guidance (25). Sonographic-guided sclerosing injections of regional

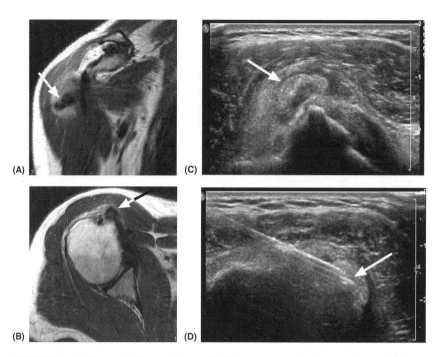

FIGURE 4   Calcific tendinitis aspiration. (**A**) Oblique coronal fast spin-echo and fat-suppressed magnetic resonance (MR) images of the far anterior margin of the shoulder in a patient with relatively acute onset shoulder pain reveals a focal, curvilinear focus of low signal intensity just anterolateral to the subscapularis tendon insertion, with moderate regional surrounding hyperintensity (*arrow*). (**B**) Axial fast spin-echo MR image, mildly motion degraded, in the same patient, demonstrates the calcific deposit just anterolateral to the subscapularis tendon insertion (*arrow*). Ultrasound-guided calcific tendinitis aspiration was requested. (**C**) Short-axis image of the anterior margin of the shoulder demonstrates the curvilinear focus of calcification as a mildly heterogeneous focus of hyperechogenicity with no posterior acoustic shadowing (*arrow*), suggesting it is relatively poorly mineralized. Regional hypoechogenicity is seen about the calcific deposit, consistent with regional inflammation and edema. (**D**) An 18-gauge needle was placed in the calcific deposit (*arrow*), and several attempts at mechanical lavage and aspiration were performed with the return of cloudy white fluid that demonstrated frank sediment in the syringe, consistent with aspirated calcium. After mechanical lavage and fragmentation, a mixture of steroid and anesthetic was injected into the pericalcific region. Patient noted significant improvement in symptomatology postprocedure.

vessels about the Achilles tendon, proposed to be implicated in the pain of Achilles tendinopathy, have also been performed with some success (26,27). Somewhat slightly more involved, sonographic-guided tendon debridements have resulted in reasonably good clinical outcomes, including ultrasound-guided percutaneous longitudinal tenotomy (28).

Sonography can be used to guide for procedures in the setting of global pain management, often stemming from irritation of peripheral nerves, perhaps from post-traumatic or postsurgical scar encasement. Nerves can be visualized with sonography as predominantly hypoechoic structures, with internal hyperechoic perineural tissue with nerve abnormalities, often demonstrating nerve enlargement (29–31). The same procedure used for tendon sheath injections can essentially be

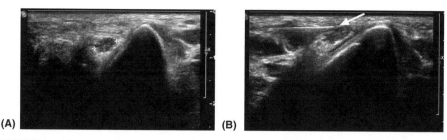

(A)   **(B)**

FIGURE 5   (**A**) Ultrasound of the cubital tunnel in a patient with ulnar nerve symptoms reveals mild enlargement of the ulnar nerve, marked with calipers, in the cubital tunnel. (**B**) Perineural injection was requested for pain relief and sonography was used for accurate delivery of the medication in an immediate perineural location (*thin arrow*). The linear echogenic needle can be seen (*thick white arrow*).

applied to perineural injections, with visualization of the nerve in short axis and directing the needle in a perineural location (32) (Fig. 5).

Posttraumatic or postsurgical collections, such as hematomas or seromas can also be addressed with sonographic-guided aspiration (33,34) (Fig. 6). Preliminary gray scale evaluation of fluid collections, such as these, can help in preprocedure

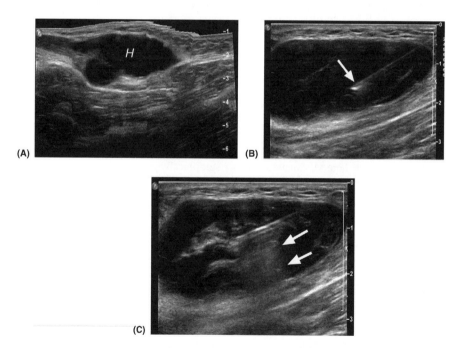

FIGURE 6   (**A**) Longitudinal extended field of view image of the thigh in a patient status post adductor strain demonstrates a mildly heterogeneous elliptical hypoechoic fluid collection, with linear internal septations and debris consistent with a hematoma (H). (**B**) Ultrasound-guided aspiration of the cyst yielded minimal return of serosanguinous fluid owing to the viscous nature of the fluid. The needle (*arrow*) can be seen within the hematoma cavity. (**C**) Ultrasound-guided lavage of the collection with a mixture of 1% lidocaine and normal saline resulted in some loosening of the thick clotting hematoma. Reverberation artifact from injection (*arrows*) of the saline/1% lidocaine mixture can be seen.

planning and providing prognostic information. The internal complexity of the collection can indicate the potential success of performing sonographic aspiration, with older, more complex and resolving hematomas, often resulting in poor yield with sonographic-guided aspiration, even with a large bore needle.

The role of sonography in guiding for articular injections throughout the musculoskeletal system, ranging from the small joints of the hands and feet to larger joints, such as the hip, traditionally performed under fluoroscopic guidance, has been documented, though is outside the scope of this chapter (1,2,6,9).

CONCLUSIONS

In summary ultrasound is a readily available, reliable, and relatively low-cost method of imaging guidance for musculoskeletal interventional procedures. The absence of ionizing radiation makes sonography a fairly universal and globally accepted imaging modality across all patient populations, including pregnant and pediatric patients. The large majority of soft-tissue structures and joints can be visualized and therefore addressed for injection with sonographic guidance. Tendons throughout the musculoskeletal system can be treated with sonographic-guided interventions. Soft-tissue masses, with appropriate preprocedure consultation with other imaging modalities and the oncologic orthopedic surgeon, can result in reliable accurate soft-tissue biopsies.

REFERENCES

1. Adler RS, Sofka CM. Percutaneous ultrasound-guided injections in the musculoskeletal system. Ultrasound Q 2003; 19(1):3–12.
2. Sofka CM, Adler RS. Ultrasound-guided interventions in the foot and ankle. Semin Musculoskelet Radiol 2002; 6(2):163–168.
3. Lin J, Jacobson JA, Fessell DP, Weadock WJ, Hayes CW. An illustrated tutorial of musculoskeletal sonography: part 4, musculoskeletal masses, sonographically guided interventions, and miscellaneous topics. AJR 2000; 175(6):1711–1719.
4. Torriani M, Etchebehere M, Amstalden E. Sonographically guided core needle biopsy of bone and soft tissue tumors. J Ultrasound Med 2002; 21(9):275–281.
5. Naredo E, Cabero F, Beneyto P, et al. A randomized comparative study of short term response to blind injection versus sonographic-guided injection of local corticosteroids in patients with painful shoulder. J Rheumatol 2004; 31(2):308–314.
6. Sofka CM, Collins AJ, Adler RS. Use of ultrasonographic guidance in interventional musculoskeletal procedures: a review from a single institution. J Ultrasound Med 2001; 20(1):21–26.
7. Adler RS, Buly R, Ambrose R, Sculco T. Diagnostic and therapeutic use of sonography-guided iliopsoas peritendinous injections. AJR 2005; 185(4):940–943.
8. Wank R, Miller TT, Shapiro JF. Sonographically guided injection of anesthetic for iliopsoas tendinopathy after total hip arthroplasty. J Clin Ultrasound 2004; 32(7):354–357.
9. Sofka CM, Saboeiro G, Adler RS. Ultrasound-guided adult hip injections. J Vasc Interv Radiol 2005; 16(8):1121–1123.
10. Fredberg U, van Overeem Hansen G, Bolvig L. Placement of intra-articular injections verified by ultrasonography and injected air as contrast medium. Ann Rheum Dis 2001; 60(5):542.
11. Breidahl WH, Adler RS. Ultrasound-guided injection of ganglia with corticosteroids. Skelet Radiol 1996; 25(7):635–638.
12. Sofka CM, Adler RS. Sonography of cubital bursitis. AJR 2004; 183(1):51–53.
13. Cooper G, Lutz GE, Adler RS. Ultrasound-guided aspiration of symptomatic rotator cuff calcific tendinitis. Am J Phys Med Rehabil 2005; 84(1):81.

14. Luchs J, Sofka CM, Adler RS. Sonographic contrast effect of combined steroid and anesthetic injections: in vitro analysis. J Ultrasound Med 2007; 26:227–231.
15. Sofka CM, Adler RS, Danon M. Sonography of the acetabular labrum: visualization of labral pathology during intraarticular injections. J Ultrasound Med 2006; 25(10): 1321–1326.
16. Breidahl WH, Newman JS, Taljanovic MS, Adler RS. Power Doppler sonography in the assessment of musculoskeletal fluid collections. AJR 1996; 166(6):1443–1446.
17. Filippucci E, Farina A, Carotti M, Salaffi F, Grassi W. Grey scale and power Doppler sonographic changes induced by intra-articular steroid injection treatment. Ann Rheum Dis 2004; 63(6):740–743.
18. Salaffi F, Carotti M, Manganelli P, Filippucci E, Giuseppetti GM, Grassi W. Contrast-enhanced power Doppler sonography of knee synovitis in rheumatoid arthritis: assessment of therapeutic response. Clin Rheumatol 2004; 23(4):285–290.
19. Batz R, Sofka CM, Adler RS, DiCarlo E, Lane J. Sonographic evaluation and diagnosis of postoperative pseudotumor of the back with histologic correlation. J Ultrasound Med 2005; 24(7):1017–1019.
20. Wu KK. Morton's interdigital neuroma: a clinical review of its etiology, treatment and results. J Foot Ankle Surg 1996; 35(2):112–119.
21. Neviaser RJ. Painful conditions affecting the shoulder. Clin Orthop Relat Res 1983; (173):63–69.
22. Farin PU, Rasanen H, Jaroma H, Harju A. Rotator cuff calcifications: treatment with ultrasound-guided percutaneous needle aspiration and lavage. Skelet Radiol 1996; 25(6):551–554.
23. Chiou HJ, Chou YH, Wu JJ, Hsu CC, Huang DY, Chang CY. Evaluation of calcific tendinitis of the rotator cuff: role of color Doppler ultrasonography. J Ultrasound Med 2002; 21(3):289–295.
24. Acevedo JI, Beskin JL. Complications of plantar fascia rupture associated with corticosteroid injection. Foot Ankle Int 1998; 19(2):91–97.
25. Jain R, Bandhu S, Sawhney S, Mittal R. Sonographically guided percutaneous sclerosis using 1% polidocanol in the treatment of vascular malformations. J Clin Ultrasound 2002; 30(7):416–423.
26. Ohberg L, Alfredson H. Ultrasound guided sclerosis of neovessels in painful chronic Achilles tendinosis: pilot study of a new treatment. Br J Sports Med 2002; 36(3): 173–175.
27. Alfredson H, Ohberg L. Neovascularization in chronic painful patellar tendinosis: promising results after sclerosing neovessels outside the tendon. Knee Surg Sports Traumatol Arthrosc 2005; 13(2):74–80.
28. Testa V, Capasso G, Maffulli N, Bifulco G. Ultrasound-guided percutaneous longitudinal tenotomy for the management of patellar tendinopathy. Med Sci Sports Exerc 1999; 31(11):1509–1515.
29. Martinoli C, Bianchi S, Derchi LE. Tendon and nerve sonography. Radiol Clin North Am 1999; 37(4):691–711, viii.
30. Gruber H, Peer S, Meirer R, Bodner G. Peroneal nerve palsy associated with knee luxation: evaluation by sonography—initial experiences. AJR 2005; 185(5):1119–1125.
31. Beekman R, van den Berg LH, Franssen H, Visser LH, van Asseldonk JT, Wokke JH. Ultrasonography shows extensive nerve enlargements in multifocal motor neuropathy. Neurology 2005; 65(2):305–307.
32. Galiano K, Obwegeser AA, Bodner G, et al. Realtime sonographic imaging for periradicular injections in the lumbar spine—a sonographic anatomic study of a new technique. J Ultrasound Med 2005; 24(1):33–38.
33. Peetrons P. Ultrasound of muscles. Eur Radiol 2002; 12(1):35–43.
34. Cardinal E, Chhem RK, Beauregard CG. Ultrasound guided interventional procedures in the musculoskeletal system. Radiol Clin North Am 1998; 36(3):597–604.

9

Musculoskeletal Percutaneous Biopsy: Techniques and Tips

William B. Morrison
Thomas Jefferson University Hospital, Philadelphia, Pennsylvania, U.S.A.

Eoin Kavanagh
Department of Musculoskeletal Radiology, University of Pittsburgh Medical Center, Pittsburgh, Pennsylvania, U.S.A.

INTRODUCTION

Image-guided percutaneous biopsy of bone and soft-tissue lesions has become an integral part of modern medical care (1–12). There are a number of advantages to this technique: first, imaging guidance increases the likelihood that the biopsy will be acquired from the lesion if small, or viable regions of the lesion if large. Imaging also enables the operator to avoid vessels, nerves, organs, and other sensitive structures during passage of the needle. Conscious sedation (or in some cases, just local anesthetic) may be used, instead of general anesthesia associated with surgery. Therefore, percutaneous biopsy can also reduce risk of complications. Percutaneous biopsy has been shown in numerous studies to be safe and effective (3–12). However, biopsy must be performed by an experienced practitioner with knowledge of equipment, use of the imaging modalities and relevant anatomy, approaches and potential complications and limitations of the procedure. This chapter will attempt to outline these issues.

EVALUATION OF THE PREBIOPSY IMAGING STUDIES

There are a number of considerations when a percutaneous biopsy is requested. These considerations are strongly influenced by findings on recent imaging exams in which the lesion was diagnosed. These exams should always be reviewed. The clinical service requesting biopsy should provide all relevant imaging exams performed, and the available radiology information system should be searched for prior studies.

EQUIPMENT
Guidance Modalities

One essential aspect to keep in mind when planning a biopsy is that the lesion should be visible on the guidance modality. Alternatively, for extensive or infiltrative lesions, the lesion itself need not be visible, but the region involved [e.g., by magnetic resonance imaging (MRI)] should be accessible on the modality. Fluoroscopy has definite advantages over other modalities: imaging is easily performed real time. The limitation of projectional radiographic imaging is not a major one considering the ease to alter the angle craniocaudally or transversely in order to acquire a different viewpoint. Biopsies using fluoroscopy are often easier to schedule as well. However, the room and configuration of the fluoroscopy equipment

(C-arm, fixed image intensifier, angiography room) can create problems with access to the biopsy area, and must be considered in advance. Many angiography units have a narrow work area which can cause problems if a long biopsy needle is used; in addition, some C-arms and angiography units cannot achieve the angulations needed for the desired approach.

For most lesions, computed tomography (CT) is the preferred guidance method. Simultaneous visualization of the lesion and soft-tissue structures, such as blood vessels, is extremely helpful for planning the approach, especially for small or deep lesions. The angle of approach can be planned to avoid vital structures, and assessment of the depth to the lesion assists in needle selection. Repeat scans can be acquired in the plane of the needle when changes in needle position are made. Computed tomographic fluoroscopy assists in speeding this process; instead of leaving the suite for each scan, the operator remains in protective lead and steps on a foot pedal to almost instantly acquire a small series of images through the needle. Disadvantages of CT include relatively high radiation dose and limitation regarding craniocaudal angulation.

Ultrasound is very versatile, and can also be used for localization of soft tissue lesions (10,11). Evidently, as ultrasound does not visualize within bone, it generally cannot be used for bone biopsy localization except for superficial lesions or those with cortical breakthrough (12). Ultrasound with Doppler easily visualizes blood vessels, and can improve the safety of the desired approach. Solid and vascular regions of soft-tissue masses can also be accurately targeted. The needle passage can be directly visualized in real time, instead of periodically, after repositioning.

Magnetic resonance imaging is used in some centers for localization, but requires special preparation (13,14). If equipment is needed (e.g., to provide sedation and monitoring), it must be MRI compatible (e.g., all components must be non-ferromagnetic). Additionally, needles must be MRI compatible, and should be made of a material that creates relatively little artifact so that the needle tract is well visualized with reference to surrounding anatomy. Magnetic resonance imaging can be useful for ablation as the destroyed tissue can be visualized (e.g., ice ball formation in cryoablation).

Needles
Fine-needle aspiration

Fine-needle aspiration needles are used for collection of cytology samples; needles are small gauge and collect groups of cells rather than core samples. The needle is placed within the lesion with stylet in place; the stylet is removed, and using an "in-and-out" motion within the lesion, changing direction each pass while pulling the stylet out collects the sample. Alternatively, a syringe can be attached to the needle hub and aspiration performed while the needle is manipulated. The sample is placed into cytology fluid; in the lab, the sample is spun down into a block and evaluated.

Fine-needle aspiration is useful, especially because low-profile needles may reduce risk of damage to adjacent tissues. However, unless real-time imaging is performed during needle manipulation (i.e., ultrasound) the in-and-out motion is performed blind, and may not be advised for lesions near vital structures. Another disadvantage is that the architecture of the lesion is altered and the sample volume is small, making it more difficult to make the diagnosis, especially for primary lesions. Nevertheless, some authors have recommended that a cytology sample be acquired in addition to the core biopsy sent to histology for increased diagnostic yield overall (15).

Diagnostic yield is highly dependent on the experience of the interpreting cytologist or pathologist. Close communication between the radiologist and pathologist is important to give feedback in both directions. The radiologist should discuss radiological findings with the pathologist, especially for atypical cases, and the pathologist should provide feedback to the radiologist regarding the quality of the samples acquired that may require a change in needle type or methodology.

Needles have a variety of configurations and tips designed to offer different advantages. As there are many needles, and vendors are continually modifying them, it is difficult to discuss the specific features of each. However, there are some general features that can be outlined with reference to their intended purpose.

Coaxial systems

These are needles intended for either soft tissue or bone that have an outer sheath and an inner cutting needle. The cutting needle extends a certain distance beyond the sheath. This is almost universally used in musculoskeletal biopsies, as it requires only one localization/placement procedure to position the sheath/stylet at the margin of the lesion, after which multiple passes can be obtained. The only situation in which a noncoaxial system may be used is a very superficial lesion that is easy to localize, and that is not near any vital structure.

Soft-tissue guns

Soft-tissue guns collect a core of tissue unlike fine aspiration needles. They are larger gauge, typically 14–18 G. Instead of a hollow cutting needle design, they incorporate a solid inner core with a recess near the tip. This portion of the needle is advanced into the lesion, after which an inner sheath "shoots" over it, cutting the tissue filling the recess; the system is withdrawn from the outer sheath and the sample is collected. Therefore two components are advanced in succession—the solid inner needle and the inner sheath. In some needles, this is automated, triggered by a button that is pressed when the needle is in position. However, it is not always desired to shoot the inner needle without feel or control; if the lesion is near a vital structure, or not as large as the "throw" of the needle, it is better to retain control of the first step. Some needles have a setting or alternate triggering mechanism that allows the radiologist to slowly advance the inner needle as far as desired; when in position, the sheath is triggered to advance.

Bone biopsy needles

Various techniques are used to cut and hold the sample in the needle. The Elson and Ackermann needles (Cook, Bloomington, Indiana, U.S.A.) have a serrated tip that is useful for cutting through cortex. Trephine needles, such as the Jamshidi type have a simple, beveled tip that facilitates purchase on bone. These needles have a straight inner bore without tapering. However, most needles have a tapered tip, in which the end of the needle is curved slightly inward. After the needle is advanced into the lesion, the end is "wobbled" or rotated in order to cut the tip of the core. The disadvantage of this is that the actual inner gauge of the needle is smaller than advertised on the package. If the needle is used as a sheath for another needle, this must be taken into account; there may be a two- to three-gauge difference in what can actually fit through the needle. The Ostycut needle (Bard, Tempe, Arizona, U.S.A.) has a threaded tip that is screwed into the lesion; altering the course and advancing further is supposed to cut the sample. A syringe can be used to provide negative pressure in the needle in order to assist retention of the core. The Traplok system (MD Tech, Gainesville, Florida, U.S.A.) has a thin, curved implement that hugs the inner margin of the needle, and is advanced around the core, "trapping" it in as the needle is withdrawn.

The Bonopty needle system (Radi, Uppsala, Sweden) is a coaxial system in which the radiologist can substitute the stylet for a small drill. The drill is slightly eccentric and "wobbles," thereby cutting a hole large enough to accommodate the sheath. The drill is excellent for accessing lesions within sclerotic bone or through thick cortex. In addition, lesions that are deep within bone (e.g., anterior vertebral body lesion approached through the pedicle) can be difficult to access coaxially with other systems. With Bonopty, the sheath/stylet is placed at the outer margin of bone, lined up with the lesion; the stylet is replaced with the drill, which creates a pathway. The sheath is advanced over the drill, and this process is continued until the lesion is reached. Subsequently, the drill is replaced with the cutting needle, and multiple samples are acquired through the sheath.

With all bone biopsy needles, the core can occlude the needle, making it difficult to advance. This is especially true when a thick cortex is penetrated. If there is difficulty advancing the needle at any point, the bore may be occluded and the needle should be withdrawn and cleared. If this is not done, the biopsy is made more difficult, and the sample can be damaged with crush artifact seen at histology.

Stylets

Stylets are kept in the needle and function to occlude the barrel (avoiding extraneous tissue damage and sampling); help guide the needle in place (for beveled stylets); and achieve "purchase," or initiation of entry into bone. Although different vendors sell a number of configurations, the point can either be in the center (diamond tip) or at the edge with a flat, tilted surface (bevel).

Diamond point tips make the needle more difficult to "steer." However, this has the advantage of being deflected less than a beveled tip by fascia and muscle. This type of tip may also be easier to achieve "purchase" in bone.

A beveled tip can be very useful to guide the needle in place by directing open aspect of bevel away from desired direction. This can be useful for deflection within bone as well (especially useful for vertebroplasty). When the desired angle of approach is achieved, some needles allow for trading out with a diamond tip stylet, facilitating straight advancement toward the lesion.

When guiding a needle into place through the soft tissue, it should be recognized that the fascia serves as a fulcrum. If proper guidance cannot be achieved and the needle continues along the same course, it may need to be pulled back beyond the primary fascia, or a deeper skin/fascial cut should be made (instead of just skin nick).

Selection of appropriate needle

The optimal needle should always be selected ahead of time, with an alternate choice kept to the side. The prebiopsy imaging is very useful for planning needle selection. Axial CT or MR images are especially useful; the angle and distance from the skin can be evaluated. The depth of the lesion within bone and thickness of the cortex should be noted (a drill-type needle may be needed). If the lesion is lytic and near the cortex, a combination of bone and soft-tissue biopsy needles can be used. For example, a large-bore bone biopsy needle can be used to punch a hole in the intact cortex positioned at the superficial margin of the lesion; the stylet is removed and a soft-tissue gun is passed coaxially into the lesion, and samples acquired. If this method is used, care should be taken not to use the automatic needle throw. Some soft-tissue guns function by cocking the needle back and pressing a button, causing the needle to shoot out 2–4 cm followed immediately by the sheath, cutting the sample. If this is done within or onto bone, the end of the needle can bend or break.

It can be difficult to acquire a solid sample from very aggressive, lytic lesions using a bone biopsy needle alone. One technique is to pass the needle completely through the lesion (assuming the opposite cortex is intact), impacting bone into the tip of the needle, holding the sample in the needle. If the lesion is lytic and the cortex is permeated or thinned, a soft-tissue gun inserted through a sheath may be the best option. The sheath of a soft-tissue gun with sylet in place can be used to punch through the weakened cortex, and the sample acquired as earlier (16,17).

Length: On the preliminary imaging studies, an estimation should be made regarding the depth of the lesion through soft tissue, and how much bone should be traversed to reach the lesion at the planned angle of approach. Obviously, the needle selected should be long enough to reach the bone. Some needles are more easily able to traverse bone than others. For lesions deep within bone, an eccentric drill system (Bonopty) is very useful; for example, a lesion in the anterior vertebral body, for which a transpedicle approach is planned. However, the needle is quite short, and this may be a limiting factor in obese patients.

Gauge/number of passes: In general, for all lesions, the larger the cores and the more cores are acquired, the better. The core sent to histology will shrink 25% to 50% during decalcification; hence, the actual sample size is smaller than the needle width would suggest. However, attention should always be given to the safety of the patient, and if the lesion is near vessels, nerves, or other important structures, a smaller-gauge needle may be a better choice. Similarly, more passes with the needle may increase potential for complications if the lesion is near a vital area. Typically three to five passes are taken.

Whenever possible, it is beneficial to have a cytologist present to verify that an adequate sample has been acquired. Although this increases the time of the procedure, it helps prevent the need for rebiopsy. The experience of the pathologist is important as well. If there is no bone pathologist at the institution, the "yield" or "success" of biopsy may be artificially low owing to hedging with a high ratio of "inadequate samples." On the other hand, the radiologist can help avoid this by providing as much relevant clinical information as possible on the request. A good pathologist will review imaging studies on cases that are not clear-cut. Similarly, for cases of infection, yield may be increased if the sample is sent for both histological and microbiological evaluation. Even if no bacteria are cultured from the sample, histological evaluation can confirm the presence of osteomyelitis (18). Lidocaine, once thought to be inhibitory toward the growth of bacteria, has been found to have no significant effect on growth (19).

LESION TYPES/APPROACHES

There have been a number of techniques and approaches described for various lesion types and locations (1–17). Needle or needle combination used is dependent on the location and the type of lesion in addition to practitioner comfort and experience (20). One general concept is that the adjacent vital structures, such as the spinal canal, the pleura, or the aorta, must be directly visualized or location easily surmised using the modality selected. For all lesions under CT

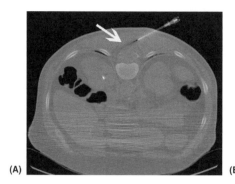 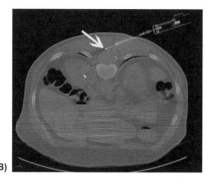

(A)   (B)

FIGURE 1 Biopsy of a superficial lesion. This 67-year-old male presented with back pain. A computed tomography (CT) scan showed an expansile and lytic lesion within the spinous process of T12, which proved to be a myelomatous deposit at histology. (**A**) Axial CT image from percutaneous biopsy of T12 lesion shows an expansile mass replacing the spinous process (*arrow*). The coaxial biopsy device has been placed adjacent to the lesion via an oblique approach so as to avoid the underlying central canal and spinal cord when deploying the soft-tissue biopsy gun. (**B**) Axial CT image from percutaneous biopsy of T12 lesion shows deployment of the soft-tissue gun via the coaxial device. The tip of the cutting portion of the biopsy gun is seen within the lesion (*arrow*).

guidance, one must always measure from the skin straight to the closest "danger point" (e.g., pleura, aorta, and the like); the needle must not be inserted beyond this point before checking position and angle.

Superficial Lesion

The problem here is that the needle flops against the skin and does not stay in line after positioning. If imaging is truly needed for localization, this can be a challenging situation. Ultrasound guidance may be the best option in this situation. If CT or fluoroscopy is used, it is helpful to use the shortest needle available (e.g., 5 cm), and park the sheath at the lesion, acquiring samples via coaxial technique (Fig. 1). If the small sheath does not stay in place, a small needle (e.g., 22 g, 1.5 inch) can be localized at the margin of the lesion by imaging, and the orientation of this needle can be used as a guide for the biopsy needle orientation. If the lesion is large enough, a coaxial technique may not be needed at all, and a simple biopsy needle can be passed repeatedly into the lesion and samples collected through the same skin site.

Rib Lesion

Rib lesions can be challenging to biopsy. The bone is small and rounded, and needles can "slip" off with pleura and lung underneath. Additionally, the ribs pass obliquely through the axial plane, making them hard to localize on CT, especially with breathing motion. Fluoroscopy can be difficult as well; a C-arm can be used to triangulate the needle tip relative to the lesion, but this technique requires some experience. If the lesion can be seen by ultrasound, this may be useful. Computed tomography is commonly used by musculoskeletal radiologists, because the pleural margin is most easily seen. Two popular approaches are directly perpendicular and tangential to the rib (Fig. 2). The tangential approach is useful to avoid the pleura but it may be more difficult to acquire a core sample. Depending

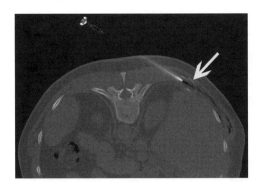

FIGURE 2 Tangential approach to rib biopsy. A 64-year-old male presented with posterior chest wall pain. Biopsy of this lesion revealed metastatic carcinoma from a primary lung carcinoma. An axial image from a biopsy of the right tenth rib shows the lytic lesion in the posterior rib (*arrow*), with the biopsy needle placed via a tangential approach.

on the location, there may be limited choice. Rib lesions under the scapula, to a certain extent, can be uncovered by changing arm position. Rib lesions present different problems in thin people (superficial location) versus obese people (deep location). In thin people, it can be tough to keep the sheath in place between sampling and scanning. As mentioned earlier, it may be helpful to place a small needle at the lesion for orientation which will remain in place better. In obese people, it can be difficult to place the needle on the rib, confident the pleural margin has not been transgressed. Measuring the depth of the pleura from the skin using the desired approach is essential, with the needle marker or block placed to prevent entry to this depth. Computed tomographic fluoroscopy can be very useful for rapid checks of needle-tip position. For CT, breath-holding during scanning can be detrimental, as the degree of inspiration varies, especially with conscious sedation, and this can move the rib out of the scanned field. It is often better to have the patient just breathe shallow and naturally.

Lesion Near Vital Structures
For lesions near vital structures (Fig. 3), careful planning of the approach is essential. Use of a smaller gauge needle is prudent. Frequent checks using the guidance modality are recommended. If a soft-tissue gun is used, the "manual throw" setting is the best; instead of the needle shooting out of the sheath, the manual throw setting allows the user to slowly push the needle out manually as far as desired. The sheath is triggered, which shoots over the needle cutting the sample. The needle tip advances no farther than manually placed.

Deep Soft-Tissue Lesion
For deep soft-tissue lesions (Fig. 4), a soft-tissue gun is generally used, and a coaxial system is essential; the outer sheath is placed at the margin of the lesion, and multiple samples can be acquired.

Deep, Small Lesion in Bone
A lesion deep within bone (Fig. 5) presents a special challenge. A coaxial system is essential, again, to allow acquisition of multiple samples through the same sheath.

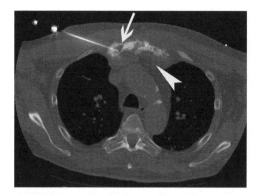

FIGURE 3 Lesion near vital structures. A 78-year-old male with osteomyelitis of the sternum (*arrow*) and a retrosternal mass (*arrowhead*). Note the close proximity of the great vessels to the area of interest. In this case, a steep oblique approach with a 20-gauge biopsy needle was used to avoid vascular injury.

However, most sheaths cannot be advanced into bone, but rather are "parked" at the outer margin of the bone, with the cutting needle placed into the lesion. With many coaxial systems, the cutting needle cannot pass a long way through the sheath, making it difficult to reach the lesion through the sheath. The radiologist must make sure the cutting needle is long enough to access the lesion with the system used. An alternative to this is the Bonopty drill system, in which an eccentric drill makes a channel larger than the sheath, allowing advancement of the sheath into bone, facilitating access of deep lesions.

Spine Lesions—Approaches
Transpedicular Approach
The transpedicular approach (Fig. 6) is very useful for lesions in the anterior vertebral body. Using this route, the radicular nerves, major blood vessels, and the

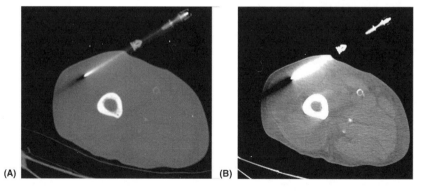

FIGURE 4 Deep soft-tissue lesion. This 68-year-old female with insulin-dependant diabetes mellitus presented with thigh pain. Biopsy showed diabetic myonecrosis. (**A**) Axial computed tomography (CT) image (bone windows) from deep soft-tissue biopsy of the thigh shows coaxial biopsy device in position. (**B**) Same axial CT image as (A) on soft-tissue windows. The low density changes and edema of diabetic myonecrosis in the quadriceps muscle can be seen.

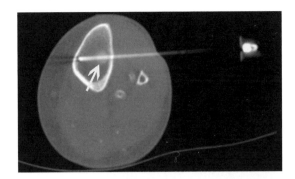

FIGURE 5 Deep, small lesion in bone. This 48-year-old female with a history of breast carcinoma presented with an incidental finding of a sclerotic lesion in the mid tibia (*arrow*). Biopsy proved this lesion to be a small bone island. Axial computed tomography (CT) image shows the coaxial biopsy device in position. A drill was used to access this deep tibial lesion.

spinal canal are avoided, Additionally, the walls of the pedicle, tangential to the needle course, tend to keep the needle/stylet on track, with the medullary cavity being the path of least resistance to needle advancement. The disadvantage is that the needle can be difficult to guide toward the lesion once in the pedicle, and unless the lesion is lined up with the pedicle, a different approach may be needed. A beveled stylet can be useful for guiding the needle once in bone. Another disadvantage is that the needle passes close to the walls of the pedicle, and if the wall is transgressed, there is a high risk of complication involving the spinal canal (medial wall) or neural foramen (superior or inferior wall). Whether CT or fluoroscopy is used, the walls of the pedicle must not be transgressed. This gets harder to accomplish the higher in the spine it is attempted, as the pedicle size diminishes significantly above the midthoracic region. In addition, in patients with kyphosis and osteoporosis, it can be difficult to visualize the upper thoracic pedicles.

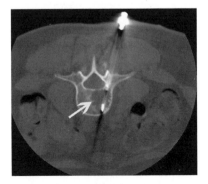

FIGURE 6 Transpedicular approach for spinal lesions using computed tomography (CT) guidance. This 60-year-old female with a history of breast carcinoma presented with back pain. Workup showed a lytic lesion in the L4 vertebral body (*arrow*), which proved to be a metastatic deposit. Axial CT image from transpedicuar biopsy shows the transpedicular approach used and the biopsy device traversing the lesion.

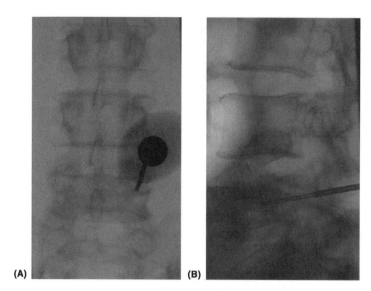

(A)   (B)

FIGURE 7 Transpedicular approach for spinal lesions using fluoroscopy. A 67-year-old male presented with back pain; imaging showed a pathological fracture of the L5 vertebral body. Biopsy revealed metastatic adenocarcinoma from a primary lung carcinoma. (**A**) Anteroposterior (AP) fluoroscopic image from L5 transpedicular biopsy shows placement of a transpedicular biopsy needle at L5 on the left. (**B**) Lateral fluoroscopic image from L5 transpedicular biopsy shows the biopsy needle tip to be in the mid L5 vertebral body.

Vertebroplasty Fluoroscopic Approach

Using fluoroscopy (Fig. 7), the vertebral body can be accessed using a transpedicle approach by means of a steep or shallow trajectory. For the steep trajectory, the vertebra is imaged in the anteroposterior (AP) plane, angled craniocaudally, so the pedicles come sharply into view. A slight degree of rotation can help visualize the pedicle on the side being accessed. The needle is advanced to the lateral margin of the pedicle, midway from top to bottom. The needle is advanced into the bone, and the correct orientation of the needle in craniocaudal direction is assessed on the lateral view. Back on the AP view, the needle is advanced further toward the center of the pedicle more medially. When the medial wall of the pedicle is approached, the lateral projection is again checked to make sure that the needle tip is at or beyond the posterior vertebral body margin. If so, the needle can be advanced into the vertebral body without the fear of traversing the spinal canal. However, if on the AP view, the tip of the needle is near the medial wall of the pedicle, and on the lateral view, it is not yet at the posterior vertebral body wall, the needle must be repositioned more laterally to avoid the canal.

Paravertebral Approach

The paravertebral approach (Fig. 8) is very straightforward. This can be started just lateral to the pedicle at the crux, or dip in the cortex between the facet joint and the pedicle. This location is excellent for achieving needle "purchase" into bone. From this location, the needle enters the lateral pedicle and then into the vertebral body. The needle can alternatively be started lateral to the facet joint, avoiding bone altogether until the posterolateral margin of the vertebral body is reached. This approach makes it easier to guide the needle toward a focal lesion in the vertebral

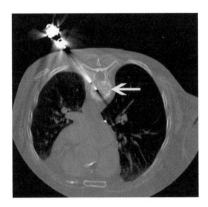

FIGURE 8 Paravertebral approach for spinal lesions. A 60-year-old male presented with back pain, and sclerotic replacement of the T9 vertebral body was noted (*arrow*). Axial computed tomography (CT) image shows Bonopty coaxial biopsy device placed via a paravertebral approach.

body, as less bone must be passed to get to the lesion. However, this approach is only feasible when there is enough paraspinal soft tissue to accommodate the needle track. In the thoracic spine, the pleural margin may prevent this approach. Some authors have reported injecting saline or air into the paraspinal soft tissues to push the pleural surface away from the needle tip.

Discographic Approach
When using fluoroscopy, the discographic approach is an excellent way to access intervertebral discs for aspiration. With the patient in prone position, the image intensifier is obliqued so that the superior articular process is near the junction of the middle and posterior thirds of the vertebral body at the level to be aspirated. Subsequently, the image intensifier is angled craniocaudally to make the disc tangential to the beam. The needle is passed straight down the beam just anterior to the superior articular process, into the center of the disc. This approach is quite straightforward in the lumbar spine, except that it may be difficult at L5-S1. Some individuals have a low L5-S1 junction, and during rotation and angulation of the image intensifier to the appropriate position, the iliac crest overlies the disc. In this case, the beam is progressively rotated to a steeper approach until a small triangle appears, bounded by the iliac bone, the superior articular process and the inferior L5 endplate. In the thoracic spine, a similar approach can be used, but the ribs and pleural margin must also be avoided.

Cervical spine
In the cervical spine, the posterior elements can be accessed using an oblique posterior approach under CT. The vertebral bodies can be difficult to access using a posterior or lateral approach, as there is little space in the soft tissues without important blood vessels or nerves. Pedicles are usually too small to use as a needle guide. The anterior approach is limited by the trachea in addition to vessels and nerves. Computed tomography is very useful for these biopsies, as the major structures can be seen. An intravenous contrast bolus can be used to delineate the major vessels prior to biopsy, but this is usually not needed. The route is determined by the location of the lesion relative to overlying structures.

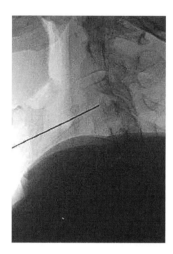

FIGURE 9   Anterior discographic approach in the cervical spine. A 49-year-old female presented with pyrexia of unknown origin. A magnetic resonance imaging (MRI) of the cervical spine (not shown) showed features suspicious for discitis/osteomyelitis at the C3/C4 level. This lateral fluoroscopic image shows placement of an aspiration needle into the C3/C4 disc space via an anterior cervical approach.

An anterior approach has been described, and is similar to the technique used for placing needles into the discs for cervical discography (Fig. 9). The carotid is palpated with the tips of the fingers of one hand, whereas the needle is held in the other. Using gentle pressure, the carotid is deflected laterally, and the needle placed just medial to it, lateral to the trachea. The thyroid may be transgressed, but this is not usually problematic and often cannot be avoided. Obviously, a coaxial needle is necessary and a small gauge needle is recommended.

Thick bone
Biopsy of a thick bone (e.g., femur) requires a coaxial system, as it often takes multiple passes at the same point to traverse the cortex into the medullary cavity (Fig. 10). A needle with serrated tip (such as the Cook Ackermann or Elson) can be helpful, as can the Radi Bonopty drill system.

Small bone
The biopsy of a small bone (e.g., toe) which is superficially located may not require a coaxial system; often the approach is fairly obvious through the same skin entry site, and initial fluoroscopic verification of needle position may be all that is needed, followed by multiple passes along the same approach. A short needle is usually desirable in this situation, because it is easier to control and position (Fig. 11).

Disc Aspiration/Biopsy
Disc aspiration (Figs. 9, 12, 13) is performed for infection. However, for aspiration alone, the yield of Gram stain/culture is quite low, in the order of 20% to 50%. If the patient is already on antibiotics, this figure drops even lower. A trial period of 48 hours off antibiotics may be used if the patient is stable enough, in order to increase yield. Similar to joint aspiration, if no fluid can be aspirated, a few cubic centimeters

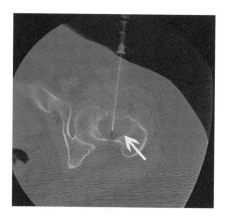

FIGURE 10 Percutaneous biopsy of a large bone. A 55-year-old man with a known history of renal carcinoma presented with left hip pain. Computed tomography (CT) showed a large lytic lesion in the left femoral neck (*arrow*), which proved to be a focus of metastatic disease. This axial CT image shows the coaxial biopsy device in good position within the lytic lesion of the left femoral neck.

of sterile saline can be injected and reaspirated immediately. This is a common practice, but it is unclear whether it is effective; in addition, similar to septic arthritis, a dry tap of a disc may imply lack of infection. To assure that the fluid present will be aspirated, a larger gauge needle (at least 18 G) must be used. The infected fluid is often very viscous, and may not be able to be drawn through smaller needles. Because of the low yield of aspiration alone, most authors advocate acquiring samples of the area of signal abnormality in the endplate as well. To accomplish this, it is useful to use a bone biopsy needle and a paravertebral approach (by

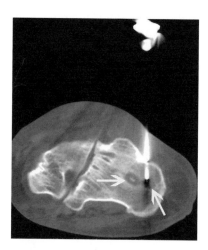

FIGURE 11 Percutaneous biopsy of a small bone. This 42-year-old male had a long history of diabetes mellitus, and presented with a heel ulcer and suspected osteomyelitis of the calcaneus. This axial computed tomography (CT) image shows the foot placed in the lateral position with perpendicular placement of the biopsy device. Note the abnormal areas of permeative bony destruction within the calcaneus (*arrows*). This biopsy confirmed osteomyelitis of the calcaneus.

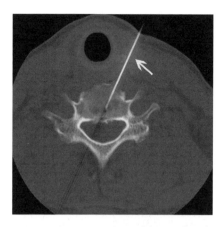

FIGURE 12   Anterior discographic approach in the cervical region. This 54-year-old lady presented with neck pain and had imaging features suggestive of discitis at the C5/C6 level. The axial computed tomography (CT) image shows placement of the aspiration needle via an anterior approach (anterior discographic approach). The needle is seen to traverse the left lobe of the thyroid gland (*arrow*). Aspiration failed to show evidence of infectious discitis.

CT, described earlier) or a discography approach (by fluoroscopy). Advantages of fluoroscopy are: (*i*) imaging to check needle position is performed more quickly; (*ii*) the plane can be more easily tilted parallel to the disc, especially useful at L5-S1; (*iii*) the needle can be observed in real time, as it is deflected toward the endplate for bone biopsy. The pleural margin is seen easily using both techniques.

Biopsying a primary tumor
Primary tumors of bone or soft tissue may require definitive surgery by a specialized bone tumor surgeon. If amputation or limb-salvage surgery is required, they may need adjacent tissue for a myocutaneous flap, covering the resected area or

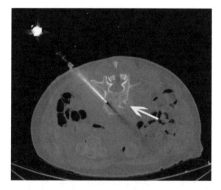

FIGURE 13   A 42-year-old male intravenous drug abuser presented with lower back pain. Imaging revealed fluid in the L3/L4 disc space with features suggestive of osteomyelitis. A computed tomography (CT)-guided biopsy was performed, which confirmed discitis. This axial CT image shows the destructive end plate changes at L3/L4 (*arrow*). In this case, a paravertebral approach was used for access.

stump. If the passage of the biopsy needle traverses this adjacent tissue, it may be considered contaminated and necessitate a more extensive surgical procedure. Therefore, it is essential for the radiologist to discuss the intended approach to a presumed primary lesion with the surgeon who would perform the definitive surgery. Often the agreed-upon approach is more technically difficult than the direct approach through the myocutaneous flap tissue.

Biopsy-assist devices
Some institutions have developed tracking software linked to preprocedure imaging which establishes fiducial markers and allows dynamic localization without frequent rescanning. These systems are predominantly used for placement of screws, but in the future may be available commercially for biopsy procedures. The SeeStar (Radi, Uppsala, Sweden) is an external guide that holds the needle in position outside the patient (preventing deflection of the needle when let go during scanning), making it very useful for biopsy of superficial lesions or for biopsy of lesions using a horizontal approach. In addition, the metallic needle guide creates a dark, linear artifact on CT images, which can be aligned to the lesion, facilitating the approach prior to needle placement.

Percutaneous needle localization
Occasionally, a lesion is in a dangerous location, or there is a lesion in the soft tissues that is hard or calcified, and a core biopsy is difficult or inadvisable. Other situations occur in which the patient is scheduled for an open surgical biopsy, but the anatomy is distorted by scar tissue, or the lesion is small enough where it may be difficult to localize at surgery, preoperative localization may be preferred (21). This is accomplished by using a hookwire-type breast localization needle. The needle is placed (within the sheath) into or adjacent to the lesion using the guidance modality. The needle tip position is verified and the sheath is withdrawn. The hook deploys as it is unsheathed, holding the needle in position. The wire extending from the skin is coiled and steri-stripped against the sterilized skin, and is covered with a sterile gauze cover. A final scan is acquired and printed for the surgeon to use for planning in the operating room.

SEDATION/MONITORING

The choice of local anesthetic only versus conscious sedation versus monitored anesthesia care (MAC) depends on a number of factors, including location of the biopsy, inherent level of sensation (e.g., diabetic neuropathy or paraplegia), cardiopulmonary status, ability to cooperate, and patient pain tolerance, among other things. For most musculoskeletal biopsies, conscious sedation is used, with a combination of versed and fentanyl. In the event of oversedation, versed can be reversed, and fentanyl is short acting. Monitoring patients is important to assess for oxygenation and heart rate and rhythm.

REFERENCES

1. Kelekis AD, Somon T, Yilmaz H, et al. Interventional spine procedures. Eur J Radiol 2005; 55(3):362–383.
2. Geremia G, Joglekar S. Percutaneous needle biopsy of the spine. Neuroimaging Clin N Am 2000; 10(3):503–533.

3. Jelinek JS, Murphey MD, Welker JA, et al. Diagnosis of primary bone tumors with image-guided percutaneous biopsy: experience with 110 tumors. Radiology 2002; 223(3): 731–737.
4. Vieillard MH, Boutry N, Chastanet P, Duquesnoy B, Cotten A, Cortet B. Contribution of percutaneous biopsy to the definite diagnosis in patients with suspected bone tumor. Joint Bone Spine 2005; 72(1):53–60.
5. Ahrar K, Himmerich JU, Herzog CE, et al. Percutaneous ultrasound-guided biopsy in the definitive diagnosis of osteosarcoma. J Vasc Interv Radiol 2004; 15(11):1329–1333.
6. Hadjipavlou AG, Kontakis GM, Gaitanis JN, Katonis PG, Lander P, Crow WN. Effectiveness and pitfalls of percutaneous transpedicle biopsy of the spine. Clin Orthop Relat Res 2003; (411):54–60.
7. Moller S, Kothe R, Wiesner L, Werner M, Ruther W, Delling G. Fluoroscopy-guided transpedicular trocar biopsy of the spine—results, review, and technical notes. Acta Orthop Belg 2001; 67(5):488–499.
8. Mathis JM, Wong W. Percutaneous vertebroplasty: technical considerations. J Vasc Interv Radiol 2003; 14(8):953–960.
9. Gangi A, Guth S, Imbert JP, Marin H, Dietemann JL. Percutaneous vertebroplasty: indications, technique, and results. Radiographics 2003; 23(2):e10.
10. Liu JC, Chiou HJ, Chen WM, et al. Sonographically guided core needle biopsy of soft tissue neoplasms. J Clin Ultrasound 2004; 32(6):294–298.
11. Gil-Sanchez S, Marco-Domenech SF, Irurzun-Lopez J, Fernandez-Garcia P, de la Iglesia-Cardena P, Ambit-Capdevila S. Ultrasound-guided skeletal biopsies. Skeletal Radiol 2001; 30(11):615–619.
12. Saifuddin A, Mitchell R, Burnett SJ, Sandison A, Pringle JA. Ultrasound-guided needle biopsy of primary bone tumours. J Bone Joint Surg [Br] 2000; 82(1):50–54.
13. Sequeiros RB, Ojala R, Kariniemi J, et al. MR-guided interventional procedures: a review. Acta Radiol 2005; 46(6):576–586.
14. Blanco Sequeiros R, Carrino JA. Musculoskeletal interventional MR imaging. Magn Reson Imaging Clin N Am 2005; 13(3):519–532.
15. Schweitzer ME, Gannon FH, Deely DM, O'Hara BJ, Juneja V. Percutaneous skeletal aspiration and core biopsy: complementary techniques. AJR 1996; 166(2):415–418.
16. White LM, Schweitzer ME, Deely DM. Coaxial percutaneous needle biopsy of osteolytic lesions with intact cortical bone. AJR 1996; 166(1):143–144.
17. Schweitzer ME, Deely DM. Percutaneous biopsy of osteolytic lesions: use of a biopsy gun. Radiology 1993; 189(2):615–616.
18. White LM, Schweitzer ME, Deely DM, Gannon F. Study of osteomyelitis: utility of combined histologic and microbiologic evaluation of percutaneous biopsy samples. Radiology 1995; 197(3):840–842.
19. Schweitzer ME, Deely DM, Beavis K, Gannon F. Does the use of lidocaine affect the culture of percutaneous bone biopsy specimens obtained to diagnose osteomyelitis? An in vitro and in vivo study. AJR 1995; 164(5):1201–1203.
20. Roberts CC, Morrison WB, Leslie KO, Carrino JA, Lozevski JL, Liu PT. Assessment of bone biopsy needles for sample size, specimen quality and ease of use. Skelet Radiol 2005; 34(6):329–335.
21. Morrison WB, Sanders TG, Parsons TW, Penrod BJ. Preoperative CT-guided hookwire needle localization of musculoskeletal lesions. AJR 2001; 176(6):1531–1533.

10

Image-Guided Thermoablation: Applications in the Musculoskeletal System

Carmine A. Grieco and Damian E. Dupuy

Department of Diagnostic Imaging, Brown University Medical School,
Rhode Island Hospital, Providence, Rhode Island, U.S.A.

INTRODUCTION

The advances in image-guided thermoablation continue to expand the treatment options for many oncology patients, reflecting the growing trend toward minimally invasive cancer therapy. Having established its efficacy for the treatment of benign osteoid osteomas, radiofrequency ablation (RFA) has become an increasingly recognized and applied alternative for malignancies affecting the musculoskeletal system. Although vastly different in terms of prognosis and therapeutic aims, the benign and malignant skeletal tumors have in common the potential for causing severe, debilitating pain throughout their course. For the typical patient diagnosed with osteoid osteoma, it is the impact of this pain on an often active, normal level of functioning that prompts early referral. For patients experiencing the pain of bone metastases, effective and durable symptom relief is similarly urgent, but in the setting of an often terminal disease. Together, these tumors represent a disease spectrum where the efficacious, minimally invasive therapy offered by thermoablation may provide the best outcomes, for local cure and palliation alike. This chapter offers a brief introduction to the percutaneous image-guided thermoablation techniques that are currently being applied within the musculoskeletal system. Radiofrequency ablation and its related modalities, including microwave ablation (MWA) and cryoablation, are discussed individually, and in the context of the traditional therapies with which they are increasingly being integrated.

BENIGN BONE TUMORS—BACKGROUND AND TRADITIONAL THERAPY

Osteomas, including osteoid osteomas and osteoblastomas, are the second most common matrix-producing tumors of bone, following the chondromas (1). First characterized in 1935 (2), osteoid osteomas account for 5% of all primary bone tumors (3) (10–12% of benign bone tumors) (3,4), being diagnosed before 25 years of age in 75% of cases (5), and showing at least a 2:1 male predominance (3). Arising within the cortex of the tibial or femoral diaphysis in over 50% of cases (6), they are also found in the intramedullary and subperiosteal zones. Although differentiated from the osteoblastomas by their smaller size (generally less than 1.5 cm) (5) and predilection for the appendicular skeleton, at least 10% of osteoid osteomas are known to occur in the spine (7,8). The severe, nocturnally worsening pain shows an often dramatic response to cyclo-oxygenase blockade, reflecting the pathophysiological role of prostaglandins elaborated by the tumor cells (9,10). Although the exceedingly low malignant potential (11) and reasonably frequent resolution over time (12) argue for an initial trial of salicylates alone, patient concerns (6,13,14) and the appearance of location-related sequelae in skeletally immature patients (4,15–18) often necessitate earlier, definitive treatment.

Surgical resection has been the standard for osteoid osteoma, since its earliest descriptions (4). Predictably, success rests on the removal of the true focus of neoplastic osteoblasts or "nidus," which can be substantially more difficult to identify grossly than the dense, reactive bone surrounding it (13,19,20). Although recurrence following pathologically confirmed removal has been reported (21,22), higher rates of recurrence, or persistence more appropriately, have been shown in series where the nidus was not identified after resection and where preoperative or intraoperative localization was not possible (16,21). Given their cortical and potentially periarticular location, the generous en bloc resection or curettage supported by these data can result in significant morbidity. More than 50% of tumors arise within the femoral head and neck in some series, increasing the risk for insufficiency, avascular necrosis, and fracture postoperatively, as a result of the cortical osteotomies and periosteal disruption (4,13,14,23).

Intraprocedural, rather than pathological localization of the nidus initially focused on preoperative labeling, using agents, such as tetracycline (24,25) and 99-Technetium (24,26), to guide resection via UV-fluorescence and intraoperative scintigraphy, respectively. These methods were gradually replaced by the range of techniques enabled by computed tomography (CT) guidance (4). Guide-wire placement prior to open resection (27), arthroscopic removal (28), and percutaneous removal using biopsy techniques (29,30,31) or drilling (32,33) were each facilitated by preprocedural or intraprocedural CT, with varied results. Localization of the nidus improved, but the size of the resulting bone defects and the associated risk of complications both remained substantial (4,29–31). Among the more recent minimally invasive interventions to have emerged, including laser interstitial thermal therapy (LITT) (34,35), magnetic resonance imaging (MRI)-guided cryoablation (36), and the augmentation of drilling techniques with percutaneous ethanol instillation (PEI) (37), RFA remains one of the most effective, well-tolerated, and best-studied technique.

HISTORY OF THERMOABLATION

The seminal concept of thermoablation, that of killing tumor cells in situ using heat, can be traced back to Hippocrates' teachings regarding alternatives to surgery (38). Controlled thermal injury first came into widespread use in modern medicine with the implementation of Bovie's electrocoagulation device in the late 1920s (39). Similar electrodes capable of thermal ablation, powered by alternating current with frequencies in the range of radiowaves (460–480 kHz) were developed in the 1950s (40). Initially used in the treatment of pain syndromes (41,42), RFA was also studied and successfully applied in place of direct current shock for the ablation of arrhythmogenic cardiac foci (43). Following early studies of its effects in porcine hepatic tissue (44,45), Tillotson et al. (46) characterized the in vivo results of RFA in canine bone, with respect to size, zonal consistency, and the expected course of healing of the thermally induced lesions. These findings within normal tissues, together with the steadily improving guidance afforded by real-time CT and ultrasound (US) imaging, heightened the growing interest in minimally invasive alternatives for what were traditionally surgical pathologies. Rosenthal et al. (47) were the first to treat osteoid osteomas using percutaneous image-guided RFA in 1992. The observed symptom resolution, achieved after a single treatment in three of their four patients, represented the first report of the successful and continually expanding applications of thermoablation in the musculoskeletal system.

RADIOFREQUENCY ABLATION: UNDERLYING PHYSICS

The independent variable affecting tumor cell death, for any thermoablation modality, is temperature (48). The bulk of the improvements in RFA technology and the challenges to its implementation have related to the effective delivery of cytotoxic heat. The threshold temperature for coagulative necrosis, which varies by tissue (48), has been defined as 50°C, sustained for 30 seconds, for osteocytes (46). The standard RFA electrode is composed of an insulated shaft, typically 21-14 gauge, and an exposed tip that is advanced into the substance of the tumor under image guidance. The radiofrequency (RF) power source is connected to this electrode and to one or more grounding pads on the patient's body. Applying alternating current sets up a circuit of ionic collisions within the surrounding tissue, causing friction and generating resistive heat (40,48). As active heat deposition decreases by a power of four with distance from the active tip, thermal conduction is essential for heating beyond this narrow zone (40). The volume of necrosis achievable by these electrodes was initially quite limited, approximately 1.6 cm at maximum (49), and with its roughly cylindrical shape, was not optimally suited for the irregular geometry of solid tumors (48,50).

Various modifications have increased the volume of thermal necrosis achievable by RF electrodes. Heat deposition has been intensified directly through the use of generators of higher power (48,51), and pulsed energy delivery (52). Although seemingly beneficial, maximal heating around the active tip can have a paradoxically restrictive effect on the diameter of the ablation zone. Sustained temperatures above 100°C cause tissue carbonization or "charring," resulting in an abrupt increase in impedance that limits additional energy deposition (49). Tissue boiling and vaporization also occur at these temperatures, producing gases that insulate the electrode and interfere with conduction. Electrodes cooled by continuous internal perfusion, designed to maintain treatment temperatures between 50°C and 100°C, have produced reliably larger volumes of coagulative necrosis (53). The size and geometry of the ablation zone have been improved further through the use of larger monopolar electrodes, electrodes with multiple deployable tines or cluster arrays, and bipolar arrays involving a nearby second electrode functioning as the ground (48). Ablation zones of approximately 5 cm using a single internally cooled electrode (54), and up to 7 cm using an internally cooled cluster probe with 0.5-cm interelectrode spacing, can be achieved (Fig. 1) (55).

Despite these advances, the periphery of the ablated volume remains vulnerable to inadequate heat deposition. Adapting the bioheat transfer equation for thermoablation points out that the diameter of necrosis achieved is dependent not only on the thermal energy delivered, but on its interactions with the properties of the tissue being heated (51). Inadequate heating owing to the convective "heat-sink" effects of nearby vessels, in addition to premature cooling owing to conductive losses, are most problematic in highly vascular organs, namely the kidney and liver (48,50). Insulation, caused by variable densities of stromal fat or interdigitating air-filled compartments, can limit the consistency of energy deposition throughout breast and lung lesions, respectively (48,50). These same factors may act beneficially to shield ablation zones from heat-sink losses, however, termed the "oven effect" in

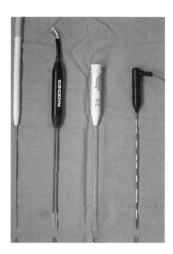

FIGURE 1   (**A**) Different thermoablation systems are currently available to clinicians in the United States. An argon-based cryoablation system with 1.7 to 2.4-mm cryoapplicators is used at the authors' institution (Endocare; Irvine, California, U.S.A.). (**B**) Multiple types of RFA electrodes have been used clinically, as detailed in the text, including those with internally cooled cluster arrays (Radionics/Valley Lab; Boulder, Colorado, U.S.A.) and (**C**) with multiple deployable tines (Boston Scientific; Boston, Massachusetts, U.S.A.). There is currently one FDA-approved system for MWA, the Vivawave system (**D**, Vivant Medical Inc; Mountain View, California, U.S.A.). *Abbreviations*: FDA, Food and Drug Administration; MWA, microwave ablation; RFA, radiofrequency ablation.

studies of RFA within areas of cirrhotic liver (56). Decreases in blood flow through the ablation zone by surgical (57–59) and pharmacological (60) means have resulted in larger and more homogenously treated RF lesions in hepatic tissue, with the drawbacks of a more invasive and dangerous procedure. Regardless of the site or sophistication of the RFA system used, intratumoral temperature monitoring provides an important gauge for assessing the adequacy of cytotoxic heating.

Bone is a unique medium for RFA, in the way of conduction properties and procedural approach, related to its structure. Bone is subject to perfusion-mediated heat dissipation via blood flow within the medullary canal, analogous to normal liver and kidney, but may also demonstrate insulative properties owing to decreased heat transmission across its substance (61), as encountered in healthy lung and fibrotic liver tissue (48,49,56). By virtue of their small size (5), osteoid osteomas are treated quite effectively within approximately 1.6 cm of thermal necrosis (49) produced by single conventional (i.e., noninternally cooled) RFA electrodes. The use of these monopolar probes has continually met with success for the treatment of osteoid osteomas, and remains the standard practice at most centers (4).

RADIOFREQUENCY ABLATION OF OSTEOID OSTEOMAS: PROCEDURE AND CLINICAL RESULTS

Minor variations exist between institutions and clinicians regarding the logistics of the RFA procedure. Percutaneous thermoablations are performed in the main radiology department at the authors' institution after medical clearance and at least one week's cessation of anti-inflammatory medications to avoid bleeding sequelae.

Conscious sedation with agents, such as midazolam and fentanyl, is the preferred mode of anesthesia. General endotracheal or laryngeal mask anesthesia is reserved for pediatric populations or patients who need deeper anesthesia for pain control during ablative therapy. Following localization of the tumor by CT, the skin is sterilely prepared over the site felt to offer the most direct and perpendicular approach that can safely avoid critical structures. Image-guided access to the nidus is initially obtained using a trephine-type biopsy needle, the outer cannula of which is then used to pass the 5- to 10-mm active tip of the electrode (4). A typical treatment lasts six minutes, with a target temperature of 90°C generally agreed upon (4,14,47,62). Additional treatments after repositioning are dictated by the size and shape of the tumor and by temperature readings.

Postprocedural pain, anecdotally reported as more severe in patients undergoing repeat RFA for recurrent symptoms (4), has been rated at 50% the severity of the pain prompting referral (14). Resolution of symptoms after a single RFA treatment has been reported in 90% to 100% of patients (62–64), falling to 60% of those being treated for pain recurrence after pervious RFA or open resection (Fig. 2) (65). At least 85% of patients would experience a substantial decrement in pain within the first three days following RFA, and importantly, equally substantial numbers will go on to report the desired improvement in function (14,64,66). Without concerns of significant bone weakening or of malignant transformation, follow-up imaging is not indicated in the absence of recurrent symptoms (4,50,62). In a retrospective study comparing the outcomes of surgical resection and RFA, Rosenthal et al. (13) found the techniques to be equivalent, in terms of clinical success, for the osteoid osteomas treated. Although recurrence was slightly higher among those treated with RFA (12% vs. 9% treated with surgery), there were two complications requiring several additional operations in the surgical group, and an average postoperative stay of 4.7 days versus 0.18 days following RFA. In addition to clearly demonstrating its equivalent efficacy, these findings reiterated the safety advantages and rapid convalescence offered by this minimally invasive alternative.

SAFETY CONSIDERATIONS

Most osteoid osteomas of the extremities are effectively and safely treated with RFA. Their occurrence within the vertebrae in roughly 10% of cases; however, often within the posterior elements, they present several unique challenges. Apart from the low but finite risk of bleeding, infection, and burns from improper grounding pad placement at any treatment site (48,50,67), RFA performed in the vicinity of critical structures risks serious iatrogenic injury (48,68). The spinal cord and nerves are especially susceptible to thermal damage, as might be encountered during RFA of a mass arising within the adjacent vertebral body or arch. Sustained temperatures above 45°C are known to cause irreversible injury to the cord and associated structures (69,70) and to peripheral nerves (71).

Following a report that the substance of the intervertebral disc could act as a heat buffer for nearby spinal nerves (72), Dupuy et al. (61) sought to investigate the vertebral bone itself for potential insulating capabilities. They demonstrated that intrathecal temperatures could remain subtoxic during RFA of a nearby vertebral body, despite using an internally cooled electrode at maximal power. The expansive plexus of epidural veins and the investing layer of cerebrospinal fluid (CSF) presenting unique features of this region were postulated to further supplement the

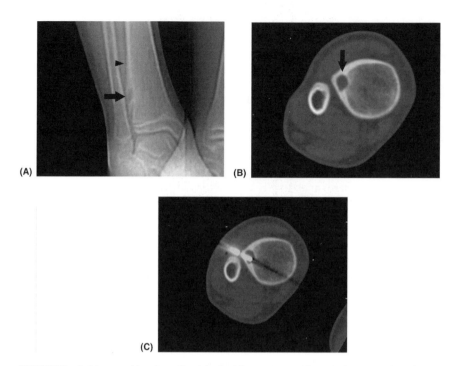

FIGURE 2 A 14-year-old male noticed the insidious onset and gradual progression of pain above his right ankle. There was no history of trauma. The pain worsened to the point that his gait became antalgic, and became less responsive to the aspirin that had previously been beneficial. He was evaluated by an orthopedic tumor specialist after plain radiographs revealed an abnormality within the right lower tibia suspicious for osteoid osteoma. The patient was referred for radiofrequency ablation. (**A**) A scout topogram of the right lower extremity shows a lucency within the cortex of the distal tibia (*arrow*) above the syndesmotic ligament, with mild periosteal reaction (*arrowhead*). (**B**) A transverse non–contrast-enhanced CT image demonstrates a lucent subcortical focus with sclerotic margins in the medial area of the distal tibia consistent with osteoid osteoma (*arrow*). Following the administration of general anesthesia, a core biopsy was performed using a 14-gauge Ackerman needle before advancement of the RFA electrode. (**C**) A transverse CT-fluoroscopy image shows placement of the RFA electrode's 1-cm active tip within the substance of the tumor (*arrow*). Two 6-minute treatments were given, each achieving a maximal temperature above 94°C, and averaging a power of 4.5 W, a current of 0.2 A, and a tissue impedance of 142 Ohms. The patient was discharged home on acetaminophen/codeine tablets. His right leg pain had effectively disappeared within 36 hours of treatment, and he remains pain free at two-month follow-up. *Abbreviations:* CT, computed tomography; RFA, radiofrequency ablation.

heat-sheltering capabilities of the intact bone. The clinical arm of this study involved RFA of an osteoid osteoma in the pedicle of T11, and of a lytic hemangio-pericytoma metastasis in a lumbar vertebral body, both of which resulted in durable pain resolution, without neurological injury (61). Importantly, the cortical bone posterior to the lumbar lesion was visibly intact in both cases. Sequelae including incomplete hemiplegia have been reported after similar procedures in which tumor had invaded the posterior cortex of the vertebral body (73).

These findings, together with additional clinical reports (64,74–77) and increasing experience with the control of ablation volumes in living bone (78)

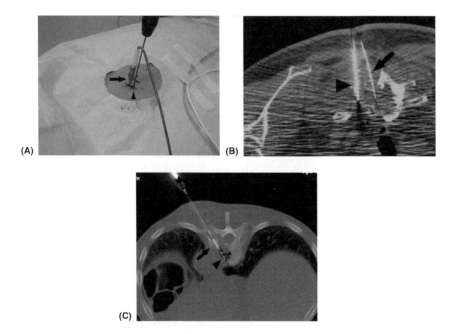

FIGURE 3 Thermoablation performed near critical structures places these structures at risk for injury. (**A**) Procedural photograph and (**B**) corresponding transverse CT-fluoroscopy image demonstrate RFA of a vertebral body metastasis from renal-cell carcinoma. Given the proximity of the electrode (*arrowhead*) to the spinal canal, an external thermocouple (*arrow*) was positioned to ensure adjacent temperatures remained below 50°C. The patient tolerated the procedure well, and had no signs or symptoms of nerve injury in the postprocedure period. (**C**) During the MWA treatment of a different patient with renal-cell carcinoma metastases, the antenna (*arrowhead*) is placed within a thoracic vertebral body at the same time as the thermocouple is directed toward the intervertebral foramen (*arrowhead*). *Abbreviations:* CT, computed tomography; RFA, radiofrequency ablation; MWA, microwave ablation.

have led to the conclusion that RFA can be performed safely when an intact layer of "shielding" bone separates the spinal canal from the electrode tip (50,61). Regardless of the sophistication of preprocedural planning and imaging, meticulous intraprocedural assessment remains essential. Intraprocedural temperature monitoring adjacent to neurovascular structures using a routine thermocouple (Fig. 3) (79) or the emerging technique of MR thermometry (80), and the titration of sedation, such that radicular symptoms can be reported, are of obvious importance.

SKELETAL METASTASES—BACKGROUND

Primary bone tumors are relatively rare (81). Bone's involvement by systemic cancer is far more common, made vulnerable by its rich vasculature and by the "seed in soil" effect of growth factors concentrated within its matrix (82,83). The skeleton is by far the most likely organ to be affected by metastases, of which more than 80% arise from a lung, breast, or prostatic primary (84,85). Skeletal metastases signify advanced disease, and almost uniformly, a prognosis where maximizing the quality of the patient's remaining time deserves priority over curative therapy. Appropriate care is directed at the expeditious relief of the most debilitating symptom, which in the vast majority of cases is intractable pain (85). Despite multidisciplinary advances, factors, such as inadequate pain assessment, communication failure, and concerns about regimen toxicity leave an estimated 50% to 70% of patients with uncontrolled pain owing to skeletal metastases (86,87).

MALIGNANT BONE PAIN: PHYSIOLOGY AND TRADITIONAL THERAPIES

In addition to the direct irritation and infiltration of afferent fibers, much of the severe pain of bone metastases is caused by microfractures and associated intrinsic motion within bone, destabilized by tumor-driven osteoclast activity (88,89). Pressure, owing to this mechanical distortion or to local hemorrhage caused by osteolysis, is a potent noxious stimulus to the periosteum, which possesses the highest density of pain fibers in the skeleton (90). Opioid analgesics, used ubiquitously and lacking many of the long-term complications of nonsteroidal anti-inflammatory drugs (NSAIDs), have shown efficacy and tolerability that are variable at best (86,91). Targeting nociception alone, their effects may become blunted by the "viscous cycle" of neural sensitization and altered neurotransmitter expression that distinguishes the pain state of bone cancer from those of inflammatory or neuropathic origins (92).

External-beam radiation therapy (XRT) is considered the standard for metastatic bone pain (87,93,94), exerting its effects through a direct decrease in tumor burden (88), and through a diminution of the inflammatory response potentiating pain (87,94,95). Generally reported as effective in 70% of cases (94), various reviews have specified that although up to 90% of patients will experience some degree of relief from palliative XRT, results approaching complete analgesia would be expected in only 40% to 60% (93,94,96). Apart from toxicity concerns, independent of benefit and often precluding retreatment, it is the potential delay of up to 12 weeks to attain maximal benefit that remains problematic (93). With pain relapse in 30% to 50% during this same period (88,96), and with the estimated survival often less than 24 weeks following the diagnosis of bone metastases (50,85), the intended result remains unattainable. In their comprehensive and widely acknowledged meta-analysis, Ratanatharathorn et al. (97) reported the treatment success, durability, and overall practices of palliative radiotherapy to be largely inadequate. Their summary finding that the "median duration of relief" was significantly shorter than the "median duration of survival" after treatment in the majority of cases is salient to the evaluation of any palliative therapy, used alone or in combination.

Hormonal- or chemotherapy-induced tumor regression can reduce the narcotic dose required, typically in the order of months, prior to the emergence of resistant clonogens (87). Adverse effects vary widely, any of which are amplified in the setting of a limited functional reserve. Bisphosphonates, now the standard for malignant hypercalcemia, act at multiple levels to inhibit osteoclastic bone resorption (95), the rate of which relates directly to the severity of bone pain (98). Having been shown to decrease the incidence of additional skeletal complications owing to metastases from multiple tumor types (95), they may also potentiate the effects of hormonal and chemotherapy in breast cancer (99). Radiopharmaceuticals, such as [89]strontium, are beneficial for widespread metastases, and lack a substantial portion of the marrow irradiation encountered with palliative XRT. They are generally not indicated for patients with one or a few painful bone lesions, however, and are contraindicated in patients with myelosuppression of any etiology or with a life expectancy less than three months (95). With benefits potentially delayed up to 12 weeks for any of these antineoplastic agents (86), a safe, effective treatment permitting rapid assessment of the desired results would have an indication independent of prognosis.

PALLIATIVE THERMOABLATION OF BONE METASTASES

Dupuy et al. (100) were the first to investigate the utility and potential analgesic benefits of RFA when applied to malignant rather than benign bone lesions. The 1998 study followed 16 patients who had undergone RFA to 18 bone metastases (1–8 cm in diameter), of various histologies and skeletal locations. Prior treatment failure had occurred with at least one traditional agent in each case, with patients rating their average day-to-day pain and worst pain at 6.5 and 8.5, respectively, by 10-point visual analog scale. Average pain ratings had fallen to 4.62 at one week ($P = 0.039$) and 4.64 at one month ($P = 0.036$). Worst pain ratings improved even further, to 6.93 ($P = 0.005$) and 5.64 ($P = 0.003$), at one week and one month, respectively, with the only adverse events referable to local inflammation, and for self-limited flu-like symptoms termed "postablation syndrome," lasting a few days after treatment. When grouped according to the preablation diameter and body region of the tumor, patients having tumors of small size and with chest wall involvement had significant relief (Fig. 4), whereas patients with larger tumors located in and around the pelvic bones did not.

Callstrom et al. (101) examined these benefits further in a group of 12 patients, each undergoing RFA to single analgesia-resistant bone metastasis (1–11 cm in diameter). Significant improvements in average and worst-pain ratings were observed at four weeks. There was also a significant reduction in perceived interference of pain with daily activities during this period, paralleling the reduction in disability reported by a group of patients who underwent RFA for painful vertebral metastases (75). The single reported complication (101) was a second-degree grounding pad burn, reiterating the importance of safety considerations, but adding to the data that such outcomes are infrequent. These early results provided an important foundation, but allowed relatively limited interpretation owing to short follow-up periods and varying study population characteristics.

Goetz et al. (76) performed a multi-institutional investigation to characterize the efficacy of RFA in further detail, for a larger number of patients who had failed or were otherwise poor candidates for standard therapy for bone metastases (1.4–18.0 cm in diameter). A total of 95% of the patients (43 of the 45 treated) experienced at least a 2-point decrease in reported pain from pre-RFA levels. Most importantly, the significance of the reported pain decrement was maintained at 12 and 24 weeks of follow-up. Complications included a burn of moderate severity at a grounding pad site, an episode of transient incontinence following RFA of a sacral lesion, and a pelvic insufficiency fracture following ablation of an acetabular metastasis. Despite the adverse events, the conclusions were a powerful argument for the effectiveness, durability, and overall safety of RFA for the palliation of painful osteolytic tumors. These data have been supported by additional positive results following RFA of painful osseous metastases, performed alone (Fig. 5) (102,103) or in conjunction with percutaneous osteoplasty (73,104), or followed by palliative surgery made feasible by the "debulking," accomplished via RFA (77).

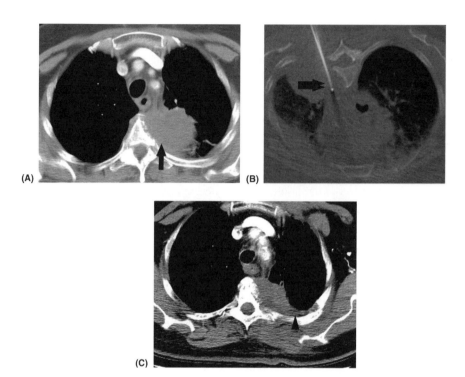

FIGURE 4   A 62-year-old female with advanced-stage adenocarcinoma of the left lung was referred for palliative thermoablation. Despite a positive intraparenchymal response to XRT and chemotherapy, the tumor went on to invade the adjacent thoracic vertebrae causing severe pain. (**A**) Transverse contrast-enhanced CT image through the thorax shows an ill-defined pleural mass eroding the body of the adjacent vertebral body (*arrow*). (**B**) Transverse CT-fluoroscopy image during the subsequent RFA procedure shows the electrode positioned within the mass (*arrow*). A total of three 4-minute treatments were given, with intratumoral temperatures exceeding 70°C in each case. Treatments averaged a current of 1.76 A, a power of 176 W, and a tissue impedance of 64 Ohms. The patient experienced dramatic relief of pain symptoms in the proceeding weeks. (**C**) Transverse contrast-enhanced CT image at 18 months post RFA shows the tumor mass to be without enhancement and regressing in size with nearby pleural thickening consistent with post-RFA changes (*arrowhead*). The patient remains pain-free and without any evidence of disease progression. *Abbreviations:* CT, computed tomography; RFA, radiofrequency ablation; XRT, external-beam radiation therapy.

PROCEDURAL OBJECTIVES: LOCALLY CURATIVE VERSUS PALLIATIVE

Compared with procedures having curative intention, palliative thermoablation has objectives that are similar at the level of the target lesion, but substantially different at the level of the patient being treated. These patients typically have a medical complexity that is markedly increased over those with osteoid osteoma that must factor into appropriate preprocedural clearance. In addition to being substantially larger than benign tumors in most cases, symptomatic metastases virtually always have some degree of involvement, if not frank invasion, of the surrounding soft tissues and neurovascular structures that must be carefully considered during treatment planning. The effects of metastases on the bony structures

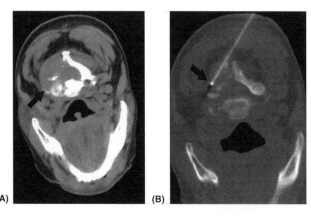

(A) (B)

FIGURE 5 A 66-year-old male with widely disseminated squamous cell lung carcinoma began to complain of increasingly severe pain and tenderness over the cervical spine accompanied by decreased range of motion. (**A**) A transverse noncontrast-enhanced CT image through the neck demonstrates an aggressive lytic mass invading the C2/C3 arch on the left side (arrow) (**B**) A CT-fluoroscopy image shows the RFA electrode advanced into the substance of the mass, through a posterior approach (*arrow*). One 2-minute and two 3-minute ablations were performed, with maximal temperatures between 58 and 68 dC. Measured parameters averaged a current of 0.90 A, a power of 66 W, and an impedance of 111 Ohms. The patient reported significant improvements in pain and range of motion after treatment. Despite rapidly progressing systemic disease, he remained without recurrence of neck symptoms prior to his death, approximately three months post RFA. *Abbreviations:* CT, computed tomography; RFA, radiofrequency ablation.

themselves are also important. Disruption of the cortex by lytic or mixed lytic blastic lesions may obviate the use of a biopsy device to gain access for the electrode. Although the approach may be simplified, such cortical discontinuity may significantly increase the risk of injury to local structures during thermoablation, owing to the loss of insulation, as detailed earlier (61,73). Curative and palliative thermoablation may vary the most with respect to the extent of thermal coagulation that is necessary. Complete tumor necrosis, mandatory for curative ablation, is obviously the ideal for cases of palliation as well. It is advocated that when size, irregularity, or proximity to neurovascular structures would make complete treatment of the metastasis dangerous, attention should be focused on areas judged to be responsible for the bulk of symptoms, such as the advancing margin or bone–soft-tissue interface (4,76,101).

Palliative thermoablation, a local therapy in the midst of systemic disease, is not performed with the expectation of increasing survival. It can be reasoned, however, that an improved level of activity, a decreased narcotic requirement, and an overall sense of improved status are far from trivial prognostic factors. Regardless, the degree of subjective improvement remains the sole measure of success in this setting. This success can be remarkable for even the latest stages of disease, as highlighted in the report of two patients who developed a reversible overuse neuropathy of the lower extremities after the dramatic analgesia obtained after RFA of pelvic metastases (103). It should be noted that the majority of patients described in the earlier studies were already facing severe therapy-resistant bone pain at the time of RFA. Treating earlier, less-advanced symptoms could yield an even higher rate of success, but has had virtually no study in this regard, owing to issues of availability and technical experience, and to current practice parameters emphasizing maximization of traditional therapy. A Phase I/II prospective trial currently underway through the American College of Radiology Imaging Network will examine analgesic responses following RFA of a single metastatic tumor, in patients with persistent bone pain. Analysis of the outcomes will provide a framework for further study of thermal ablation as a primary rather than delayed treatment alternative.

MICROWAVE ABLATION

Microwave ablation, one of the more recently studied thermoablation modalities, has identical principles but multiple mechanistic advantages over RFA. The high frequencies of microwaves, at or above 900 MHz (105), act on the permanent dipoles within a tissue's water molecules, causing rapid oscillation and the production of intense heat. Heat is actively generated throughout a field, rather than being focused immediately adjacent to the probe as with RFA. Thus, MWA is not dependent on conduction, and grounding pads are unnecessary. Microwave ablation achieves consistently higher intratumoral temperatures over larger volumes (106,107), in a shorter time (108). As a result, partially cystic and air-filled tumors are coagulated more reliably, as are tumors bordering large blood vessels, with heat-sink effects largely eliminated (107,108). Thus, temperatures need only be monitored, via external thermocouple, when the tumor mass is abutting critical neurovascular structures (Fig. 3C). Multiple antennae can be run simultaneously, when dictated by tumor size or geometry. Reports of successful hepatobiliary applications of MWA are accumulating (109–111), and its potential efficacy for pulmonary tumors is being investigated.

Clinical experience with MWA has been limited in general, particularly so for bone tumors. Although lacking formal study, it is unlikely that attempting to treat osteoid osteomas with MWA would improve on the predictable and largely favorable outcomes achieved using RFA. High rates of local control have been reported using intraoperative MWA for a variety of skeletal tumors, but were qualified by several postprocedure fractures (112). At our institution, several patients have undergone palliation of bone metastases using percutaneous MWA. One was an 84-year-old man with resistant pain in the region of T10 and L1 owing to metastases from renal cell carcinoma. He underwent uncomplicated MWA of both lesions, followed by vertebroplasty, and reported improved pain at two months post-treatment (Fig. 6). Another patient, aged 70 years, underwent successful MWA of a severely painful transitional-cell carcinoma metastasis to the acetabular rim. He remains pain- and complication free at 1.5 years of follow-up.

CRYOABLATION

Cryoablation, applied in various forms to many pathologies over the last century (113,114), has come into widespread use for the treatment of liver tumors (115). It was considered a strictly intraoperative modality in its earlier forms, given the large-caliber, incompletely insulated probes and the difficulty of controlling the liquid nitrogen being applied (116). Modern cryoablation generates thermal injury using the extreme cold of argon gas decompression, with cryoapplicators adapted for percutaneous use. Real-time visualization of the hypoechoic frozen region or "ice ball" (117) and reports of decreased procedural pain (118)

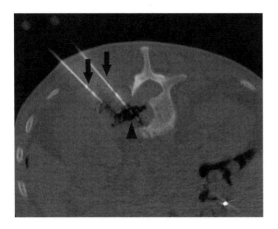

FIGURE 6 An 85-year-old male with known T11 and L2 metastases from renal cell carcinoma was referred for possible thermoablation after his back pain became intolerable, despite radiation therapy. A transverse CT-fluoroscopy image during MWA of the L2 lesion shows two of the three microwave antennae placed within the mass for simultaneous treatment (*arrows*). Gas is visible within the lesion (*arrowhead*), released by the vaporization of tissue during treatment. One 10-minute and one 4-minute MWA were performed, at 45 W of power. A single MWA antenna was advanced into the T11 lesion, and one 4-minute treatment was performed at 45 W (not shown). The antennae were then removed, and vertebroplasty was performed at both levels. Postprocedure plain film demonstrates appropriate placement of the cranioplast material at the T11 site (*arrow*). The patient experienced substantial pain relief and without vertebral sequelae. and remained pain free before succumbing to complications of systemic disease. *Abbreviations:* CT, computed tomography; MWA, microwave ablation.

are some of the noted advantages over RFA. In addition to frostbite injury and potential skin necrosis surrounding the treatment sites, serious complications have been reported at a higher frequency than with equivalent RFA procedures in hepatic tissue, including hemorrhage (116), infection (113), and rarely, death (113). These have not detracted from additional studies, however, and successful applications for liver (119), kidney (120), and lung neoplasms (121) continue to be reported.

Cryoablation, in the form of cryosurgery, has long been studied as a potentially curative therapy for various bone tumors. Usually performed after curettage or operative exposure, cryoablation has seen gradual improvements in safety profile and in the observed rates of success over time (122). After following a group of over 300 patients treated with cryosurgery for primary bone tumors, Dutch researchers concluded that combining cryosurgery with intralesional excision could yield local control outcomes equivalent to those of marginal excision for many tumors, including grade I chondrosarcoma (114). As with the other studies, the variability of the protocols and of the combinations with other percutaneous or open procedures prevents more than a cursory comparison between RFA and cryoablation procedures intended for cure. Recent studies noting the beneficial results of palliative cryoablation have included case reports (123) and an ongoing prospective trial following 14 patients after undergoing cryoablation for painful lytic metastases (124). Preliminary results have been positive, with a significant decrement in worst pain reported at one month postprocedure, and 50% of patients reporting complete disappearance of pain symptoms.

Of interest, in the setting of pain palliation, is the preservation of the connective tissue and myelin sheath of local sensory axons during the cryoablation process, as documented by postprocedure histology (125). To the analgesia and cytoreduction offered by RFA and MWA, cryoablation thus adds the potential for regeneration of sensory afferents following eradication, in theory, of the malignant stimulus. On the order of time of the typical patient's life expectancy with bone metastases, the latter effect may be inconsequential. In the case of patients with a small number of symptomatic lesions amid reasonably preserved health, however, there is the potential for remarkable benefit. As with the other thermal ablation procedures, skeletal cryoablation may be carried out in conjunction with biopsy, osteoplasty, or even operative stabilization (114,124), if the latter is supported by sufficiently low surgical risk and evidence of impending fracture that would negate the analgesia achieved.

ADDITIONAL THERMOABLATION MODALITIES

The additional thermoablation modalities have various advantages and shortcomings with respect to RFA, but have had very limited comparative study (113). Laser ablation, noted briefly earlier as an alternative for osteoid osteoma (34,35), maintains the minimally invasive nature of RFA, but offers precise control over the photo-coagulated area, allowing a finer delineation between tumor and normal tissue (126). The fine lesion size requires that multiple overlapping treatments be performed for larger tumors, which would add further to the inhomogeneity in heating caused by irregular vascularization, as experienced with RFA. Further, the equipment and procedures are costly, and have no proven benefits over RFA, as of yet (113). High-intensity focused US (127) is gaining momentum as another method for minimally invasive thermoablation, particularly since its integration with MR guidance, for breast and brain tumors, and for tumors arising within the pelvis (128). The utility of US waves capable of penetrating deep within tissues, guided by superior imaging, has raised interest in HIFU for several benign and malignant disease processes. To date, experience in the musculoskeletal system has been minimal, and its efficacy remains to be demonstrated (113).

COMBINED THERAPY

Thermoablation has typically been studied as one step or stage amid the sequence of traditional treatments for cancer, rather than as an isolated, prospectively investigated therapy. Given the unlikely event that a single modality will achieve a 100% cure rate, for any malignancy, interest has been growing in regard to the intentional combination of thermoablation with traditional modalities (48). The objective driving such investigations has been the achievement of synergistic results, without similarly compounded morbidity. Synergism between chemotherapy and thermoablation would be especially relevant to patients with late-stage disease, who may experience a greater benefit from palliative thermoablation of bone metastases when performed at a particular time during further systemic therapy. The benefits of combining chemotherapy (129,130) with controlled hyperthermia (42–45°C) have been previously reported, leading to studies substituting RFA as the source of potentially sensitizing thermal injury. Synergistically larger ablation volumes have been demonstrated by performing RFA within 30 minutes of intratumoral doxorubicin injection (131), or immediately following PEI in an animal tumor model (132). The postulated mechanisms relate to improved thermal conduction through chemically manipulated tissue. Percutaneous ethanol instillation has met with success, but limited the acceptance for the treatment of osteoid osteoma (37). Given the favorable outcomes of osteoid osteomas treated with RFA alone, PEI may prove more beneficial in combined therapy for the larger malignant lesions.

As with chemotherapy, radiation therapy has been increasingly studied in temporal and spatial combination with thermoablation, with proposed complimentarity based on tumor biology and tissue properties. One case study has reported achieving a larger RFA volume in liver tissue previously treated with XRT than in the nonirradiated area, in the same patient (133). More recently, synergistically increased rates of local control and survival were noted, in an animal tumor model, after combined treatment with XRT and RFA, over either modality alone (134). It is known that tumor oxygenation is directly related to radiation sensitivity, and that the central, irregularly vascularized and often necrotic region of many solid tumors is less radiosensitive. This zone harbors increasingly resistant clonogens that may contribute to treatment failure and tumor cell repopulation over time (135,136). As detailed earlier, the well-vascularized periphery of such tumors is often inadequately heated by RFA (48). The zones of reciprocal efficacy of these modalities suggest a potential complementarity when they are temporally combined. Further study must determine if the theoretical advantages are observed clinically, in the way of local control and symptom palliation. Regardless of the specifics of the regimen selected, regular follow-up assessments and imaging after combined treatment will maximize on the crucial utility of repeating thermoablation, without any increased risk or summation of tissue toxicity, in the event of progression or symptom recurrence.

FUTURE APPLICATIONS

Image-guided thermoablation has reshaped the treatment options for benign and malignant skeletal tumors. Its safety and reproducibility may support an analogous but largely unexplored role for non-neoplastic disorders of the musculoskeletal system. Radiofrequency ablation has already had substantial study for the treatment of nonmalignant bone pain, being functionally equivalent to a rhizotomy, for spine pain of discogenic and post-traumatic origin (4). In contrast, its effects on the bone growth and remodeling have had very little study. Manipulation and artificial arrest of longitudinal bone growth through various means directed at the physis, termed epiphysiodesis, have become well-accepted treatments for the disorders of skeletal development, such as limb-length discrepancy and angular deformity (137). Disruption of the physis and contiguous bone through a percutaneous approach, resulting in subsequent fusion, has achieved high rates of success (138,139), but this method carries with it the risk of significant operative and postoperative complications, including insufficiency and fracture. A pilot study at the authors' institution has investigated image-guided RFA as an alternative method for percutaneous epiphysiodesis (Fig. 7). In the weeks following RFA of the proximal tibial physis in rabbits, there was a significantly decreased rate of growth in the treated limb compared with the contralateral control limb, and a complete cessation of longitudinal growth in the treated limbs at two months postprocedure. Analyses

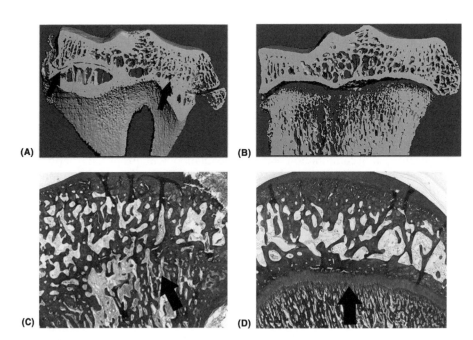

FIGURE 7 The efficacy of percutaneous radiofrequency ablation (RFA) for epiphysiodesis was investigated in a rabbit model by a group at the authors' institution. In the period following experimental RFA of the proximal tibial physis, treated limbs demonstrated a significantly decreased rate of growth, and ultimately a premature cessation of longitudinal growth, compared with the contralateral control limbs. (**A,B**) After 10 weeks, high-resolution three-dimensional volume images of the physes were obtained using compact fan-beam tomography (μCT 40; Scanco Medical, Bassersdorf, Switzerland). Radiofrequency ablation-treated specimens showed the bony bridging typical of fused physes (*arrowhead*), with cartilage being replaced by trabecular bone. The sham-treated physes were normal and open in appearance, without any significant derangement of the surrounding anatomy (*arrowhead*). These findings were consistent with subsequent histological examination of the RFA-treated physes (**C**, *arrowhead*) and sham-treated physes (**D**, *arrowhead*). *Source*: Photographs courtesy of F. Nickisch, M.D. and D. Moore, M.S., Department of Orthopedics, Brown Medical School and Rhode Island Hospital, Providence, Rhode Island, U.S.A.

via histological section and micro-CT demonstrated ossification of the RF-ablated physes, with essentially normal bone surrounding the treated areas. A great deal of study will obviously separate these preliminary findings from clinical testing. The potential for replacing current operative and percutaneous methods with RFA-epiphysiodesis is representative of the prominent place thermoablation will hold for the future of musculoskeletal pathology.

CONCLUSION

Ever since its initial study within the musculoskeletal system, percutaneous image-guided thermoablation has been increasing in applicability and in rates of clinical success for a wide variety of benign and malignant tumors. By virtue of the encouraging safety profile, minimal hospitalization, and rapid convalescence these techniques offer, thermoablation truly allows the patient, rather than the disease process, to be the immediate focus of these benefits. Radiofrequency ablation has proven itself as the preferred treatment for virtually all extraspinal osteoid osteomas, and for those centered in the vertebrae that are adequately shielded from adjacent neurovascular structures by intact bone. The implications of an equally primary role for the palliation of skeletal metastases are enormous, as the survival and proportion of cancer patients affected by these and other morbidities continue to rise. The expansion of long-term follow-up data and the continued collaboration among oncologic subspecialists will guide the selection of patients and the planning of the thermoablation treatments that will benefit them the most.

REFERENCES

1. Rosenberg A. Bones, joints, and soft tissue tumors. In: Cotran RS, Kumar V, Collins T, eds. Robbins Pathological Basis of Disease, 6th ed. Philadelphia: Saunders, 1999: 1216–1268.
2. Jaffe HL. Osteoid-osteoma: a benign osteoblastic tumor composed of osteoid and atypical bone. Arch Surg 1935; 31:709–728.
3. Schajowicz F. Bone forming tumors. In: Schajowicz F, ed. Tumors and Tumor-Like Lesions of Bones and Joints. New York: Springer, 1982:36–47.
4. Kirkland WD, Choi JJ, Blankenbaker DG. Radiofrequency ablation in the musculoskeletal system. Semin Roentgenol 2004; 39(1):129–144.
5. Unni KK. Benign osteoblastoma. In: Unni KK, ed. Dahlin's Bone Tumors: General Aspects and Data on 11,087 Cases, 5th ed. Philadelphia: Lippincott-Raven, 1996:131–142.
6. Cantwell CP, Obyrne J, Eustace S. Current trends in treatment of osteoid osteoma with an emphasis on radiofrequency ablation. Eur Radiol 2004; 14(4):607–617.
7. Ozaki T, Liljenqvist U, Hillmann A. Osteoid osteoma and osteoblastoma of the spine: experience with 22 patients. Clin Orthop Relat Res 2002; 397:394–402.
8. Zileli M, Cagli S, Basdemir G, et al. Osteoid osteomas and osteoblastomas of the spine. Neurosurg Focus 2003; 15(5):E5.
9. Makley JT, Dunn MJ. Prostaglandin synthesis by osteoid osteoma [letter]. Lancet 1982; 2:42.
10. Ciabattoni G, Tamburrelli F, Greco F. Increased prostacyclin biosynthesis in patients with osteoid osteoma. Eicosanoids 1991; 3:165–167.
11. Pieterse AS, Vernon-Roberts B, Paterson DC, et al. Osteoid osteoma transforming to aggressive (low-grade malignant) osteoblastoma: a case report and literature review. Histopathology 1983; 7:789–800.
12. Kneisl JS, Simon MA. Medical management compared with operative treatment for osteoid osteoma. J Bone Joint Surg 1992; 74A:179–185.
13. Rosenthal DI, Hornicek FJ, Wolfe MW, et al. Percutaneous radiofrequency coagulation of osteoid osteoma compared with operative treatment. J Bone Joint Surg 1998; 80A:815–821.
14. Barei DP, Moreau G, Scarborough MT, Neel MD. Percutaneous radiofrequency ablation of osteoid osteoma. Clin Orthop Rel Res 2000; 373:115–124.
15. Haibach H, Farrell C, Gaines RW. Osteoid osteoma of the spine: surgically correctable cause of painful scoliosis. Can Med Assoc J 1986; 135:895–899.
16. Greenspan A. Benign bone-forming lesions: osteoma, osteoid osteoma, osteoblastoma —clinical, imaging, pathologic and differential considerations. Skelet Radiol 1993; 22:485–500.
17. Saifuddin A, Sherazi Z, Shaikh MI, et al. Spinal osteoblastoma: relationship between paravertebral muscle e abnormalities and scoliosis. Skelet Radiol 1996; 25:531–535.
18. Norman A, Abdelwahab IF, Buyon J, Matzkin E. Osteoid osteoma of the hip stimulating an early onset of osteoarthritis. Radiology 1986; 158:410–417.
19. Sim FH, Dahlin DC, Beabout JW. Osteoid-osteoma: diagnostic problems. J Bone Joint Surg 1975; 57A:154–159.

20. Doyle T, King K. Percutaneous removal of osteoid osteomas using CT control. Clin Radiol 1989; 40:514–517.
21. Norman A. Persistence or recurrence of pain: a sign of surgical failure in osteoid-osteoma. Clin Orthop 1978; 130:263–266.
22. Worland RL, Ryder CT, Johnston AD. Recurrent osteoid-osteoma—report of a case. J Bone Joint Surg 1975; 57A:277–278.
23. Sluga M, Windhager R, Pfeiffer M, et al. Peripheral osteoid osteoma: is there still place for surgery? J Bone Joint Surg 2002; 84B:249–251.
24. Lee DH, Malawer MM. Staging and treatment of primary and persistent (recurrent) osteoid osteoma—evaluation of intraoperative nuclear scanning, tetracycline fluorescence, and tomography. Clin Orthop 1992; 281:229–238.
25. Ayala AG, Murray JA, Erling MA, et al. Osteoid-osteoma: intraoperative tetracycline fluorescence demonstrating the nidus. J Bone Joint Surg 1986; 68A:747–751.
26. Kirchner B, Hillmann A, Lottes G, et al. Intraoperative probe-guided curettage of osteoid osteoma. Eur J Nucl Med 1993; 20:609–613.
27. Steinberg GG, Coumas JM, Breen T. Preoperative localization of osteoid osteoma: a new technique that uses CT. AJR 1990; 155:883–885.
28. Resnick RB, Jarolem KL, Sheskier SC, et al. Arthroscopic removal of an osteoid osteoma of the talus: a case report. Foot Ankle Int 1995; 16:212–215.
29. Assoun J, Railhac JJ, Bonnevialle P, et al. Osteoid osteoma: percutaneous resection with CT guidance. Radiology 1993; 188:541–547.
30. Towbin R, Kaye R, Meza MP, et al. Osteoid osteoma: percutaneous excision using a CT-guided coaxial technique. AJR 1995; 164:945–949.
31. Sans N, Galy-Fourcade D, Assoun J, et al. Osteoid osteoma: percutaneous resection and follow-up in 38 patients. Radiology 1999; 212:687–692.
32. Klose KC, Forst R, Vorwerk D, Guenther RW. The percutaneous removal of osteoid osteomas via CT-guided drilling. Fortschr Geb Rontgenstr 1991; 155: 532–537.
33. Kohler R, Rubini J, Postec F, et al. Treatment of osteoid osteoma by CT-controlled percutaneous drill resection: apropos of 27 cases. Rev Chir Orthop Reparatrice Appar Mot 1995; 81:317–325.
34. Gangi A, Dietemann JL, Clavert JM, et al. Treatment of osteoid osteoma using laser photo-coagulation—apropos of 28 cases. Rev Chir Orthop Reparatrice Appar Mot 1998; 84:676–684.
35. Gangi A, Dietemann JL, Guth S, et al. Percutaneous laser photocoagulation of spinal osteoid osteomas under CT guidance. AJNR 1998; 19:1955–1958.
36. Skeldal S, Lilleas F, Folleras G, et al. Real time MRI-guided excision and cryo-treatment of osteoid osteoma in os ischii: a case report. Acta Orthop Scand 2000; 71(6):637–638.
37. Adam G, Keulers P, Vorwerk D, et al. The percutaneous CT-guided treatment of osteoid osteomas: a combined procedure with a biopsy drill and subsequent ethanol injection. Fortschr Geb Rontgenstr 1995; 162:232–235.
38. Dupuy DE. Tumor ablation: treatment and palliation using image-guided therapy. Oncology 2005(suppl); 19:4–5.
39. Cushing H, Bovie WT. Electrosurgery as an aid to the removal of intracranial tumors. Surg Gynecol Obstet 1928; 47:751–784.
40. Cosman ER, Nashold BS, Ovelman-Levitt J. Theoretical aspects of radiofrequency lesions in the dorsal root entry zone. Neurosurgery 1984; 15:945–950.
41. Sweet WH, Wepsic JG. Controlled thermo coagulation of trigeminal ganglion and rootlets for differential destruction of pain fibers. J Neurosurg 1974; 39:143–156.
42. Pagura JR, Schnapp M, Passarelli P. Percutaneous radiofrequency glossopharyngeal rhizotomy for cancer pain. Appl Neurophysiol 1983; 46:154–159.
43. Jackman WM, Wang X, Friday KJ, et al. Catheter ablation of accessory atrioventricular pathways (Wolff-Parkinson-White syndrome) by radiofrequency current. N Engl J Med 1991; 324:1605–1611.
44. McGahan JP, Browning PD, Brook JM, et al. Hepatic ablation using radiofrequency electrocautery. Invest Radiol 1990; 25:267–270.

45. Rossi S, Fornari F, Pathles C, et al. Thermal lesions induced by 480 KHz localized current field in guinea pig and pig liver. Tumori 1990; 76:54–57.
46. Tillotson CL, Rosenberg AE, Rosenthal DI. Controlled thermal injury of bone: report of a percutaneous technique using radiofrequency electrode and generator. Invest Radiol 1989; 24:888–892.
47. Rosenthal DI, Alexander A, Rosenberg AE, et al. Ablation of osteoid osteomas with a percutaneously placed electrode: a new procedure. Radiology 1992; 183:29–33.
48. Goldberg SN, Dupuy DE. Image-guided radiofrequency tumor ablation: challenges and opportunities—part I. J Vasc Interv Radiol 2001; 12:1021–1032.
49. Goldberg SN, Gazelle GS, Halpern EF, et al. Radiofrequency tissue ablation: importance of local temperature along the electrode tip exposure in determining lesion shape and size. Acad Radiol 1996; 3:212–218.
50. Dupuy DE, Goldberg SN. Image-guided radiofrequency tumor ablation: challenges and—part II. J Vasc Interv Radiol 2001; 12:1135–1148.
51. Goldberg SN, Gazelle GS, Mueller PR. Thermal ablation therapy for focal malignancy: a unified approach to underlying principles, techniques, and diagnostic imaging guidance. AJR 2000; 174:323–331.
52. Goldberg SN, Stein M, Gazelle GS, et al. Percutaneous radiofrequency tissue ablation: optimization of pulsed-RF technique to increase coagulation necrosis. J Vasc Interv Radiol 1999; 10:907–916.
53. Lorentzen T. A cooled needle electrode for radiofrequency tissue ablation: thermodynamic aspects of improved performance compared with conventional needle design. Acad Radiol 1996; 3:556–563.
54. Goldberg SN, Gazelle GS, Solbiati L. Radiofrequency tissue ablation: increased lesion diameter with a perfusion electrode. Acad Radiol 1996; 3:636–644.
55. Goldberg SN, Solbiati L, Hahn PF. Large-volume tissue ablation with radiofrequency by using a clustered, internally cooled electrode technique: laboratory and clinical experience in liver metastases. Radiology 1998; 209:371–379.
56. Livraghi T, Goldberg SN, Meloni F. Hepatocellular carcinoma: comparison of efficacy between percutaneous ethanol instillation and radiofrequency. Radiology 1999; 210:655–661.
57. Goldberg SN, Gazelle GS, Compton CC, et al. Treatment of intrahepatic malignancy with radiofrequency ablation: radiologic–pathologic correlation. Cancer 2000; 88:2452.
58. Rossi S, Garbagnati F, Lencioni R, et al. Percutaneous radiofrequency ablation of nonresectable hepatocellular carcinoma after occlusion of tumor blood supply. Radiology 2000; 217:119–126.
59. Chang I, Mikityansky I, Wray-Chan D, et al. Effects of perfusion on radiofrequency ablation in swine kidneys. Radiology 2004; 231:500–505.
60. Horkan C, Ahmed M, Liu Z, et al. Radiofrequency ablation: effect of pharmacological modulation of hepatic and renal blood flow on coagulation diameter in a VX2 tumor model. J Vasc Interv Radiol 2004; 15:269–274.
61. Dupuy DE, Hong R, Oliver B, et al. Radiofrequency ablation of spinal tumors: temperature distribution in the spinal canal. AJR 2000; 175:1263–1266.
62. Lindner NJ, Roedl OR, Gosheger G, et al. Percutaneous radiofrequency ablation in osteoid osteoma. J Bone Joint Surg 2001; 83B:391–396.
63. Rosenthal DI, Springfield DS, Gebhardt MC, et al. Osteoid osteoma: percutaneous radiofrequency ablation. Radiology 1995; 197:451–454.
64. Woertler K, Vestring T, Boettner F, et al. Osteoid osteoma: CT-guided percutaneous radiofrequency ablation and follow-up in 47 patients. J Vasc Interv Radiol 2001; 12(6):717–722.
65. Rosenthal DI, Hornicek FJ, Torriani M, et al. Osteoid osteoma: percutaneous treatment with radiofrequency energy. Radiology 2003; 229:171–175.
66. Bjorn M, Carsten G, Georg G, et al. Percutaneous radiofrequency ablation of an osteoid osteoma of the scapula: a case report. J Shoulder Elbow Surg 2005; 14:447–449.
67. Goldberg SN, Solbiati L, Halpern EF, et al. Variables affecting proper system grounding for radiofrequency ablation in an animal model. J Vasc Interv Radiol 2000; 11:1069–1075.

68. Livraghi T, Solbiati L, Meloni MF, et al. Treatment of focal liver tumors with radiofrequency ablation: complications encountered in a multicenter study. Radiology 2003; 226:441–451.
69. Froese G, Das RM, Dunscombe PB. The sensitivity of the thoracolumbar spinal cord of the mouse to hyperthermia. Radiat Res 1991; 125:173–180.
70. Yamane T, Tateishi A, Cho S, et al. The effects of hyperthermia on the spinal cord. Spine 1992; 17:1386–1391.
71. Letcher FS, Goldring S. The effect of radiofrequency current and heat on peripheral nerve action potential in the cat. J Neurosurg 1968; 29:42–47.
72. Houpt TC. Experimental study of temperature distributions and thermal transport during radiofrequency current therapy of the intervertebral disc. Spine 1996; 21:108.
73. Nakatsuka A, Yamakado K, Maeda M, et al. Radiofrequency ablation combined with bone cement injection for the treatment of bone malignancies. J Vasc Interv Radiol 2004; 15:707–712.
74. Osti OL, Sebben R. High-frequency radio-wave ablation of osteoid osteoma in the lumbar spine. Eur Spine J 1998; 7:422–425.
75. Gronemeyer DH, Gevargez A, Schirp S. Image-guided radiofrequency ablation of spinal tumors: preliminary experience with an expandable array electrode. Cancer J 2002; 8:33–39.
76. Goetz MP, Callstrom MR, Charboneau JW, et al. Percutaneous image-guided radiofrequency ablation of painful metastases involving bone: a multicenter study. J Clin Oncol 2004; 22:300–306.
77. Posteraro AF, Dupuy DE, Mayo-Smith WW. Radiofrequency ablation of bony metastatic disease. Clin Radiol 2004; 59:803–811.
78. Lee JM, Choi SH, Park HS. Radiofrequency thermal ablation in canine femur: evaluation of coagulation necrosis reproducibility and MRI-histopathologic correlation. AJR 2005; 185:661–667.
79. Wood BJ. Feasibility of thermal ablation of lytic vertebral metastases with radiofrequency current. Cancer J 2002; 8:26–29.
80. Oshiro T, Sinha U, Lu D, et al. Reduction of electronic noise from radiofrequency generator during radiofrequency ablation in interventional MRI. JCAT 2002; 26:308–316.
81. American Cancer Society. Cancer Facts and Figures 2005. Atlanta, GA: American Cancer Society.
82. Paget S. The distribution of secondary growths in cancer of the breast. Lancet 1889; 1:571–573.
83. Roodman, DG. Mechanism of bone metastasis. N Engl J Med 2004; 350:1655–1664.
84. Rubens RD, Coleman RE. Bone metastases. In: Abeloff MD, Armitage JO, Lichter AS, et al., eds. Clinical Oncology. New York: Churchill Livingstone, 1995:643–665.
85. Coleman RE. Skeletal complications of malignancy. Cancer 1997; 80(suppl 8): 1588–1594.
86. Janjan NA, Payne R, Gillis T, et al. Presenting symptoms in patients referred to a multidisciplinary clinic for bone metastases. J Pain Symptom Manag 1998; 16: 171–178.
87. Janjan NA. Bone metastases: approaches to management. Semin Oncol 2001; 28: 28–34.
88. Clohisy DR, Mantyh PW. Bone cancer pain. Clin Orthop Rel Res 2003; 415(suppl): 279–288.
89. Clohisy DR, Ramnaraine ML. Osteoclasts are required for bone tumors to grow and destroy bone. J Orthop Res 1998; 16:660–666.
90. Mach DB, Rogers SD, Sabino MAC, et al. Origins of skeletal pain: sensory and sympathetic innervation of the mouse femur. Neuroscience 2002; 113:156–166.
91. Janjan NA. Management of pain. In: Perez C, Brady L, eds. Principles and Practice of Radiation Oncology, 3rd ed. New York: JB Lippincott, 1997:2227–2241.
92. Honore P, Rogers SD, Schwei MJ, et al. Murine models of inflammatory, neuropathic, and cancer pain each generates a unique set of neurochemical changes in the spinal cord and sensory neurons. Neuroscience 2000; 98:585–598.

93. Janjan NA. Radiation for bone metastases: conventional techniques and the role of systemic radiopharmaceuticals. Cancer 1997; 80(suppl):1628–1645.
94. Frassica DA. General principles of external beam radiation therapy for skeletal metastases. Clin Orthop Relat Res 2003; 415(suppl):158–164.
95. Pandit-Taskar N, Batraki M, Divgi CR. Radiopharmaceutical therapy for palliation of bone pain from osseous metastases. J Nucl Med 2004; 45:1358–1365.
96. Tong D, Gillick L, Hendrickson FR. The palliation of symptomatic osseous metastases: final results of the study by the radiation therapy oncology group. Cancer 1982; 50: 893–899.
97. Ratanatharathorn V, Powers WE, Moss WT, et al. Bone metastasis: review and critical analysis of random allocation trials of local field treatment. Int J Rad Oncol Biol Phys 1999; 44:1–18.
98. Vinholes JJ, Purohit OP, Abbey ME, et al. Relationships between biochemical and symptomatic response in double-blinded trial of pamidronate for metastatic bone disease. Ann Oncol 1997; 8:1243–1250.
99. Hillner BE, Ingle JN, Berenson JR, et al. American society of clinical oncology guideline on the role of bisphosphonates in breast cancer. American society of clinical oncology bisphosphonates expert panel. J Clin Oncol 2000; 18:1378–1391.
100. Dupuy DE, Safran H, Mayo-Smith WW, et al. Radiofrequency ablation of painful osseous metastatic disease [abstract]. Radiology 2000; 209:389.
101. Callstrom MR, Charboneau JW, Goetz MP, et al. Painful metastases involving bone: feasibility of percutaneous CT- and US-guided radio-frequency ablation. Radiology 2002; 224:87–97.
102. Van Sonnenberg E, Shankar S, Morrison P, et al. Radiofrequency ablation of thoracic lesions: part II, initial clinical experience—technical and multidisciplinary considerations in 30 patients. AJR 2005; 184:381.
103. Glaiberman CB, Brown DB. Reversible neuropathy caused by overuse following radiofrequency ablation of metastatic pelvic lesions. J Vasc Interv Radiol 2004; 15:1307–1310.
104. Stang A, Celebcioglu S, Keles H, et al. Minimally-invasive regional treatment of symptomatic ischial metastasis using radiofrequency ablation and osteoplasty. Dtsch Med Wochenschr 2005; 130:1195–1198.
105. Shibata T, Iimuro Y, Yamamoto Y, et al. Small hepatocellular carcinoma: comparison of radio-frequency ablation and percutaneous microwave coagulation therapy. Radiology 2002; 223:331–337.
106. Skinner MG, Iizuka MN, Kolios MC, et al. A theoretical comparison of energy sources—microwave, ultrasound, and laser—for interstitial thermal therapy. Phys Med Biol 1998; 43:3535–3547.
107. Wright AS, Lee FT, Mahvi DM. Hepatic microwave ablation with multiple antennae results in synergistically larger zones of coagulation necrosis. Ann Surg Oncol 2003; 10:275–283.
108. Shock SA, Meredith K, Warner TF, et al. Microwave ablation with loop antenna: in vivo porcine liver model. Radiology 2004; 231:143–149.
109. Yu NC, Lu DSK, Dupuy DE, et al. Microwave ablation of hepatocellular carcinoma: preliminary evaluation of novel antennae designs. Radiology 2005. In press.
110. Jain S, Sacchi M, Vrachnos P, et al. Recent advances in the treatment of colorectal liver metastases. Hepatogastroenterology 2005; 52:1567–1584.
111. Ichikwawa T, Uenishi T, Hirohashi K, et al. A case of a small intrahepatic cholangiocarcinoma treated with microwave coagulation therapy. Nippon Shokakibyo Gakkai Zasshi 2005; 102:1299–1304.
112. Fan QY, Ma BA, Qlu XC, et al. Preliminary report on treatment of bone tumors with microwave-induced hyperthermia. Bioelectromagnetics 1996; 17:218–222.
113. Mirza AN, Fornage BD, Sneige N, et al. Radiofrequency ablation of solid tumors. Cancer J 2001; 7:95–104.
114. Profrene V, Schreduer B, van Beem H, et al. Cryosurgery in aggressive, benign, and low-grade malignant bone tumors. Lancet Oncol 2005; 6:25–34.

115. Weber SM, Lee FT. Expanded treatment of hepatic tumors with radiofrequency ablation and cryoablation. Oncology 2005; (suppl):19, 27–32.
116. De Sanctis JT, Goldberg SN, Mueller PR. Percutaneous treatment of hepatic neoplasms: a review of current techniques. Cardiovasc Intervent Radiol 1998; 21:273–296.
117. Lee FT Jr., Chosy SG, Littrup JP, et al. CT-monitored percutaneous cryoablation in a pig liver model: pilot study. Radiology 1999; 211:687–692.
118. Allaf ME, Varkarakis IM, Bhayani SB, et al. Pain control requirements for percutaneous ablation of renal tumors: cryoablation versus radiofrequency ablation. Radiology 2005; 237:366–370.
119. Yan DB, Clingan P, Morris DL. Hepatic cryotherapy and regional chemotherapy with or without resection for liver metastases from colorectal carcinoma—how many are too many? Cancer 2003; 98:320–330.
120. Shingleton WB, Sewell PE Jr. Percutaneous renal cryoablation of renal tumors in patients with von Hippel-Lindau disease. J Urol 2002; 167:1268–1270.
121. Wang H, Littrup PJ, Duan Y, et al. Thoracic masses treated with percutaneous cryotherapy: initial experience with more than 200 procedures. Radiology 2005; 235:289–298.
122. Popken F, Meschede P, Von Smekal U, et al. Rate of perioperative complications in thermal ablation of bone: an animal trial. Arch Orthop Trauma Surg 2004; 124:326–330.
123. Beland MD, Dupuy DE, Mayo-Smith WW. Percutaneous cryoablation of symptomatic extra-abdominal metastatic disease: preliminary results. AJR 2005; 184:926–930.
124. Callstrom MR, Charboneau JW. Percutaneous ablation: safe, effective treatment of bone tumors. Oncology 2005; (suppl):19, 22–26.
125. Maiwand MO. The role of cryosurgery in palliation of tracheo-bronchial carcinoma. Eur J Cardiothoracic Surg 1999; 15:764–768.
126. Amin Z, Donald JJ, Masters A, et al. Hepatic metastases: interstitial laser photocoagulation with real-time US monitoring and dynamic CT evaluation of treatment. Radiology 1993; 187:339–347.
127. Chen W, Wang Z, Wu F. High intensity focused ultrasound in the treatment of primary malignant bone tumors. Zhonghua Zhong Liu Za Zhi 2002; 24:612–615.
128. Jolesz FA, Hynynen K, McDannold N, et al. MR imaging-controlled focused ultrasound ablation: a noninvasive image-guided surgery. Magn Reson Imaging Clin N Am 2005; 13:545–560.
129. Seegenschmiedt MH, Brady LW, Sauer R. Interstitial thermoradiotherapy: review on technical and clinical aspects. Am J Clin Oncol 1990; 13:352–363.
130. Trembley BS, Ryan TP, Strehbehn JW. Interstitial hyperthermia: physics, biology, and clinical aspects. In: Urano M, Double E, eds. Physics of Microwave Hyperthermia in Hyperthermia and Oncology. Vol. 3. Utrecht: Verlag Springer, 1992:11–98.
131. Goldberg SN, Saldinger PF, Gazelle GS, et al. Percutaneous tumor ablation: increased necrosis with combined radiofrequency ablation and intratumoral doxorubicin injection in a rat breast tumor model. Radiology 2001; 220:420–427.
132. Goldberg SN, Kruskal JB, Oliver BS, et al. Percutaneous tumor ablation: increased coagulation by combining radio-frequency ablation and ethanol instillation in a rat breast tumor model. Radiology 2000; 217:827–831.
133. Friedman MA, Altemus R, Wood BJ. Radiofrequency ablation in a previously irradiated liver. J Vasc Interv Radiol 2003; 14:1345–1348.
134. Horkan C, Dalal K, Coderre JA, et al. Reduced tumor growth with combined radiofrequency ablation and radiation therapy in a rat breast tumor model. Radiology 2005; 235:81–88.
135. Hall E. Radiobiology for the radiologist. 5th ed. Philadelphia: Lippincott, Williams, and Wilkins, 2000:91–111, 288–313, 377–396, 495–520.
136. DiPetrillo TA, Dupuy DE. Radiofrequency ablation and radiotherapy: complimenting treatments for solid tumors. Semin Interven Radiol 2003; 20:341–345.

137. Timperlake RW, Bowen JR, Guille JT. Prospective evaluation of fifty-three consecutive percutaneous epiphysiodeses of the distal femur and proximal tibia and fibula. J Pediatr Orthop 1991; 11:350–357.
138. Metaizeau JP, Wong-Chung J, Bertrand H, et al. Percutaneous epiphysiodesis using transphyseal screws (PETS). J Pediatr Orthop 1998; 18:363–369.
139. Nouth F, Kuo LA. Percutaneous epiphysiodesis using transphyseal screws (PETS): prospective case study and review. J Pediatr Orthop 2004; 24:721–725.

11 Sacroiliac Joint Injections

Theodore D. Conliffe, Jr.
Rothman Institute, Thomas Jefferson University Hospital, Philadelphia, Pennsylvania, U.S.A.

SACROILIAC JOINT INJECTIONS

Sacroiliac (SI) joint syndrome has been considered to be a source of low back pain for approximately 100 years (1,2). Prior to the work of Mixter and Barr (3) in 1934, which identified the intervertebral disc as a principal etiology of low back pain, the SI joint was believed to be the primary pain generator. Studies utilizing injection techniques for diagnosis have dramatically altered the diagnosis and treatment of SI joint syndrome. This chapter introduces the techniques of fluoroscopically guided SI injections, and discusses the indications, contraindications, complications, and evidence-based literature regarding this procedure.

Patients with SI joint pain typically complain of deep aching low back pain, buttock pain, thigh pain or groin pain of variable duration. Symptoms are commonly one-sided, but may be bilateral. The mechanism of injury is usually unknown, although there can be a description of minor trauma. Symptoms are not accompanied by neurological deficits and can be exacerbated by prolonged sitting or standing. This pain can radiate down the leg past the knee at times, but typically stops at the knee. Patients may achieve temporary relief by changing positions, using modalities, such as heat and anti-inflammatory medications.

Physical exam findings in SI joint syndrome are unreliable (4). Patients commonly exhibit tenderness over the sacral sulcus and buttocks on the symptomatic side. Provocative maneuvers which compress the joint space can reproduce pain around the posterior superior iliac spine. Motions to the hips, such as flexion, external rotation, abduction, and extension may reproduce pain, but are not specific to the SI joint.

The differential diagnosis of SI joint syndrome is extensive. It includes lumbar disc disease, piriformis syndrome, zygapophyseal joint pain, degenerative joint disease of the hip, spinal metastases, gluteal bursitis, ischiorectal abscess, myofascial pain syndrome, fibromyalgia, ankylosing spondylitis, sacral fractures and spondylolysis, and pelvic inflammatory disease.

Presently, there are no diagnostic tests useful in the diagnosis of SI joint syndrome (5). Two recent studies examined the efficacy of computed tomography (CT) scans and bone scans to diagnose SI dysfunction. Both studies failed to show any correlation between radiographic findings and clinical symptoms or signs (6,7).

Sacroiliac joint injections have become an invaluable tool in confirming the diagnosis of SI joint syndrome. Many recent studies have questioned the adequacy of physical examination and radiographic studies in support of clinical diagnosis (4–6). Most recently, a study by Laslett's group (8) reaffirmed previous work by Fortin (9) and Schwarzer (10), stating that pain relief with SI injections under fluoroscopic guidance remains the gold standard for diagnosis of this condition.

ANATOMY

The SI joint lies at the junction of the sacral bone and the iliacus bones. It is initially described as an L-shaped joint, with its long arm oriented caudally and its short arm cranially (5). As humans mature into adulthood, the joint becomes nearly C-shaped in appearance.

In 1920, Lynch reported that the SI joint is a true synovial joint, based on a work by eighteenth-century anatomists Bernhard Albinus and William Hunter (11). It contains synovial fluid, has two opposing joint surfaces, and the articulating bones possess ligamentous connections (12). There are six ligaments which span the articular surfaces of the SI joint. These include the interosseous SI ligament, the ventral SI ligament, the long dorsal SI ligament, the sacrotuberous ligament, the sacrospinous and the iliolumbar ligaments.

There are several important changes that occur in the joints with aging. The articular surfaces become rough after puberty. The joints also develop cavitations which increase friction and enhance joint stability. Finally, with aging, the joint surfaces erode and narrowing of the joint space occurs, although ankylosis of the joints is rare.

The SI joint is unique in that it is covered by two different types of cartilage. The sacral surface is covered by a hyaline cartilage and the iliac surface is covered by a fibrocartilage.

The joint is innervated on its posterior surface by lateral branches of the posterior ramus from L4 to S3. There may also be a ventral contribution to the innervation. This remains controversial following the recent work by Fortin in 1999 (13). Because of the diverse innervation, the pain referral patterns can easily be confused with radicular symptoms between L4 and S1. The most common patient complaints remain buttock, lateral hip, groin, and posterior thigh pain. Sacroiliac pain is rarely seen above the iliac crest.

PATIENT SELECTION

Injections are performed to minimize low back pain and to confirm the diagnosis of SI joint syndrome. Specific indications for diagnostic and/or therapeutic SI injections include discomfort at and below the iliac crest. The distribution of discomfort secondary to SI dysfunction was mapped by Fortin in a landmark work (14). Other indications for the procedure include patients with low back pain and MRIs negative for disc pathology or facet arthropathy. Prior to performing injections, patients have generally failed other conservative treatments for at least four weeks. Conservative treatments for this condition include physical therapy, medication, SI belts, and spinal manipulation.

CONTRAINDICATIONS

Absolute contraindications for this procedure include patients with systemic infections. Patients with localized infection near the injection site should also be excluded. Patients should be afebrile and off all antibiotics prior to the injection. Other patients precluded from the procedure include those with bleeding diatheses or chronic anticoagulation. Those patients on anticoagulants should have their medication held and prothrombin time (PT) rechecked to minimize bleeding risks. Patients who are pregnant should not receive SI injections because of exposure to fluoroscopy.

Sacroiliac joint blocks should be performed cautiously in patients with known allergies to contrast media or iodine, local anesthetics, and corticosteroids. These patients will need prophylaxis against allergic reaction prior to the procedure. Relative contraindications to the performance of SI injections include poorly controlled diabetes and labile congestive heart failure if steroids are to be utilized. Aspirin can be stopped one week before the procedure and nonsteroidal anti-inflammatory drugs (NSAIDs), except for cyclo-oxygenase-2 (COX-2) inhibitors can be held for three days before the injection. However, this is not critical. Finally, the physician should be aware of any potential latex allergy prior to the procedure.

TECHNIQUE

There are several techniques described in the medical literature. The first technique was described by Miskew in 1979, for aspiration of an infected joint (15). The technique was then simplified in 1982 by Hendrix (16), and is still commonly performed. This technique involved superimposing the anterior and superior joint surfaces.

After informed consent is obtained, the patient is brought into the fluoroscopy suite and placed on the examination table in the prone position. The C-arm fluoroscope is positioned obliquely to superimpose the anterior and posterior joint surfaces of the SI joints. The patient's contralateral hip is raised slightly to an angle of 10° to 30° to allow optimal views of the joint to be injected. The patient's skin is then sterilely prepped and draped in the usual fashion. The skin and soft tissues overlying the joint surface are anesthetized with a local anesthetic. Using intermittent fluoroscopy, a sterile 22-gauge spinal needle is then inserted into the lower one-third of the SI joint. Hendrix (16) described increased resistance as the needle passes through the posterior SI ligament and decreased resistance as the needle pops into the joint. The needle may appear to bend slightly at its tip upon entrance into the joint space. Needle placement within the joint is then confirmed by injection of 0.5–1 ml of water-soluble contrast. The contrast spreads in a cephalad direction from the

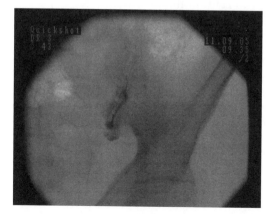

FIGURE 1   Fluoroscopic image of arthrogram of right sacroiliac (SI) joint utilizing the technique of Hendrix as described in 1982. The anterior and posterior joint margins are superimposed by rotation of the fluoroscope image obliquely. The spinal needle is observed in the bottom third of the joint about 1 cm from the caudal-most segment. Contrast spreads superiorly in the joint space.

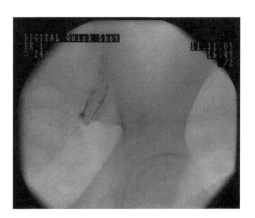

FIGURE 2   Fluoroscopic image of arthrogram of right sacroiliac (SI) joint utilizing the technique described by Fortin in 1994. The anterior and posterior joint margins are clearly separated and the spinal needle is observed in the posterior joint margin. The needle is positioned in the bottom third of the joint 1–2 cm above the caudal-most segment of the joint. Contrast spreads superiorly in the joint space away from the needle. Contrast is also observed in the anterior joint margin (lateral position).

inferior aspect of the joint. Pictures should be obtained and printed to be placed on the patient chart (Fig. 1). After satisfactory arthrogram is obtained, a solution of local anesthetic and corticosteroid is injected into the joint. The volume of the injectate should be less than 3 ml, because the joint can only hold maximum 2–5 ml (10,14).

During this immediate postinjection period, the patient should be encouraged to perform activities that previously elicited the pain response. A pain diary may be kept by the patient at various intervals following the procedure to record the degree of pain relief. Typically, a significantly positive response to the injection is at least a 75% reduction in pain immediately following the injection during the period of analgesia provided by the specific anesthetic (8,17,18). On another occasion, a second injection should be performed to confirm the diagnosis of the SI joint as the pain generator. This eliminates the possibility of a false positive response to an initially successful diagnostic injection.

An alternative to this procedure was proposed by Fortin in 1994 (9), and modified by Dussault (19) in 2000. The technique is varied to separate the anterior and posterior joint surfaces by rotation of the C-arm either obliquely with the hips elevated minimally, as described by Fortin, or by angling the C-arm by 20° to 25° in a cephalad position (Dussault). This procedure allows easier cannulation of the posterior joint surface. The posterior joint margin is observed medially with this technique. The optimal injection site would be seen when the posterior joint surface develops a hyperlucent appearance, described as a medial silhouette (20). The procedure would then be conducted as described earlier, with the entry point for the needle in the inferior portion of the joint space (Fig. 2).

COMPLICATIONS

Bleeding, bruising, and discomfort at the injection site are uncommon, but may occur. Local and systemic infections are also rare complications observed with a sterile technique. Potentially fatal anaphylactic reactions can occur with unknown allergies to latex, contrast media, local anesthetics, and steroids.

EVIDENCE-BASED LITERATURE

Medical science has studied fluoroscopic SI injections for approximately 25 years. To date, there have been no random assigned double-blinded controlled studies of this procedure in patients without known seronegative spondyloarthropathy (21). Rosenberg (22) in 2000 determined that nonfluoroscopic injections rarely enter the SI joint. This study determined that only 22% of these blind injections actually entered the joint space. Fortin previously established pain referral maps in 1994 to diagnose suspected SI joint syndrome (9,14). After diagnosis, he found that 14 out of the 16 patients studied had improvement with fluoroscopic SI injections. Schwarzer et al. (10) studied 43 patients with idiopathic low back pain below L5 and found that 30% of this group improved with this procedure. Maigne prospectively studied 54 patients with suspected SI joint pain and using a double-block paradigm determined that 18.5% had significant improvement after two blocks.

Slipman (17) performed a retrospective study of 31 patients with SI joint syndrome in 2001. These patients underwent fluoroscopic injections after failing conservative treatments for four weeks. His group found statistically significant improvements in the Visual Analog Scale, Oswestry Disability Scores, and work status following therapeutic SI injections.

Current medical literature is quite favorable regarding the use of fluoroscopic SI injections for the diagnosis of SI joint syndrome. History and physical examination alone are not sufficient to diagnose SI dysfunction. Further randomized, controlled research is necessary to establish that therapeutic SI injections are beneficial to our patients. This research should include a double-block paradigm to minimize the placebo effect of a single positive injection.

REFERENCES

1. Goldwaite GE, Osgood RB. A consideration of the pelvic articulations from an anatomical, pathological, and clinical standpoint. Boston Med Surg J 1905;152:593–601.
2. Slipman CW, Whyte II WS, Chow DW, et al. Sacroiliac joint syndrome. Pain Physician 2001; 4(2):143–152.
3. Mixter WJ, Barr JS. Rupture of the intervertebral disc with involvement of the spinal canal. NEJM 1934; 211:210–215.
4. Dreyfuss P, Michaelsen M, Pauza K, et al. The value of medical history and physical examination in diagnosing sacroiliac joint pain. Spine 1996; 21(22):2594–2602.
5. Beal MC. The sacroiliac problem: review of anatomy, mechanics, and diagnosis. Am Osteopath Assoc 1982; 81:667–679.
6. Slipman CW, Sterenfeld EB, Chou LH, et al. The value of radionuclide imaging in the diagnosis of sacroiliac joint syndrome. Spine 1996; 21(19):2251–2254.
7. Elgafy H, Semaan HB, Ebraheim NA, et al. Computed tomography findings in patients with sacroiliac pain. Clin Orthop 2001; 382:112–118.
8. Laslett M, Aprill CN, McDonald B, et al. Diagnosis of sacroiliac joint pain: validity of individual provocation tests and composites of tests. Manual Ther 2005; 10(3):207–218.
9. Fortin JD, Aprill CN, Ponthieux B, et al. Sacroiliac joint: pain referral maps upon applying a new injection/arthrography technique. Part II: Clinical evaluation. Spine 1994; 19(13):1483–1489.
10. Schwarzer AC, Aprill CN, Bogduk N. The sacroiliac joint in chronic low back pain. Spine 1995; 20(1):31–37.
11. Lee D, ed. Anatomy. The Pelvic Girdle. 3rd ed. Edinburgh: Churchill Livingstone, 2004:15–39.
12. Mooney V. Understanding, examining for, and treating sacroiliac pain. Musculoskelet Med 1993; 10(7):37–49.
13. Fortin JD, Kissling RO, O'Connor BL, et al. Sacroiliac joint innervation and pain. Am J Orthop 1999; 28:687–690.

14. Fortin JD, Dwyer AP, West S, et al. Sacroiliac joint: pain referral maps upon applying a new injection/arthrography technique, Part I: Asymptomatic volunteers. Spine 1994; 19(13):1475–1482.
15. Miskew DB, Block RA, Witt PF. Aspiration of infected sacroiliac joints. JBJS 1979; 61A(7):1071–1072.
16. Hendrix RW, Lin PP, Kane WJ, et al. JBJS 1982; 64A(8):1249–1252.
17. Slipman CW, Lipertz JS, Plastaras CT, et al. Flouroscopically guided therapeutic sacroiliac joint injections for sacroiliac joint syndrome. Am J Phys Med Rehab 2001; 80: 425–432.
18. Maigne JY, Aivaliklis A, Pfefer F. Results of sacroiliac double block and value of sacroiliac pain provocation tests in 54 patients with low back pain. Spine 1996; 21(16): 1889–1892.
19. Dussault RG, Kaplan PA, Anderson MW. Flouroscopy-guided sacroiliac joint injections. Radiology 2000; 214:273–277.
20. Dreyfuss P, Cole AJ, Pauza K. Sacroiliac joint injection techniques. Phys Med Rehab Clin North Am 1995; 6(4):785–813.
21. Dreyfuss P, Dreyer SJ, Cole A, et al. Sacroiliac joint pain. Am Acad Orthop Surg 2004; 12:255–265.
22. Rosenberg JM, Quint DJ, de Rosayro AM. Computerized tomographic localization of clinically-guided sacroiliac joint injections. Clin J Pain 2000; 16:18–21.

12 Cervical and Lumbar Zygapophyseal Joint Disease and Interventions

Ira Kornbluth

Center for Pain Management, Glen Burnie, Maryland, U.S.A.

Jeremy Simon

Orthopedic and Spine Specialists, Physical Medicine and Rehabilitation, Bowie, Maryland, U.S.A.

INTRODUCTION

Neck and low back pain are common, yet challenging problems affecting many patients. The differential diagnosis is quite large and the pain generator(s) may be difficult to tease out from the history, physical, and routine diagnostic studies. Reasons for pain are often multifactorial, and when related to degenerative changes, often involve multiple structures in the spine simultaneously. Diagnosis and treatment is complicated, as numerous studies have shown a poor correlation between imaging findings and patient symptoms (1,2,3). This chapter will discuss the diagnosis and the treatments of cervical and lumbar zygapophyseal (Z) joints of the spine. Zygapophyseal joints have also been implicated as a cause of thoracic pain. We opted to focus this chapter on the cervical and lumbar Z joints as they have been investigated more in these spine segments.

BACKGROUND

In 1911, Goldwaith first postulated that the "facet" joints (the term used in older references) could be a source of low back pain (4). A study from Putti in 1927 first documented osteoarthritis in the facet joints of cadaveric specimens who were over 40 years of age (5). Ghormley coined the term "facet syndrome" in 1933 in reference to low back pain caused by osteophytosis of these joints with subsequent lumbar nerve root entrapment (6). In 1963, Hirsch gave credence to the facet joint as a pain generator in and of itself (7). He and his colleagues injected the lumbar facet joints of volunteers with hypertonic saline, and were able to induce pain in the upper back and thighs.

The term "facet," although still popular in the literature and amongst many clinicians, is nonspecific. There are numerous facet joints in the human body, and therefore, when one is referring to the spine, the more descriptive and preferred term is zygapophyseal joint or Z joint. Zygapophyseal joint syndrome or facet syndrome refers to the irritation of one or more of these joints, and may occur unilaterally or bilaterally, and at one, or more commonly, multiple levels.

EPIDEMIOLOGY

Studies have quoted the overall frequency of neck pain to be as high as 34%, with the duration and development of chronic pain increasing with age (8). In a study of

500 patients presenting to a pain clinic with chronic, nonspecific spinal pain, the prevalence of the Z joint as a generator was determined using diagnostic medial branch blocks. The Z joint was implicated in 55% of those with cervical pain, 42% of thoracic pain, and 31% in lumbar pain (9).

Studies of cervical pain after whiplash injuries implicate the Z joint as a pain generator in nearly 60% of patients (10) and the C2-3 and C5-6 joints were found to be most commonly involved (11,12). These patients often develop significant alterations in their perception of health (13). In a Finnish study of whiplash patients three years postinjury, 11.8% of patients reported that symptoms related to the injury caused their health to deteriorate significantly (14).

Low back pain is an extremely common problem encountered by clinicians of nearly every specialty. In fact, it is second only to the common cold as the leading cause of worker absenteeism, and results in more lost productivity than any other medical condition (15). Up to 90% of adults experience low back pain at some time in their lives (16).

Studies utilizing medial branch blocks as the gold standard for diagnosis indicate the prevalence of lumbar Z-joint pain in patients with chronic low back pain to range from 15% to 40% (9,15). A prevalence of 15% was noted in young, injured workers, and 40% was noted in elderly patients. There may be a higher incidence of z-joint pain with increasing age.

ANATOMY OF THE ZYGAPOPHYSEAL JOINT

The Z joint is a true synovial joint with a fibrous hyaline capsule, articular cartilage menisci, and synovial lining. It lies between the inferior articular process of the vertebrae above and the superior articular process of vertebrae below (Figs. 1–3). The superior aspect of the Z joint faces anterolaterally, and the inferior portion faces posteromedially. The Z joints' menisci help distribute loads over greater articular areas and provide stability.

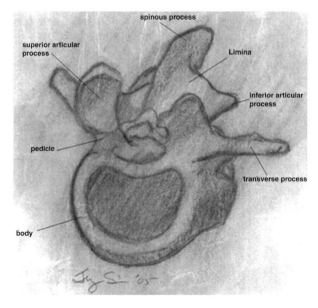

FIGURE 1 Lumbar vertebra (axial-oblique view).

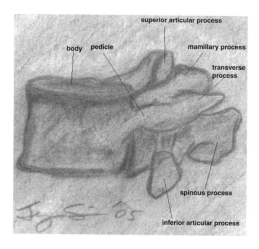

FIGURE 2   Lumbar vertebra (sagittal view).

The capsule of the Z joint is richly innervated by the medial sensory branches of the dorsal rami from the same level and from the level above it. The innervation of the C2-3 joint is different. The C2-3 joint is innervated by C3 (lesser occipital nerve), which crosses the C2-3 Z joint and a communicating branch from C2. In addition to innervating the Z joints, the medial branches also innervate the multifidi, interspinous muscles, and the interspinous ligaments. They contain nocioceptive fibers that can be triggered by capsular stretch and local pressure.

The angles of the Z joints in the cervical, thoracic, and lumbar vertebrae restrict or allow different motions. In the cervical spine, the Z joints are approximately at 45° angles to the coronal or sagittal planes. They also are obliquely oriented in the cephalocaudad direction. The thoracic Z joints approximate the coronal plane, thus limiting shear forces on the thoracic spine. The upper lumbar Z joints are in a predominantly sagittal plane, and develop a more coronal orientation down the spine, with the L5/S1 segment lying most coronal. This orientation allows the upper portion of the lumbar spine to resist rotation, whereas the lower portions resist forward displacement (16). The sagittal lumbar facet orientation permits the facet joints to glide anteroposteriorly, and help facilitate the flexion and extension movements of the lower back (16).

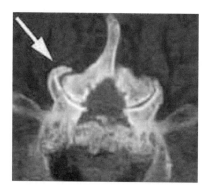

FIGURE 3   Computed tomography with good view of the lumbar zygapophyseal (Z) joint (*arrow*).

PATHOPHYSIOLOGY

The spine is a magnificent structure. Its functions include protection of the spinal cord, attachment sites for various muscles of the neck and back, permission and restriction of various spinal movements, load bearing, and maintenance of an upright posture. This is achieved through an elegant interaction between discs, bones, joints, and ligaments in the spine. When any of these structures are compromised, the result can be a disruption to the entire spinal system. It is for this reason that one cannot discuss disorders of the Z joint without additionally considering the other structures in the spine.

In the normal spine, the intervertebral disc and anterior segment bear 80% of the vertical load. Only 20% of this force is transmitted through the posterior segment, including the Z joints (17). The segments also diminish increasing axial loads in progressively caudal segments. This load reaches 12% to 25% in the lumbar spine. Both the anterior and posterior segments are interdependent, and thus, if the integrity of one segment is disrupted, stress or dysfunction may occur in the other.

The division of labor in the spine is such that the anterior segment primarily serves the functions of weight bearing, shock absorbing, and flexibility. The role of the posterior elements is primarily the protection of the neural elements, restriction and permission of movements, and they act as a fulcrum for movements (17). When the intervertebral disc is desiccated, the posterior elements, including the Z joints, are forced to bear more weight.

There are many possible explanations as to why Z joints can become painful. Theories include joint microtrauma, systemic or focal arthritic processes, synovitis, meniscoid entrapment, synovial impingement, and joint chondromalacia.

HISTORY

The history in patients with Z-joint pain is often nonspecific. It is important to consider other causes of back pain before coming to the diagnosis. Patients with Z-joint pain syndromes classically report pain in the spinal region affected, which is worse with extension and torsional loads. However, increased pain upon extension is certainly not sufficient to formulate a diagnosis of Z-joint pain. Z-joint pain is not associated with motor or sensory loss.

When radiation is present, it does not follow, but may mimic, a radicular distribution. Although there is variation in the referral zones for a given affected Z joint, investigators have found common patterns (18). It is important to keep in mind that often times there are more than one Z joints that is a pain generator. Evaluation and treatment may need to encompass multiple joints.

The C2-3 joint is often implicated in pain that radiates to the head causing occipital headaches. The C3-4 and C4-5 joints have similar distributions, and typically cause pain in the mid-cervical spine that may extend to the lower cervical spine and/or upper trapezius region. It may be particularly difficult to distinguish pain distributions from the C3-4 and C4-5 joints. Referred pattern from the C5-6 joint extends to the ipsilateral shoulder and the cephald third of the scapula. The C6-7 referral pattern is distinguished from the C5-6, as the C6-7 referral pattern is considerably larger and extends to encompass almost the entire scapula, whereas the C5-6 joint usually does not refer below the spine of the scapula (18,19).

Pain owing to stimulation of the L1-2 joint is confined to the lumbar region, whereas referred pain from the L2-3 joint can be experienced at the greater trochanter, lateral thigh and gluteals. The L3-4, L4-5, and L5-S1 joints, all may refer pain that extends from the lumbar region to the gluteals, groin, the great trochanter, posterior and lateral thigh. Buttock pain originates fairly often from the lumbar Z joints, and is most likely from the L4-5 and/or L5-S1 joints (20).

As there is significant overlap in referred distribution from Z joints, it can be hard to determine which joint(s) is a pain generator. Patients often describe Z-joint pain as deep, dull, and aching in quality, frequently localized to the paravertebral area. Pain may be aggravated by twisting movements, stretching, and lateral bending. Pain may be worse in the morning and improve throughout the day.

Often, patients describe an inciting event. In the cervical spine, this is most frequently a rear-end collision resulting in "whiplash." The whiplash syndrome often involves the cervical Z joints (11). The thoracic and lumbar Z joints may similarly be compromised in an extension or rotation-type injury.

Red flags in the history for serious disease include fever, unintentional weight loss, fatigue, saddle anesthesia, progressive neurologic deficits, difficulty in swallowing, progressive gait dysfunction, difficulty with sexual function, bowel and/or bladder incontinence or hesitancy, intractable pain, and night pain.

PHYSICAL EXAMINATION

The physical examination begins when the patient walks into the examining room. The clinician should pay close attention to the patient's gait, noting any lurching, pelvic tilt, the lack or presence of lordosis, and any other altered gait biomechanics. The alignment of the spine and the presence of scoliosis should be noted. In chronic Z-joint disease, the patient may lose the normal cervical or lumbar lordotic curvature.

Palpation should include the paraspinal muscles, and bony elements, including vertebrae. In low back pain, the sacroiliac joint and sacrum should also be palpated. Range of motion may suggest a facetogenic component to the patient's pain. In cervical pain, lateral rotation is often limited on the side of facetogenic pain. In lumbar pain, extension may be limited. A comprehensive neurological examination must be performed, and should include reflexes, muscle strength, and sensory testing (21).

There is a poor correlation between physical examination and the diagnosis of Z-joint-related pain. Although some maneuvers are suggestive, none are specific to this entity. Schwarzer reported up to a 45% false-positive rate when compared with medial branch blocks (15). In evaluating the patient for Z-joint disease, it is also important to rule out other entities that could cause pain in the neck or back.

GENERAL CONSIDERATIONS OF INTERVENTIONAL ZYGAPOPHYSEAL-JOINT PROCEDURES

Informed consent is required before all invasive procedures. Prior to any interventional procedure, the clinician should discuss risks and expected outcome. Sedative anesthesia is often not necessary, but if needed, should be performed with cardiorespiratory monitoring. Intravenous midazolam 1.0 to 2.0 mg is often used for this purpose, as it has a quick onset and is short acting. It is important that the patient not be asleep or incoherent from sedation. Sedation has been shown to adversely affect the validity of diagnostic zygapophyseal-joint injections (22). Excess sedation would prevent the patient from communicating if relief is obtained, pain is experienced from the procedure, and if a perceived new neurologic deficit or other complication has occurred. A driver or escort should accompany the patient upon discharge. To optimize diagnostic injections, patients are instructed to stop pain medications on the procedure day. It is crucial that computed tomography (CT) guidance or fluoroscopy is utilized for these procedures.

Selecting the level(s) which is more challenging is largely based upon a combination of the physician's clinical experience and pain referral patterns. It is important to keep in mind that each Z joint (with the exception of the C2-3 joint) is innervated by two medial branches, and that each medial branch innervates two Z joints. For instance, the L4-5 Z joint is innervated by the L3 and L4 medial branches, and blockade should be performed at the L4 and L5 transverse processes. In the cervical spine, the C4-5 Z joint is innervated by the C4 and C5 medial branches at the C4 and C5 articular pillars. Performing the procedure at one level is not sufficient as only half the joint's innervation is anesthetized (23).

Interpretation of diagnostic tests is based on the patient's subjective pain response prior to and after the procedure. Pain is subjective; utility of the test is largely dependent on the reliability of the patient's subjective response. Patients should be asked about pain level on a numerical scale prior to and after the procedure in addition to what percentage relief (if any) was obtained. Many interventionalists use a minimum of 70% relief on two separate diagnostic tests to warrant proceeding with rhizotomy (19). Some use a more stringent criteria of 80% benefit in order to proceed with rhizotomy (9,24). Patients should attempt to reproduce activity, such as standing and/or lumbar extension that usually provokes pain, and see if this has changed after a diagnostic procedure. The authors typically prefer medial branch blocks to intra-articular injections, as the response tends to be more immediate and easier for the patient to interpret.

Reasons for false-positive responses to diagnostic injections include too much anesthetic used and placebo response. The placebo response is significant as the more invasive the procedure, the higher the placebo response (25). Reasons for false-negative responses include incorrect needle position, vascular injection, and wrong level(s) injected.

Contrast is used to assure proper needle placement. The proximity of a needle to the Z joint or injection itself may reproduce pain. Prior to injection or rhizotomy, the fluoroscope should be rotated to ensure that the needle is not too far medial or anterior. Intra-articular contrast should flow in an arc-like configuration if placement is ideal.

Zygapophyseal joints may develop cysts for unclear reasons. Although not all Z-joint cysts are symptomatic, they can become inflamed and can grow to be fairly large. The cysts themselves can extend to compress the thecal sac or encroach upon exiting nerve roots in the nearby the neural foramen, causing a neurological deficit and/or pain (26).

Findings on CT, X-ray, magnetic resonance imaging (MRI), and other forms of imaging are nonspecific, and cannot be used to establish the Z joints as a source of pain (9,11). Because of the ambiguity in determining whether there is a prominent Z-joint component to the pain complaint based on history, physical examination, and imaging, medial branch blocks are the gold standard in diagnosis. Diagnostic Z-joint injections are indicated if the clinician has a suspicion of a significant Z-joint etiology to the patient's pain.

CONTRAINDICATIONS TO ZYGAPOPHYSEAL-JOINT PROCEDURES

All interventional Z-joint procedures require extensive physician training, and should not be taken lightly, as complications may be disastrous. Erroneous needle positioning is the most likely reason for a bad patient outcome. For instance, if the needle is too far anterior, structures in the neural foramen, such as the dorsal rami, may be lesioned during rhizotomy, and the patient could end up with weakness or deafferentation syndrome. Possible complications need to be discussed with and understood by the patient prior to the procedure and include infection, weakness, deafferentation pain syndrome, thecal sac puncture, and bleeding complications. Patients should be advised to stop anticoagulants in sufficient time prior to the procedure to diminish the chance of an epidural hematoma. In the cervical spine, vasovagal responses and ataxia may occur (27).

The procedures should not be carried out if the patient has difficulty lying prone, infection or suspicion of infection, psychological factors that would affect interpretation of results, the patient is on anticoagulants, or anatomy prevents clear visualization of the Z joints to be targeted by injection. It is more likely that the epidural space, intervertebral foramen, and vertebral artery may be inadvertently entered when attempting an intra-articular joint injection than medial branch block as depth is more difficult to gauge with intra-articular injections. This could have disastrous consequences, particularly in the cervical spine.

INTRA-ARTICULAR ZYGAPOPHYSEAL-JOINT INJECTIONS
General Overview

Intra-articular Z-joint injections provide diagnostic information, and impart therapeutic benefit. A pure diagnostic injection can be performed with a local anesthetic agent alone. In diagnostic injections, a small volume (1 cc or less) is essential to avoid inadvertent extravasation of anesthetic to nearby spinal structures, reducing diagnostic accuracy. Steroid, if used, may well provide protracted relief of pain pertaining to the injected joint. It is always important to keep the possibility of a false-positive response in mind when interpreting diagnostic information from invasive procedures. If pain persists and the diagnosis is not firmly established, another intra-articular injection or medial branch block should be performed, as a reproducible beneficial result lessens the chance of a false-positive response.

Anesthetics of different durations can be used for diagnostic purposes. A prolonged response is expected with a longer-acting anesthetic agent with a briefer response to the anesthetic from a shorter-acting agent. The normal Z joint will accommodate 1.0 to 1.5 mL of injectate. A typical diagnostic injection will utilize 0.5–1.0 mL of 1–2% lidocaine or 0.25% to 0.5% bupivacaine. A typical therapeutic injection will consist of 0.5 to 1.0 mL of lidocaine or bupivicaine and 0.5 mL of steroid. It is important to ask the patient if the injection causes concordant pain, as this information may aid in diagnosis.

Lumbar Intra-articular Zygapophyseal-Joint Injection
Procedure

The patient is placed on the fluoroscopy table in the prone position. The skin area is prepared in a sterile fashion. The C-arm is placed in an oblique position at 10–45° from the anteroposterior (AP) view to obtain the optimal angle of needle insertion into the joint space. The ideal entry point is at the inferolateral edge of the inferior articulating process, as this is the largest area for injection (Fig. 4). Once the target is

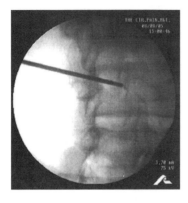

FIGURE 4 Target entry site (*pointer*) at inferior aspect of lumbar zygapophyseal joint.

identified, 1% lidocaine is injected subcutaneously for local anesthesia. A 22- or 25-gauge spinal needle is advanced through the facet capsule. When the Z-joint capsule is entered, the interventionalist typically feels a loss of needle resistance (Figs. 5 and 6). After the joint is penetrated, a small amount of contrast should be injected into the capsule (Fig. 7) to assure the needle is not in a vessel and is indeed in the Z joint. Once proper placement is confirmed, the injectate is slowly delivered with attention to joint capacity.

Cervical Zygapophyseal-Joint Injection
Procedure
The patient is positioned in the lateral decubitus position with the painful side facing upward. The neck is supported with a folded towel or small pillow so as to keep the head in line with the table. It is more difficult to judge needle positioning and gain joint entry when the procedure is done from a posterior approach with the patient prone, and thus we advise that the patient be in the lateral decubitus position. The cervical area is prepared in a sterile fashion and the C-arm is positioned to locate the suspected Z joint(s). A local injection of 1% lidocaine is instilled subcutaneously. Then, a 25-gauge spinal needle is advanced toward the target Z joint, with spot films taken periodically to ensure the proper approach. A 22-gauge needle can also be used, but we utilize a 25-gauge needle as it is less uncomfortable for the patient. The needle is advanced under fluoroscopy toward

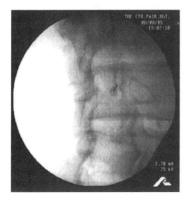

FIGURE 5 Twenty-five-gauge needle entering the zygapophyseal joint. Often, the interventionalist can "feel" entry into the joint. This patient had a joint cyst that was aspirated and her condition improved significantly thereafter.

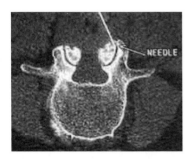

FIGURE 6 Computed tomography showing needle entry into lumbar zygapophyseal joint.

the targeted joint until bony contact is made. The needle is then withdrawn slightly and redirected into the joint. After the joint is penetrated, a small amount of contrast should be injected into the capsule (Fig. 8) to assure that the needle is not in a vessel and is indeed in the Z joint. Once proper placement is confirmed, the injectate is slowly delivered with attention to joint capacity.

Zygapophyseal Joint Cyst Aspiration
Procedure
The treatment of the cysts can be quite challenging. Cysts can be aspirated using a small-gauge needle, although often very little or no fluid is appreciated. Even if adequate synovial fluid is aspirated, cysts may reaccumulate.

Intra-articular steroid injection and cyst distension achieved excellent pain relief in 75% with complete cyst regression in 67% in a case series of 12 patients. If the referral pattern related to the cyst is radicular, a transforaminal epidural steroid injection may be beneficial (28). In another case series of 18 patients with radicular pain related to a Z-joint cyst, transforaminal epidural injections were combined with cyst aspiration. Fifty percent of these patients had significant long-term pain relief (29).

Medial Branch Blocks
Procedure
The patient lies prone on the procedure table for lumbar medial branch blocks, and can be in a lateral or prone position for cervical medical branch blocks. We prefer placing the patient in a lateral position with the painful side up for cervical medial branch blocks. The advantage of the lateral approach is that the articular

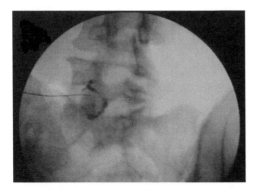

FIGURE 7 Excellent flow of contrast into a zygapophyseal joint. Notice the arc-like configuration.

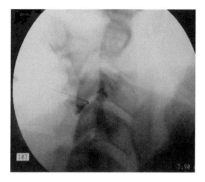

FIGURE 8 Twenty-five-gauge needle in cervical zyga-pophyseal joint with contrast confirming joint spread with no vascular uptake.

pillar can be well visualized, and definite bony contact with the pillar can be made. It is more difficult to judge needle positioning in the AP plane from a posterior approach, and needle placement too far anterior can be catastrophic.

The skin is thoroughly cleansed. The physician uses lidocaine to numb a small area of skin overlying the target. From L1-4, the medial branch lies at the intersection of the superior articular process and transverse process (Fig. 9). At the sacral groove, the L5 dorsal ramus is just adjacent to the sacral superior articular process (Fig. 10). The C3-7 Z joints are similarly innervated by medial branches that run along the articular pillar in the cervical spine, varying in height and position along the vertebral body. The C2-3 joint is unique as the needle should be placed just lateral to the joint at the location of the large third occipital nerve that innervates the joint (Fig. 11).

Once the needle contacts the bone and appears to be in excellent position, a small amount of contrast should be used to confirm injection is not vascular. A small amount of anesthetic is then used to numb the targeted medial branch (Figs. 12–14). The authors use 0.3 to 0.5 cc of 2% lidocaine at each medial branch. It is important to not exceed 1 cc, as excess volume can spread to other structures, such as the nearby dorsal rami.

Radiofrequency Ablation
Indications
If the patient reports profound pain relief on two separate occasions after diagnostic Z-joint procedures, the clinician can proceed to rhizotomy of the involved joints and

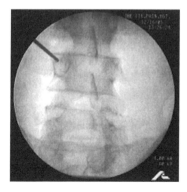

FIGURE 9 A pointer marking the target for injection of the medial branch at the intersection of the superior articular process and transverse process.

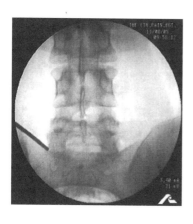

FIGURE 10   A pointer marking the target for injection of the L5 dorsa rami just adjacent to the sacral superior articular process.

expect substantial symptomatic improvement. Diagnostic medial branch injections on two separate occasions or one intra-articular injection and one diagnostic Z-joint injection can be used to firmly establish the Z joints as a significant pain generator. One diagnostic injection does not suffice in firmly establishing the Z joints as a pain generator owing to the high level of false-positive responses. Schwarzer noted a 38% false-positive response rate with one lumbar medial branch block. The sensitivity of a single uncontrolled cervical medial branch block has been estimated to be 95%, and the specificity is 73% (30). Because of the high false positive rate of diagnostic medial branch blocks, a placebo can be utilized to increase diagnostic accuracy (31).

The patient should be made aware that benefit should be long lasting, but pain may return as the medial branch grows back. Pain from ablated Z joints may not return for up to nine months but may be short lived (32). The procedure involves minimum risk in the hands of an experienced physician and little or no sedation should be used.

Procedure

A grounding pad should be placed on the patient and skin overlying the target area prepped and draped appropriately. The C-arm is rotated so the target is clearly in focus. The authors use direct AP C-arm positioning in the cervical spine and an AP view with 5–10° of oblique C-arm angulation in the lumbar spine. The authors use straight needles in the cervical spine and needles with a slight degree bend in the

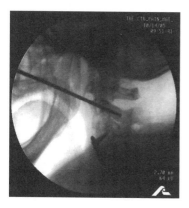

FIGURE 11   A pointer marking the target for injection of the cervical medial branch. Note the cervical fusion below the targeted medial branch. Fusions may increase biomechanical forces across adjacent zygapophyseal joints and accelerate painful spondylytic changes.

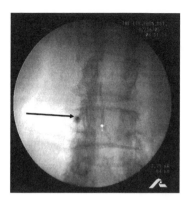

FIGURE 12 Needle in excellent position for lumbar medial branch injection. Note a slight oblique view being used.

lumbar spine. The slight bend is used as it allows easier steering of the needle, and because the authors feel a better lesion is created. Needles should be placed in the same position as they were during the diagnostic medial branch blocks.

In the cervical spine, the radiofrequency (RF) needle is directed ventrally to the location of the medial branch along the articular pillar. Definite contact must be made with the articular pillar. A lateral view should confirm proper placement, ensuring that the needle is not too far anterior. Some clinicians perform rhizotomy from a lateral approach. However, these authors believe a better lesion is created when the procedure is done from a posterior approach, as the RF ablation (RFA) needle can best approximate the medial branch from this method.

The medial branch tends to vary in location along the vertebral pillars. For instance, the C7 medial branch tends to be more cephalad than the remaining vertebral levels where the medial branch is in the mid-substance of the pillars. More than one lesion must be done along the C2-3 Z joint to ensure adequate lesioning of the sizeable occipital nerve.

Once the needle appears to be well positioned, motor and sensory testing are performed. The patient should be told in advance that the machine which will create the lesion will be used to confirm proper needle placement and that the patient will be asked to report any sensation during testing. Most often, patients will report a thumping, throbbing, aching, or pressure-like sensation. Any motor or sensory symptoms in the extremities reported during testing should guide the

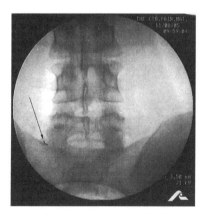

FIGURE 13 Needle in excellent position for injection of the L5 dorsal rami. A straight anteroposterior (AP) view was used for this level.

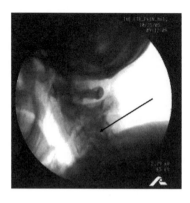

FIGURE 14 Needle in excellent position for cervical medial branch injection. Note a lateral view being used.

physician to reposition the needle and retest before lesioning. Sensory testing is done at 50 Hz, with the voltage slowly increased from 0 to 1 V. Motor testing is done at 2 Hz, with the voltage slowly increased from 0 to 1 V. If the patient experiences axial symptoms at a low voltage, the needle is probably very close to the medial branch as desired. The patient should report axial and not radicular sensations. During motor testing, a thumping sensation is commonly reported by the patient and seen by the physician. The thumping sensation reflects shared innervation with the multifidi, and suggests good needle placement.

Upon confirmation of ideal needle placement using fluoroscopic visualization, sensory and motor testing, the physician can proceed to RF lesioning. Prior to lesioning, the authors advocate using a local anesthetic to numb the medial branch. We use 1 cc of 2% lidocaine. These authors lesion at 80°C for 60 seconds. During lesioning, the patient should be questioned about the presence of radicular symptoms, and the procedure should be terminated if radicular symptoms are reported. Radiofrequency ablation should not be a very painful procedure; significant pain should prompt the physician to consider whether to continue.

CONCLUSIONS

Zygapophyseal joint syndrome can be a challenging diagnosis to make and to treat. This is a common diagnosis, and should be considered in patients with axial back and neck pain. If the physician is confident that the pain generator is the Z joint and noninvasive strategies have failed, consideration should be given to interventional procedures. Once the involved level(s) is identified using diagnostic medial branch blocks and/or intra-articular Z-joint injections on two occasions, strong consideration for RFA should be given. Spinal procedures should only be performed by a trained physician and under fluoroscopic or CT guidance. This reduces accidental injuries and ensures needles are placed in their intended targets. These procedures are not a panacea. Pain may not be relieved completely as multiple structures can contribute to painful conditions.

REFERENCES

1. Boden SD, Davis DO, Dina TS, et al. Abnormal magnetic resonance scans of the lumbar spine in asymptomatic subjects: a prospective investigation. J Bone Joint Surg Am 1990; 72:403–408.

2. Jensen MC, Brant-Zawadzki MN, Obuchowski N, et al. Magnetic resononance imaging of the lumbar spine in people without back pain. N Engl J Med 1994; 331:69–73.
3. Borenstein DG, O'Mara J Jr, Boden SD, et al. The value of magnetic resonance imaging of the lumbar spine to predict low back pain in asymptomatic subjects: a seven-year follow-up study. J Bone Joint Surg Am 2001; 83:1306–1311.
4. Goldwaith JE. The lumbosacral articulation: an explanation of many cases of lumbago, sciatica, and paraplegia. Boston Med Surg J 1911; 164:365–372.
5. Putti V. New conceptions in the pathogenesis of sciatic pain. Lancet 1927; 2:53.
6. Ghormley RK. Low back pain with special reference to the articular facets, with presentation of an operative procedure. JAMA 1933; 101:773.
7. Hirsch C, Inglemark BE, Miller M. The anatomical basis for low back pain. Studies on the presence of sensory nerve endings in ligamentous, capsular and intervertebral disc structures in the human lumbar spine. Acta Orthop Scand 1963; 33:1–17.
8. Bovim G, Schrader H, Sand T. Neck pain in the general population. Spine 1994; 19(12): 1307–1309.
9. Manchikanti L, Boswell MV, Singh V, et al. Prevalence of facet joint pain in chronic spinal pain of cervical, thoracic, and lumbar regions. BMC Musculoskeletal Disorders 2004; 5(15):1–7.
10. Barnsley L, Lord S, Bogduk N. Whiplash injury. Pain 1994; 58(3):283–307.
11. Borenstein DG, Wiesel SW, Boden SD. In: Borenstein DG, Wiesel SW, Boden SD, eds. Low Back and Neck Pain: Comprehensive Diagnosis and Management, 3rd ed. Philadelphia, PA: W.B. Saunders Company, 2004:37–57.
12. Lord SM. Barnsley L. Wallis BJ. Bogduk N. Chronic cervical zygapophysial joint pain after whiplash. A placebo-controlled prevalence study. Spine1996; 21(15):1737–1744.
13. Westerling D, Jonsson BG. Pain from the neck-shoulder region and sick leave. Scand J Soc Med 1980; 8:131–136.
14. Miettinen T, Leino E, Airaksinen O, Lindgren KA. Whiplash injuries in Finland: the situation 3 years later. European Spine Journal 2004; 13(5):415–418.
15. Schwarzer AC, Aprill CN, Derby R, et al. The false-positive rate of uncontrolled diagnostic blocks of the lumbar zygapophyseal joints. Pain 1994; 58:195–200.
16. Braddom RL, et al. In Braddom RL ed. Physical Medicine and Rehabilitation 2nd ed. Philadelphia, PA: W.B. Saunders Company, 2000:854–856.
17. Nachemson A. Lumbar intradiscal pressure: experimental studies on post-mortem material. Acta Othop Scand Suppl 1960; 43:1.
18. Dwyer A, Aprill C, Bogduk N. Cervical zygapophyseal joint pain patterns I. A study in normal volunteers. Spine 1990; 15:456.
19. Fukui S, Ohesto K, Shiotani M, et al. Referred pain distribution of the cervical zygapophyseal joints and cervical dorsal rami. Pain 1996; 68(1):79–83.
20. McCall IW, Park WM, O'Brien JP. Induced pain referral from posterior lumbar elements in normal subjects. Spine 1979; 4(5):441–446.
21. Dvorak J. Epidemiology, physical examination, and neurodiagnostics. Spine 1998; 23(24):2663–2673.
22. Manchikanti L, Pampati V, et al. A randomized, prospective, double-blind, placebo-controlled evaluation of the effect of sedation on diagnostic validity of cervical facet joint pain. Pain Physician 2004; 7:301–309.
23. Fenton DS, Czervionke LF. In: Fenton DS, ed. Image-Guided Spine Intervention Philadelphia, PA: W.B. Saunders Company, 2003:9–72.
24. Dreyfuss P, Halbrook B, Pauza K, et al. Efficacy and validity of radiofrequency neurotomy for chronic lumbar zygapophysial joint pain. Spine 2000; 25(10):1270–1277.
25. Turner J, Deyo RA, Loesser J, Van Korff M, Fordyce WE. The importance of placebo effects in pain treatment and research. JAMA 1994; 271(20):1609–1614.
26. Bureau NJ, Kaplan PA, Dussault RG. Lumbar facet joint synovial cyst: percutaneous treatment with steroid injections and distention–clinical and imaging follow-up in 12 patients. Radiology 2001; 221(1):179–185.
27. Freedman M, Broyer Z, Kornbluth I. Complications of Spinal Injection Therapy and Discography. In: Vacarro A, ed. Complications of Pediatric and Adult Spinal Surgery. New York: Marcel Dekker, 2004:573–592.

28. Slipman CW, Lipetz JS, Wakeshima Y, Jackson HB. Nonsurgical treatment of zygapophyseal joint cyst-induced radicular pain. Archives of Physical Medicine & Rehabilitation 2000; 81(7):973–977.

29. Sabers SR, Ross SR, Grogg BE, et al. Procedure-based nonsurgical management of lumbar zygapophyseal joint cyst–induced radicular pain. Arch Phys Med Rehab 2005; 86(9):1767–1771.

30. Barnsley L, Lord S, Bogduk N. Comparative local anaesthetic blocks in the diagnosis of cervical zygapophysial joint pain. Pain 1993; 55(1):99–106.

31. Niemistö L, Kalso E, Malmivaara A. Radiofrequency denervation for neck and back pain: a systematic review within the framework of the Cochrane Collaboration back review group. Spine 2003; 28(16):1877–1888.

32. Lord SM, Barnsley L, Wallis BJ, McDonald GJ, Bogduk N. Percutaneous radio-frequency neurotomy for chronic cervical zygapophyseal-joint pain. New England Journal of Medicine 1996; 335(23):1721–1726.

13 Epidural Steroid Injections

Kenneth P. Botwin, Beth Palmisano, and Vishal Kancherla
Florida Spine Institute, Clearwater, Florida, U.S.A.

INTRODUCTION

Epidural steroid injections are commonly utilized in treating cervical and lumbosacral pain syndromes. There are two routes to perform cervical epidural injections; these are interlaminar and transforaminal. In the lumbar spine, epidural steroid injections are performed via interlaminar, transforaminal, and the caudal routes.

RATIONALE

Corticosteroid injections have become an integral part of the management of patients with cervical and lumbar pain syndromes. The placement of corticosteroids as close as possible to an inflamed nerve root in patients with sciatic symptoms related to inflammation from disc herniation, spinal stenosis, or chemical sensitivity should help lead to relief of pain (1–3).

ANATOMY

The spine is divided anatomically into three compartments. These compartments have been defined as the anterior, neuroaxial, and posterior compartments (4). The anterior compartment is comprised of the vertebral body and the intervertebral disc. The structures within the epidural space and neural pathways form the neuroaxial compartment and the posterior compartment is composed of the posterior lamina and zygapophyseal joints along with the bony vertebral arch structures. The neuroaxial compartment consists of all structures within the osseous and ligamentous boundaries of the spinal canal. Within this compartment is found the epidural space. The epidural space contains fat, epidural veins, epidural arteries, and lymphatics.

The most common constituent of the epidural space is epidural fat (5). The epidural fat acts as a shock absorber in order to protect the contents of the epidural space and can also act as a depot for drugs and anesthetics injected into the epidural space.

The epidural veins are primarily localized in the anterior lateral portion of the epidural space; the veins themselves can change with an increase in intra-abdominal pressure (5,6). Epidural arteries are also present in the epidural space and supply the surrounding bone and ligamentous structures as well as the spinal cord. Segmental radicular vessels enter the epidural space through the intervertebral foramina (7). These segmental arteries are derived from the aorta, subclavian, and iliac arteries. On entering the spinal canal, the radicular arteries pass through the dura into the intervertebral foramen at the region of the dural cuff. The anterior spinal artery receives most of its blood via these segmental radicular arteries. These radicular arteries can be quite large and the largest of these has been termed the artery of Adamkiewicz.

This artery enters the spinal canal through the intervertebral foramen usually between T8 and L3 and is localized along the left side 78% of the time (8).

The epidural space extends from the foramen magnum to the end of the dural sac at S2. The actual size of the posterior epidural space varies greatly. It expands to 5 to 6 mm at its greatest width in the mid-lumbar spine and gradually decreases to about 3 mm at the S1 level; the diameter is 1.5 to 2.0 mm at C7, 3.0 to 4.0 mm at T-2, and 3.0 to 5.0 mm in the mid-thoracic region (5,9). It is widest in the midline and narrows beneath the zygapophyseal joint.

The epidural space surrounds the dural sac. It is bordered posteriorly by the ligamentum flavum and periosteum and anteriorly by the posterior longitudinal ligament (PLL) and vertebral bodies. Laterally, it is bordered by the pedicles and intervertebral foramina.

The ligamentum flavum has been proposed to be joined in the midline. There appears to be a paired nature to the ligament having both right and left portions (10,11). When a needle is placed in the direct midline area it may actually penetrate through the ligamentum flavum, which may be thin in the midline and thus may lead to a false loss of resistance (LOR). This maybe one of the reported benefits of a paramedian approach compared with a direct midline approach for epidural needle placement (12).

The actual size and shape of the epidural space is determined by the manner of attachment of the dural sac to the walls of the spinal canal. There have been multiple studies that have actually demonstrated a dorsomedian connective tissue band in the epidural space (13). The posterior epidural space is divided by this dorsomedian connective tissue band (plica median dorsalis) and additional transverse connective tissue bands. Thus, the space is compartmentalized which can account for the limitation of flow of the injected substances.

Very few studies have actually been performed to anatomically dissect the lateral and anterior epidural space. The lateral epidural compartments contain nerves and fat, and the anterior compartment contains veins and fat. Hogan (14) evaluated the cryomicrotome appearance of the anterior epidural space and described that the anterior space appears to be filled with veins, which rarely cross the midplane of the PLL and its lateral membrane. The epidural space is filled by a thin layer of areolar connective tissue termed the epidural membrane (15). This membrane surrounds the dural sac and lines the surface of the lamina and pedicles posteriorly and laterally. Ventrally it lines the vertebral bodies and also passes medially deep to the PLL (15). The epidural membrane is drawn laterally to form a circumneural sheath around the dural sleeve of the nerve roots and spinal nerve. An anterior midline septum has been identified, which divides the anterior compartment.

PATHOPHYSIOLOGY

The pathophysiologic mechanisms of action upon which corticosteroids seem to benefit patients with radicular pain remain controversial. There have been several proposed mechanisms of action, which include anti-inflammatory, direct neuromembrane stabilization effects, and modulation of peripheral nocieptor input.

The most common conditions for which epidural steroids are given include spondylosis and herniated nucleus pulposus (HNP). In spondylotic patients, symptoms maybe a result of ischemic neuritis of the cauda equina or nerve root. Impaired epidural venous return can result from an increase in cerebrospinal fluid (CSF) pressure below the level of compression, or disruption of nerve root microcirculation when standing (16–18).

Nerve root edema can result from microvascular injury inside the nerve roots. Edema has been noted to produce pain in nerve roots (19). In patients with stenotic nerve root canals there can also be mechanical compression of an exiting nerve root. The nerve roots have a poorly developed epineurium as they exit the intervertebral foramen rendering them particularly vulnerable to mechanical and chemical injuries (18).

Compression of the large venous plexus within the intervertebral foramen may occur, leading to congestion, ischemia, intraneural edema, and increased intraneural pressure (16).

Patients with degenerative disc disease of the lumbar spine with annular disruption and herniation could have leakage of neurotoxic substances. Multiple studies have demonstrated the adverse histologic and electrophysiologic effects of discogenic inflammatory mediators on neural structures (17,20–22).

The discovery of elevated levels of phospholipase A_2 at the neural interface with herniated disc material by Saal et al. (21), in 1990 helped confirm the role of inflammation in painful lumbar conditions. Phospholipase A_2, an enzyme found in high concentration in the disc material, is responsible for initiating the arachidonic acid cascade, which results in production of leukotrienes, prostaglandins, and other inflammatory mediators (21). The role of these inflammatory mediators in the genesis of discogenic and neurogenic pain syndrome is well accepted. Corticosteroids have been noted to have potent anti-inflammatory properties (23,24). These effects are a result of inhibition of specific leukocyte function including inhibition of leukocyte migration, prevention of the granulation of granulocytes, mast cells, and macrophages, along with stabilization of lysosomal membranes (25).

Corticosteroids have been shown to block nocieptor C-fiber conduction (26) and also inhibit prostaglandin synthesis (27). Another mechanism of action through which corticosteroids achieve pain relief is the inhibition of nerve root edema with resultant improved microcirculation. They may also reduce ischemia and decrease the sensitivity of the prostaglandin-sensitized dorsal horn neurons by inhibiting inflammatory mediators such as phospholipase A_2. A direct inhibition of C-fiber neuro-membrane excitation can occur as well.

Another proposed mechanism by which corticosteroids may act is to interact with norepinephrine and 5-hydroxytryptamine neurons within the dorsal horn substantial gelantinosa, which are known to be involved in the transmission of pain (28,29). This then would suggest that epidural steroids may also modulate nociceptive input from peripheral nociceptors as well.

Overwhelming evidence seems to support that epidural steroids have a substantial role in eliminating the inflammatory reactions, which are presumed responsible for the sensory symptoms associated with radiculopathy (30,31). Studies have been performed in order to assess the effect of corticosteroids on inflamed neural tissue and on the nucleus pulposus with good inhibition of inflammatory mediators (32–34). Thus far, the evidence overwhelmingly seems to support an inflammatory-mediated process, which appears to be controlled with corticosteroids. There seems to also appear to be a direct mechanism of action on peripheral nociceptors.

OUTCOMES/EFFICACY
Cervical Epidural Injections (Interlaminar/Transforaminal)
Review of the literature (Medline/PubMed) has revealed no published randomized controlled studies of cervical epidural steroid injections. However, there have been

other studies evaluating the effectiveness of cervical epidural injections, which warrant review and analysis (35–48) (Table 1).

One randomized trial (44) evaluated the effectiveness of cervical interlaminar epidural steroid injections and showed a positive response in treating cervical radicular pain. There have been few studies evaluating the effectiveness of cervical transforaminal epidural steroid injections. The few studies performed appear to show evidence they are helpful in treating cervical radicular pain (48,49) (Table 2).

Lumbar Epidural Injections

The use of epidural steroid injections in the treatment of lumbar pain syndromes has been extensively studied. There have been many systematic reviews of the procedure and its efficacy in treating the patient with radiculopathy (50–63) (Table 3).

Review of the literature (Medline/Pubmed) has revealed several published randomized controlled studies of lumbar interlaminar epidural corticosteroid injections (64–69) (Table 4).

Four of these studies showed a short-term relief (less than three months) (65–67,70). One study by Dilke et al. (64) did show long-term relief of three months or longer. Two of these studies were randomized and double blinded (67,69). In Cuckler's study in 1985 (69), pain relief was observed only once in 24 hours following the epidural steroid injections, deemed by many as too brief in order to evaluate their full effectiveness.

TABLE 1   Studies on Cervical Interlaminar Epidural Steroid Injection

Study	Number of patients	Injectate	Benefit
Shulman 1984 (35)	136	80–160 mg methylprednisolone	76% had complete or fair relief
Rowlingson 1986 (36)	25	50 mg triamcinolone	64% had complete or >75% relief
Purkis 1986 (37)	58	120 mg triamcinolone or methylprednisolone	65% overall improvement
Warfield 1988 (38)	16	80 mg methylprednisolone	25% relief after six months 62% decreased analgesics
Cicala 1989 (39)	58	80 mg methylprednisolone	70% excellent to good relief
Proano 1990 (40)	61	80 mg methylprednisolone	63% of patients had a 50% reduction in pain
Mangar 1991 (41)	40	80 mg methylprednisolone	75% of patients with HNP had at least 50% relief
Stav 1993 (42)[a]	42	Group 1: 80 mg methylprednisolone epidurally Group 2: 80 mg intramuscular	At one year, 68% of ESI group had relief vs. 11.8% in intramuscular injection group
Ferrante 1993 (43)	100	80 mg methylprednisolone 50 mg triamcinolone	62% of patients with radicular pain had 50% or more relief
Castagnera 1994 (44)[a]	54	Group 1: 10 mg triamcinolone Group 2: 10 mg triamcinolone + 2.5 mg morphine	Overall 79% positive response rate at 3, 6, and 12 mos.
Klein 2000 (47)[b]	62	80 mg methylprednisolone	71% of patients had positive response rate

Note: All studies retrospective unless indicated.
[a]Randomized prospective.
[b]Fluoroscopically-guided epidural injection.
Abbreviations: ESI, epidural steroid injection; HNP, herniated nucleus pulposus.

TABLE 2   Nonrandomized Studies of Cervical Transforaminal Epidural Steroid Injection

Study	Number of patients	Injectate	Benefit
Prospective independent clinical review (48)	68 neck pain and radiculopathy	40 mg triamcinolone acetonide 1 ml 1% lidocaine	93% of patients had good relief for up to seven months
Retrospective analysis (46)	15 spondylitic radicular pain	6–9 mg betamethasone 0.5 ml 1% lidocaine	60% of patients had good to excellent benefits up to 20.7 mo
Retrospective analysis (49)	30 of which were: 16 foraminal stenosis 14 HNP	15 mg dexamethasone	60% of patients had good relief at two weeks and six months

Note: All fluoroscopic-guided except Cyteval et al. (49), which utilized computed tomographic guidance
Abbreviation: HNP, herniated nucleus pulposus.

It should be noted that none of these randomized controlled trials were performed utilizing fluoroscopic guidance, which has been advocated in order to completely assure that the placement of medication is indeed within the epidural space. These studies, however, seem to concur that there appears to be short-term benefits from corticosteroid epidural injections in patients with radicular pain.

Other studies of significant note on interlaminar lumbar epidural steroid injections have shown short-term benefit (71–73).

Kolsi et al. (74) did a pilot prospective randomized double-blind study comparing lumbar transforaminal epidural steroid injections with fluoroscopically guided lumbar interlaminar epidural steroid injections in patients with radicular pain and found no significant difference between the two groups.

Lumbar transforaminal epidural injections have been utilized in the treatment of radicular pain with proven success in the treatment of patients with HNP or lumbar spinal stenosis (LSS) (75–80). There have been several randomized trials studying the effectiveness of lumbar transforaminal epidural steroid injections (76–81) (Table 5).

TABLE 3   Review of Systemic Reviews on Lumbar Epidural Injections

Study	Comments
Kepes 1985 (50)	Average response to 60%
Rapp 1994 (51)	14% positive treatment over placebo
Bogduk 1994 (52)	Only 4 out of 4000 papers against use
Watts 1995 (53)	Effective in both short- and long-term
Koes 1995 (54)	Benefit in short-term only
VanTulder 1997 (56)	Moderate evidence not effective for chronic low back pain without radicular symptoms
McQuay 1998 (57)	Effective for up to 3 mos.
Rosenberg 1999 (58)[a]	Not able to determine effectiveness
Vroomen 2000 (59)	Helped patients with nerve root compression
Nelmans 2001 (60)[a]	Not effective for chronic low back pain or radicular pain
Manchikanti 2001 (61) and Manchikanti 2003 (62)	Favorable evidence for caudal and transforaminal injections
Boswell 2003 (63)	Strong evidence for transforaminal and caudal injections helped manage radicular pain

[a]Concluded not beneficial in chronic low back pain.

TABLE 4 Randomized Controlled Studies of Lumbar Interlaminar Steroid Injections

Study	Number of Patients	Injectate	Benefit
Dilke et al. 1973 (64)	100 with low back pain and sciatica one week to two year duration	Experimental group $n = 51$, 10 ml saline + 80 mg methylprednisolone Control group: $n = 48$	60% of patients in treatment group had improvement vs. 31% in control group. A greater proportion of actively treated patients improved at three months
Snoek et al. 1997 (65)	51 with sciatic symptoms compression documented on myelography	Experimental group: $n = 27$, 80 mg methylprednisolone Control group: $n = 24$, 2 ml saline single injection	No significant difference in both groups at three days and at 14 mo in low back pain, SLR, subjective improvement, and surgery
Cuckler et al. 1985 (69)	73 with low back pain from HNP or stenosis symptom more than six weeks	Experimental group: $n = 42$, 5 ml 1% procaine + 80 mg methylprednisolone Control group: $n = 31$, 2 ml saline + 5 ml 1% procaine	No significant short- or long-term improvement both groups
Ridley et al. 1988 (66)	35 with low back pain and sciatica symptoms on average of eight months	Experimental group: $n = 19$, 10 ml saline + 80 mg methylprednisolone Control group: $n = 16$, 2 ml saline in interspinous ligament	90% in control group improved at one week, two weeks, and 12 wk. At 24 wks, relief returned to pretreatment levels
Rogers et al. 1992 (70)	30 with low back pain	Experimental group: $n = 15$ Control group: $n = 15$	Experimental group had better results than control group
Carette et al. 1997 (67)	158 with sciatica because of HNP	Experimental group: $n = 78$, 8 ml saline + 80 mg methylprednisolone acetate Control group: $n = 80$, 1 ml saline, 3 injections, three weeks apart	Six weeks the experimental group had more significant reduction in leg pain. No difference at three months
McDonald et al. 2005 (68)	92 with sciatic pain Minimum six-week duration MRI consistent with HNP or stenosis	Experimental group: $n = 44$, 8 ml 0.5% bupivacaine + 80 mg methylprednisolone Control group: $n = 48$, intramuscular steroid and 80 mg methylprednisolone	Significant reduction in pain. 10–35 days following injection. No difference long-term between groups

Abbreviations: MRI, magnetic resonance imaging; HNP, herniated nucleus pulposus; SLR, straight leg raise.

TABLE 5   Randomized Studies of Lumbar Transforaminal Epidural Steroid Injection Studies

Study	Number of patients	Injectate	Benefit
Randomized double-blind (78)	55 patients HNP or spinal stenosis 28 experimental group 27 control group	Experimental group: 6 mg betamethasone, 1 ml 0.25% bupivacaine Control group: 1 ml 0.25% bupivacaine	20/28 decided not to have surgery 9/27 decided not to have surgery
Randomized double-blind (82)	160 patients with radicular pain	Experimental group: 2–3 ml bupivacaine, 40 mg methylprednisolone Control group: normal saline	Improvement in both groups in one-year follow up No significant difference
Randomized prospective (77)	48 patients with HNP or radicular pain	Experimental group: 1.5 ml 2% Xylocaine®, 9 mg betamethasone Control group: saline trigger point injections	Transforaminal epidural steroid injection had 84% success Trigger point has a 48% success
Randomized double-blind (81)	31 patients with radicular pain	Experimental group: transforaminal epidural steroid injection, 5 mg betamethasone acetate Control group: interspinous (blind) epidural steroid injection, 5 mg dexamethasone acetate, 2 ml saline	At six days transforaminal epidural steroid injection group significantly better as well as at 30 days and six months
Randomized double-blind (76)	49 patients with radicular symptoms, 24 in steroid group, 25 in normal saline group	Experimential group: 10 mg triamcinolone Control group: paravertebral local anesthetic and intramuscular corticosteroid	Epidural injections more effective than paravertebral injections Epidural perineural injection more effective than interlaminar epidural injections

Abbreviation: HNP, herniated nucleus pulposus.

All these studies reviewed the effect of the injections on radicular pain from HNP. Riew (78), however, did also include patients with central and/or lateral stenosis. All studies showed effectiveness except the Karppinen (82) study.

Randomized studies on caudal epidural injections have been performed (8,83–89). The details of these studies can be seen in Table 6. Upon review of these trials it was noted that four showed positive short-term pain relief (83,84,86,87) and four showed long-term relief (8,83,84,87). Of these studies, three were performed on patients with radiculopathy/sciatica (8,83,86), two studied post-lumbar laminectomy syndrome (86,87), and the other a mixed population (84). Of the studies performed on radiculopathy two were positive (83,86) and one was negative (8) for pain relief. Among the studies on postlumbar laminectomy pain syndrome, one study showed both short- and long-term positive relief (87). Based on two systematic reviews of the literature (90,91), evidence for caudal epidural injections reducing radicular pain is strong for short-term and moderate

TABLE 6 Randomized Studies of Caudal Epidural Steroid Injections

Study	Number of patients	Injectate	Benefit
Randomized double-blind (83)	35 patients with back and sciatic pain: duration several months to several years	Experimental group $n = 16$, 20 ml bupivacaine 0.25%, 80 mg depomethyl-prednisolone Control group $n = 19$, 20 ml bupivacaine, 0.25% 100 ml saline	56% reported considerable relief in experimental group compared with 26% in control group
Double-blind with cross-over (84)	69 patients back and sciatic pain. 26 out of 69 had prior surgery for HNP duration for five to eight months	Two injectates: 1.80 mg depomethylprednisolone bupivacaine and normal saline; if no better after three injections received other injectate	34 out of 58 (54%) patients who received caudal steroid injection had significant improvement 12 out of 49 (25%) who had bupivacaine and saline improved
Double-blind (8)	57 patients with sciatica, median duration four weeks	Exerimental group $n = 23$, 20 ml 0.125% bupivacaine, 80 mg methylprednisolene acetate Control group $n = 34$, 2 ml lidocaine over sacral hiatus	No difference between groups with short-term relief. At three months, experimental group was significantly more pain free
Randomized double blind (86)	23 patients with lumbar root compromise	Experimental group $n = 12$, 80 mg triamcinolone, 23 ml 0.5% procaine Control group $n = 11$, two injections first on admission to trial, then again at two weeks	Significant pain relief and straight leg raise in experimental group short-term. Long-term improved straight leg raise in experimental randomized trial group
Randomized trial (87)	60 patients post lumbar laminectomy with chronic low back pain	Experimental group $n = 29$, 125 mg prednisolone acetate, 40 ml normal saline Control group $n = 31$, 125 mg prednisolone acetate	49% of patients in experimental group improved sciatic symptoms vs. 19% in control group
Randomized trial paralled group (88)	47 postlumbar laminectomy pain patients and long-term	Experimental group: 20 ml normal saline $\pm$ 125 mg prednisolone acetate Control group: 125 mg prednisolone acetate given once a month for three months	No significant difference in both short- and long-term

(Continued)

TABLE 6 Randomized Studies of Caudal Epidural Steroid Injections (*Continued*)

Study	Number of patients	Injectate	Benefit
Randomized (89)	36 patients with low back pain and leg pain	Caudal epidural vs. Lumbar epidural	No significant improvement. No difference between both techniques
		Caudal epidural injection $n = 19$, 15 ml 0.5% bupivaccine $+10$ ml saline 100 mg hydrocortisone Lumbar epidural injection $n = 17$, 10 ml 0.25% bupivacaine $+ 5$ ml saline	

Abbreviation: HNP, herniated nucleus pulposus.

for long-term relief. These authors also showed that there is limited evidence in managing chronic postlumbar laminectomy syndrome, chronic low back pain without radiculopathy, and LSS.

INDICATIONS

Proper patient selection for epidural corticosteroid injection is important in order to optimize outcome and clinical benefit. Essential to the selection process is a through physical examination and review of imaging findings in order to make an accurate assessment of the possibility that the epidural corticosteroids may aid the patient in their functional improvement. Based on the review of imaging studies, the appropriate technique and route of administration of the epidural injection can be planned.

There are several indications for epidural corticosteroids in the cervical and lumbar spine (Table 7). Indications include acute pain, chronic benign pain, and cancer-related pain. Specific indications include lumbosacral radiculopathy, lower back pain syndrome, spondylosis, postlaminectomy syndrome, phantom limb pain, vertebral compression fractures, diabetic polyneuropathy, chemotherapy-related

TABLE 7 Indications for Epidural Steroid Injections

Radiculopathy
Spondylosis/stenosis
Disc herniation
Lower back pain/neck pain
Postlaminectomy syndrome
Vertebral compression fractures
Phantom limb pain
Diabetic polyneuropathy
Chemotherapy-related peripheral neuropathy
Postherpetic neuralgia
Complex regional pain syndrome
Orchalgia/proctalgia
Pelvic pain syndrome
Tension headache

peripheral neuropathy, postherpetic neuralgia, complex regional pain syndrome or
orchalgia, proctalgia, and pelvic pain syndrome (91,92). Studies have shown lumbar
epidural administration of anesthetics combined with steroid and/or opioid are
useful in the palliation of cancer-related lower abdominal, groin, back, pelvic, perineal,
and rectal pain (93). Epidural injections have also been utilized in the treatment
of acute herpes zoster (94). Patients with LSS may also benefit from epidural steroid
(95–100).

Jamison et al. in 1991 (101) described several features, which they believed
resulted in poor response to epidural injections. These include numerous prior
treatments for pain without any improvement, present use of multiple medications,
and back pain, which did not increase with activity.

The number of epidural injections performed depends on the clinical
response observed in the patient being treated. Some patients may require
several epidural injections. However, if a patient has received multiple epidural
injections and receives no significant relief then repeated injections may not be recommended (102,103).

CONTRAINDICATIONS

These can be divided into both absolute and relative contraindications (Table 8).
Absolute contraindications include patient unwillingness to consent to the procedure, known true anaphylactic reaction, and/or allergy to any constituent of
the epidural injection (steroid, anesthetic, or contrast agent), cauda equina
syndrome, anticoagulation, coagulopathy (INR >1.5 or platelets <100,000), and
suspected local or systemic infection (104). Hypovolemia along with uncontrolled
diabetes mellitus and uncontrolled glaucoma are relative contraindications.
Patients who are pregnant cannot have injections utilizing fluoroscopy.

Cervical injections should be withheld if the midline sagittal diameter of the
cervical spinal canal is less than 8 mm. It is suggested that aspirin or aspirin-based
products should be withheld 7 to 10 days prior to procedure and nonsteroidal anti-
inflammatories should be halted three to five days prior to the injection. Sedation
can be administered but should not be to the point that the patient becomes
unaware or nonresponsive (105).

TABLE 8 Contraindications for Epidural Steroid Injections

Absolute contraindications
Unwillingness to consent
True anaphylactic reaction/allergy to injectates
Anticoagulant medications
Coagulopathy
Local infection
Sepsis
Relative contraindications
Hypovolemia
Uncontrolled diabetes mellitus
Glaucoma
Injection through a posterior laminectomy site
Congestive heart failure
Pregnancy cannot use fluoroscopy

FLUOROSCOPIC RATIONALE

Proponents for fluoroscopic guidance in epidural steroid injections advocate utilizing it in order to assure that medications reach the appropriate and desired intervertebral space (106,107). Advocates of fluoroscopic guidance also point to several studies, which have shown that 13% to 30% of the time during lumbar epidural injections and 30% to 40% during caudal epidural injections, experienced injectionists have misidentified the epidural space (104,108–111). El Khoury et al. (104) found that the incidence of incorrect placement of a needle during caudal epidural injections was reduced to 2.5% when fluoroscopy is utilized. Friedman et al. (111) has shown in patients with failed back surgery syndrome that steroids reached the level of pathology only in 26% of the cases when epidural steroid injections were performed without fluoroscopic guidance.

Stojanovic et al. (112) performed a study of 38 interlaminar cervical epidural steroid injections in 31 patients using LOR technique to localize the epidural space. Multiple contrast-enhanced fluoroscopic views were assessed to confirm a satisfactory needle placement. They found a 53% rate of false LOR during the first attempt to enter the epidural space and thus suggested that using fluoroscopy can improve the accuracy of needle placement and medication delivery. They did find that the success rate improved to 75% after second and third repositioning attempts.

Another significant benefit of fluoroscopic guidance is to avoid potential intravascular injections, which can occur in 9.2% of cases despite negative aspiration of blood (108). Sullivan et al. (113) found a similar overall incidence of 8.5% intravascular uptake in lumbar spinal injections with the use of fluoroscopic guidance. Sullivan also found that intravascular uptake was twice as likely to occur in patients over 50 years of age.

The caudal and lumbar transforaminal routes revealed incidence of intravascular uptake of 10.9% and 10.8% at the time while the lumbar interlaminar route had a 1.9% incidence of intravascular injection (113). Furman et al. (114) described the incidence of intravascular injection in lumbar transforaminal epidural injections to be 11.2% and 19.4% in cervical transforaminal injections. Among the lumbar transforaminal injections, there is an incidence of intravascular injection at the S1 level of up to 21.3% (113,114).

TECHNIQUE
Patient Preparation, Procedural and Postprocedural Management, and Care

Preinjection protocol should include patient education regarding the procedure including its risks versus benefits. Informed consent, nothing per OS (NPO) status, and intravenous access may be indicated. Patient evaluation must look at hemodynamic status, noting cardiac, respiratory, and systemic comorbidities, allergies, and screening for any procedural contraindications. Preprocedural preparation includes patient positioning, attachment of cardio-respiratory monitoring equipment, sterile preparation and draping, supplemental intravenous fluids/antibiotics, and oxygen if needed. Postprocedural patient care includes monitoring of vital signs and brief neurological examination to rule out any significant changes. Clinical observation following a spinal injection should take place until the patient is deemed to be stable prior to discharge. Procedure-specific discharge instructions should be verbalized along with a written copy given to all patients. Routine use of all these steps in patients may help minimize potential complications.

Needles

There are numerous needles of different gauges and lengths, which are appropriate to perform interlaminar and caudal epidural injections. These needles may range in size from 17 to 22 gauge (ga). The needles usually utilized are Tuohy (Kimberly Clark, Roswell, Georgia, U.S.A.) needles (Fig. 1). Usually a $3\frac{1}{2}$-in needle is sufficient, however, in large patients a 5- or 6-in needle maybe needed. The Tuohy needle is specifically designed to allow easier passage of a catheter through the needle into the epidural space. Winged Tuohy needles are best utilized when performing the hanging drop technique, which allows the needle to be held with the fingers away from the fluid, placed up to the needle hub during this technique (115). Some physicians may choose to use a standard spinal needle (Quincke-Babcock, BD Medical, Franklin Lakes, New Jersey, U.S.A.) for transforaminal, caudal, and interlaminar approaches. However, it should be noted that this needle may result in higher risk of dural puncture whereas blunt-tip needles such as the Tuohy or other rounded needles such as the Green or Whitacre needles can decrease the risk of dural puncture and headache after accidental dural puncture (116). Smaller needle diameter has also been implicated in lessening the chances of locating the epidural space (117).

Identification of the Epidural Space for the Interlaminar Technique

Two separate techniques exist to help gain access to the epidural space. The first of these techniques is the loss of resistance (LOR) technique. This technique has been described as being performed with a lubricated glass syringe partially filled with air or saline. Some have stated saline is better than air. Potential complications associated with the LOR air technique are pneumocephalus, subcutaneous emphysema, or venous air embolism (118).

Once the spinal needle enters the epidural space, the hub should be observed for any fluid dripping back from the needle, which could indicate a dural puncture with CSF drainage. The drainage of fluid back from the needle, contrast media, local anesthetic, or saline can occur owing to poor compliance of the epidural space, which can worsen by a rapid rate or increased volume of injection (119). This dripping back of fluids, if not CSF, will usually cease within 30 seconds as the epidural pressure re-equlibrates.

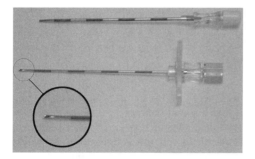

FIGURE 1   Eighteen-gauge nonwinged (*top*) and winged (*bottom*) Tuohy, needle with centimeter graduations.

Volume and Rate of Injection

The volume of the injectate in cervical interlaminar injections can vary from 1.5 to 5 ml of the injectate (35–37,44). However, Cicala et al. (39) have described utilizing 10 to 15 cc in the cervical spine without a noticeable increase in complications.

The spread of injectate in the cervical spine has been evaluated by Stojanovic et al. (112). They found in a study using 2 ml of contrast that the area covered on average was 3.14 cervical vertebral levels. Patients who did have prior cervical laminectomy did have a significant reduction in the number of levels of spread compared with those without a history of prior surgery (2.51 vs. 3.14). Volume of injectate can vary from as little as 3 ml up to 10 ml using the lumbar interlaminar technique (120). Harley (121) stated that 10 ml of dye injected at the L4-5 interspace usually spreads from the L1 to the S5 level. Volume of injectate in caudal injections can be up to 50 ml and transforaminal injection is 1 to 4 ml.

Cyriax (122) reported on the use of 50 ml of procaine following 50,000 caudal injections and had only five adverse effects; one case of hypersensitivity, two cases of transient paraplegia, and two cases of chemical meningitis. All these recovered without any residual damage. Bogduk (123) suggested volumes of 10 ml and 15 ml of epidural injectate are adequate to reach L5 and L4 levels, respectively, during a caudal approach. Bryan et al. (124) found that contrast reaches the L4–5 intervertebral level in 85% of patients with a volume of <8 ml during caudal approach.

A prospective evaluation of epidurography contrast patterns in fluoroscopically guided lumbar interlaminar epidural injections showed that dorsal contrast spread occurred in all patients and 36% of patients had ventral spread; the mean number of levels of spread cephalad was 1.28 and 0.88 levels caudally (125).

Contrast flow in transforaminal epidural injections is ventral and unilateral (125). The rate at which an injection is performed does not alter the pattern of contrast flow (126). An injection administered more rapidly may increase a patient's pain (64).

Cervical Interlaminar Epidural Injection Technique

The patient can be in the seated, lateral, or prone position during the cervical interlaminar epidural injection. The patient is usually placed in the prone position, as this is easier for the C-arm fluoroscopic unit to be maneuvered. The spinal interventionalist identifies the desired interlaminar space (Fig. 2). The injection can be performed with either a midline or a paramedian technique. The midline technique is usually performed at the C7-T1 interspace but can be performed at C6-7 if necessary. Using a guiding needle, the C-arm is situated so that the midline of the interlaminar space is correctly identified. The skin is then anesthetized with 1% lidocaine without preservative or epinephrine. Then the needle (preferred Touhy with or without wing tip) is placed in the direct midline position. For the right-handed operator, the needle hub is held with the left thumb and index finger; and this hand should rest on the patient's back in order to provide stability (Fig. 3A–C). Continuous pressure is applied on the syringe plunger with the other hand, and the needle is advanced. Intermittent use of spot pictures on the fluoroscope can be useful in assuring proper placement and advancement of the needle in the anteroposterior (AP) position. As the needle is advanced through the interspinous ligament and is noted to be in direct midline, the fluoroscope is positioned in a lateral view in order to ascertain the needle depth. The needle is then advanced into the epidural space. Once the needle has reached the epidural space with appropriate LOR to either air or saline, 1 to 3 ml of nonionic contrast (Omnipaque®, GE Healthcare, Princeton, New Jersey, U.S.A. or

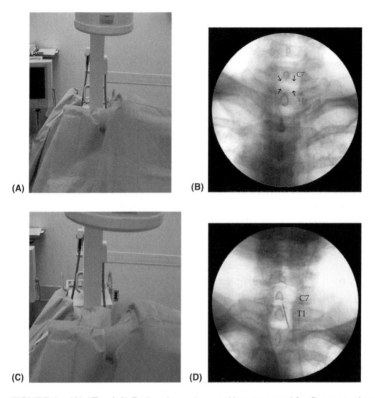

FIGURE 2 (**A**) (*Top left*) Patient in supine position prepared for fluoroscopic cervical interlaminar epidural injection with fluoroscope in anteroposterior position. (**B**) (*Top right*) Anteroposterior fluoroscopic image localizing the C7/T1 interlaminar space. (**C**) (*Bottom left*) An 18-gauge needle used as a skin marker to help localize the targeted interlaminar space. (**D**) (*Bottom right*) An anteroposterior fluoroscopic image of skin marker over C7/T1 interlaminar space.

Isovue®, Bracco Diagnostic Inc, Princeton, New Jersey, U.S.A.) is injected to confirm epidural placement. A lateral fluoroscopic image is obtained (Fig. 3D) and an AP image as well (Fig. 3D). The contrast spread has an areolar appearance. If no intravascular or soft-tissue contrast pattern is seen an injectate of local anesthetic and steroid can be placed into the epidural space. The constituents of the injectate can vary considerably. A combination of local anesthetic and steroid are usually utilized. A common injectate is 3 to 5 ml of 0.5 or 1% lidocaine without preservative or epinephrine and 1.0 to 2.0 ml of corticosteroid. Commonly used corticosteroids are 6 to 12 mg of betamethasone acetate (Celestone®, Schering Corporation, Kenilworth, New Jersey, U.S.A.), triamcinolone acetate (Kenalog®, Bristol-Myers Squibb Company, Princeton, New Jersey, U.S.A.), 40 to 80 mg of methylprednisolone acetate (Depomedrol®, Pharmacia and Upjohn Corporation, Kalamazoo, Michigan, U.S.A.), or 4 to 8 mg of dexamethasone sodium phosphate (Decadron®, Merck & Co Inc., Whitehouse Station, New Jersey, U.S.A.).

The cervical paramedian technique is identical to the midline approach except for the specific site of injection. A paramedian approach can be best utilized in patients with unilateral radicular pain syndromes. Using the fluoroscope the needle is advanced to contact the upper edge of the inferior lamina at the target interspace. The needle is subsequently then walked off superiorly into the

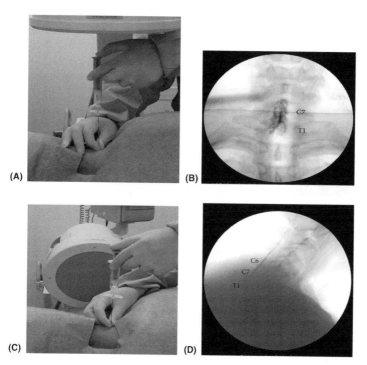

FIGURE 3 (**A**) An 18-gauge winged Tuohy needle being advanced toward targeted interlaminar space utilizing loss of resistance technique with fluoroscope in anteroposterior position. (**B**) Anteroposterior fluoroscopic paramedian cervical interlaminar epidurogram at C7/T1 level. *Note*: The characteristic areolar appearance of contrast media. (**C**) An 18-gauge winged Tuohy needle being advanced toward targeted interlaminar space utilizing loss of resistance technique with C-arm in lateral position. (**D**) Lateral fluoroscopic cervical interlaminar epidurogram at C7/T1 level.

ligamentum flavum and subsequently into the epidural space again utilizing a LOR technique. Following negative aspiration and no drip back of fluid, nonionic contract (Omnipaque® or Isovue®) is then injected to confirm epidural placement. Following this, the injectate can again be slowly injected.

Cervical Transforaminal Epidural Technique
The procedure is carried out utilizing an oblique radiologic view of the targeted intervertebral foramen. This oblique view is obtained by placing the patient either in a supine position or in a slightly oblique position. The patient can be placed in an oblique position by elevating the side being injected with pillows underneath the ipsilateral shoulder and back. After the neck is prepped with iodine-based antiseptic solution and an alcohol solution the targeted neural foraminal level is identified. The C2-3 foramen is the largest utilized in order to count down to the appropriate level to be injected. Once the targeted foramen is identified the skin is anesthetized with 1% lidocaine without preservative or epinephrine. A 25-ga $3\frac{1}{2}$- or a 2-in sterile needle is advanced to the posterior-inferior edge of the foramen until bone is contacted. The needle is then redirected and slowly walked off the bone into the foramen and advanced only a few more millimeters.

Needle depth is checked utilizing both AP views and lateral views. In the AP view, the needle tip should not extend further medially than the midpoint of the

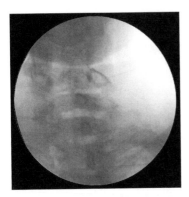

FIGURE 4 An anteroposterior fluoroscopic image of a C5-6 transforaminal epidural injection with Isovue® contrast in the epidural space.

adjacent pedicle. Once the needle is localized in the appropriate position, 0.5 ml of nonionic contrast is introduced through microbare tubing under live fluoroscopy (Fig. 4). If there is no intrasvascular or soft-tissue contrast pattern, then 1 to 2 ml of 0.5 or 1% lidocaine without preservative or epinephrine is injected followed by 1 to 2 ml of corticosteroid such as that listed previously are injected.

Lumbar Interlaminar Epidural Injection

When performing a fluoroscopic lumbar interlaminar epidural injection the patient can be in the seated, lateral, or prone position. The patient is usually placed in the prone position, as it is easier for the C-arm fluoroscopic unit to be maneuvered. Once the patient is in a proper position and is comfortable, the spinal intervention-alist identifies the desired interlaminar space (Fig. 5A and B). The injection can be performed with either a midline or a paramedian technique. The midline technique is performed at the interspace most closely associated with the patients' level of pain. Using a guiding needle placed on the skin, the C-arm is situated, so that the midline of the interlaminar space is correctly identified (Fig. 5C and D). The skin is then anesthetized with 1% lidocaine without preservative or epinephrine. Then the needle (preferred Touhy with or without wing tip) is placed in the direct midline position (Fig. 6A and B). For the right-handed operator the needle hub is held with the left thumb and index finger; and this hand should rest on the patient's back in order to provide stability (Fig. 6C and D). Continuous pressure is applied on the syringe plunger with the other hand, and the needle is advanced. Intermittent use of spot pictures on the fluoroscope can be useful in assuring proper placement and advancement of the needle in the AP position. As the needle is advanced through the interspinous ligament and is noted to be in direct midline, the fluoroscope is positioned in a lateral view in order to ascertain the needle depth (Fig. 6D). The needle is then advanced into the ligamentum flavum and subsequently into the epidural space while intermittent lateral fluoroscopic views are obtained. Once the needle has reached the epidural space with appropriate LOR to either air or saline, 1 to 3 ml of nonionic contrast (Omnipaque® or Isovue®) is injected to confirm epidural placement. A lateral fluoroscopic image is obtained (Fig. 7B) as well as an AP image (Fig. 7A). The contrast spread has an

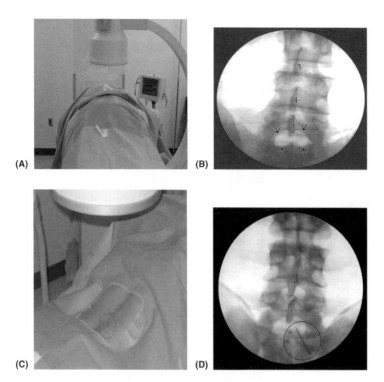

FIGURE 5 (**A**) Patient in supine position prepared for interlaminar epidural steroid injection with fluoroscope in anteroposterior position. (**B**) An anteroposterior fluoroscopic image depicting the targeted interlaminar space. (**C**) An 18-gauge needle used as skin marker over the to help localize the targeted interlaminar space. (**D**) An anteroposterior fluoroscopic image of 18-gauge needle over the L5/S1 interlaminar space.

areolar appearance. If no intravascular or soft-tissue contrast pattern is seen with 1 to 3 ml of contrast an injectate of local anesthetic and steroid can then be placed into the epidural space. The constituents of the injectate can vary considerably. A combination of local anesthetic and steroid is injected as indicated in the previous section on cervical interlaminar injections. The lumbar paramedian technique is similar to the cervical paramedian technique already described.

Lumbar Transforaminal Epidural Technique

Patients are placed in the prone position on a radiology table. Their back is prepped with an iodine-based antiseptic solution and an alcohol solution. The desired intervertebral foramen is identified and the skin is anesthetized with 1% lidocaine without preservative or epinephrine; then, by using a fluoroscope a 22-ga 3.5-inch/90-mm spinal needle or blunt-tipped needle is guided under fluoroscopic guidance to the dorsal/ventral aspect of the neural foramen at the suspected symptomatic radicular level. An AP fluoroscopic view (Fig. 8) is obtained to assure that the needle is directed to approximate the 5:30 position on the right and the 6:30 position on the left, using the pedicle as a clock face. A lateral fluoroscopic view (Fig. 8) is obtained to confirm that the needle is positioned just beneath the pedicle on the anterior epidural space. Aspirations are routinely performed. If

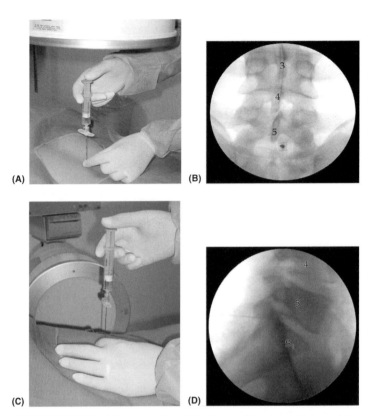

FIGURE 6 (**A**) An 18-gauge winged Tuohy needle advanced toward the targeted interlaminar space utilizing loss of resistance technique with fluoroscope in anteroposterior position. (**B**) An anteroposterior fluoroscopic image of 18-gauge Tuohy needle being advanced in (paramedian technique) to targeted L5/S1 interlaminar space. (**C**) An 18-gauge winged Tuohy needle being advanced using loss of resistance technique with fluoroscope in the lateral position. (**D**) Lateral fluoroscopic image of 18-gauge needle being advance toward the epidural space at the L5/S1 level.

negative for aspirate, 1 to 2 ml of nonionic contrast is injected under real-time fluoroscopic guidance through microbore tubing to confirm epidural flow of the injectate and to rule out intravascular, intrathecal, or soft-tissue penetration. Once the epidurogram/extradural myelogram is obtained, an AP and lateral radiographs are then obtained by a radiologic technician. An injectate of 1 to 2 ml of preservative-free lidocaine and 1 to 2 ml of corticosteroid such as that listed previously are injected.

S1 Transforaminal Epidural Injection Technique

The fluoroscope is positioned over the S1 intervertebral foramen, which will appear as a radiolucent circle under the S1 pedicle. The fluoroscope is adjusted in a lightly cephalo-caudal position with a slightly ipsilateral oblique position in order to superimpose both the anterior and posterior S1 intervertebral foramina. After the targeted foramina are identified, a 3.5-in 25- or 22-ga spinal needle is advanced toward the middle of the caudal border of the anterior path of the S1 pedicle. Lateral view of the sacrum is obtained in order to access the exact location of the

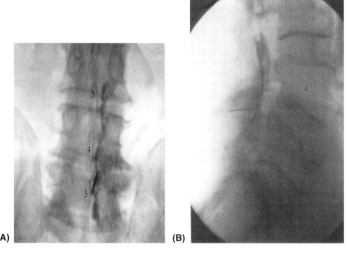

FIGURE 7 (**A**) An anteroposterior fluoroscopic image of a paramedian lumbar interlaminar epidurogram at the L5/S1 level. *Note*: The characteristic areolar appearance of contrast media. (**B**) Lateral fluoroscopic image of a lumbar interlaminar epidurogram at the L5/S1 level.

needle tip. This is taken to be sure that the needle does not enter the pelvic cavity. Once the appropriate target point has been reached, up to 2.5 ml of nonionic contrast is introduced through tubing under real-time fluoroscopic guidance in order to rule out intrathecal or intravascular placement (Fig. 9). Once appropriate epidural placement is achieved, then an injectate of 1 to 2 ml of 1% lidocaine

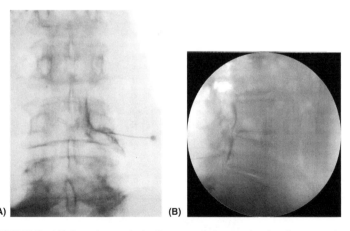

FIGURE 8 (**A**) An anteroposterior fluoroscopic image showing the proper location of the needle at base of L4 pedicle. Isovue® contrast demonstrates the epidural flow medial to the pedicle. (**B**) A lateral fluoroscopic image showing needle positioned in the ventral/superior aspect of the intervertebral foramen at L4-5 with Isovue® (Bracco Diagnostics, Princeton, New Jersey, U.S.A.) contrast demonstrating flow into the anterior epidural space.

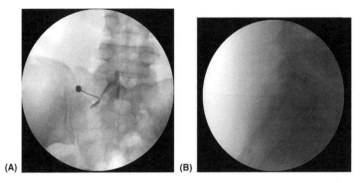

FIGURE 9 (**A**) An anteroposterior fluoroscopic image showing the proper location of the needle at the S1 foramen. Isovue® contrast demonstrates the epidural flow. (**B**) A lateral fluoroscopic image showing the proper location of the needle when performing S1 transforaminal injection.

without preservative or epinephrine and 1 to 2 ml of corticosteroid such as that listed previously are injected.

Caudal Technique
Patients are placed in the prone position on a radiology table. A wedge-shaped pillow is placed under the hips to tilt the pelvis and bring the sacral hiatus into greater prominence. The sacrococcygeal areas are prepared using an iodine-based antiseptic solution, and an alcohol solution. The interventionalist then used the sterile-gloved middle finger of the dominant hand and localized the tip of the coccyx through palpation. In this position, the area under the proximal interphalangeal joint was marked. Using a fluoroscope, a 22-ga, 3.5-inch/90-mm spinal needle or a 20-ga Tuohy needle is guided under intermittent fluoroscopic guidance to the midline of the sacral hiatus (Fig. 10). A lateral fluoroscopic view (Fig. 10) is used to

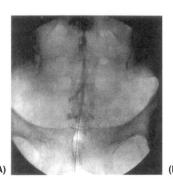
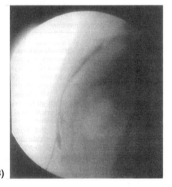

FIGURE 10 (**A**) An anteroposterior fluoroscopic image showing the proper location of the needle in the sacral hiatus. Isovue® contrast demonstrates epidural flow within the epidural space. (**B**) A lateral fluoroscopic view showing needle position in the caudal epidural space with Isovue® contrast delineating an epidural flow pattern.

confirm that the needle was in the caudal epidural space. Aspirations are routinely performed. If negative for aspirate, Isovue® M-300, 1 to 2 ml is instilled to confirm epidural flow of the injectate and to rule out intravascular, intrathecal, and/or soft-tissue infiltration. Once an epidurogram myelogram is obtained, a solution of 10 to 30 ml of 0.5% preservative-free Xylocaine® and 1 to 2 ml of corticosteroid such as that listed previously are injected. Plain radiographs in the AP and lateral views are taken after all injections to document both the contrast pattern and needle placement.

COMPLICATIONS/ADVERSE EFFECTS (TABLE 9)

Infectious complications can arise from epidural steroid injections. These complications can include epidural abscess (127–129), meningitis (130–132), and osteomyelits/discitis (133). Epidural hematoma may be the most serious of the epidural injection complications. Epidural hematomas can develop spontaneously and in patients without evidence of any bleeding tendency, anticoagulation, or traumatic needle insertion (134,135). In a review of epidural steroid injections in 65 published series with a total of 69,047 patients receiving one or more epidural injections, there was only one case of an epidural hematoma (136). Hematomas have been described in the cervical spine (137). Subdural hematoma has occurred after cervical epidural injection (138). Symptoms will vary depending on the location and size of the hematoma. The presentation can be immediate or delayed up to several days (139,140). Magnetic resonance imaging (MRI) is the

TABLE 9 Common Complications for Epidural Steroid Injections

Infections
Epidural abscess
Meningitis
Osteomyelitis/discitis
Neurologic
Nerve injury
Paresthesias
Seizures
Increased sciatic pain
Headaches
Complex regional pain syndrome
Opthalmologic
Retinal hemorrhage
Acute retinal necrosis
Respiratory
Pneumothorax
Recurrent laryngeal injury
Hoarseness of voice
Dysphenia
Dural puncture
Epidural hematoma
Pain at injection site
Anaphylaxis
Dysphonia
Cerebrospinal fluid—cutaneous fistula
Adverse effects from corticosteroids, anesthetics, and contrast media

most sensitive modality in order to diagnose a hematoma, define the extent of its spread, and distinguish it from other space-occupying lesions (139,140). Once identified, treatment of the hematoma can involve high-dose corticosteroid therapy and/or emergency decompressive surgery in order to prevent further compromise of neurologic function.

Neurological injury is an uncommon complication, which can occur when performing epidural steroid injections. Several studies have shown prospectively that the incidence of neurological injuries are approximately 0.002% to 0.7% and are usually self-limiting (141–144). Neurological compromise can also occur from spinal infection such as epidural abscess or epidural hematoma. Several studies have shown prospectively that the incidence of neurological injuries are approximately 0.002% to 0.7% and are usually self-limiting (142–144). There have been case reports of upper limb weakness and nerve root injury as well as intrinsic spinal cord damage from cervical epidural injections (145–148). Complex regional pain syndrome has been reported following cervical epidural steroid injection (149). There have been case reports of transient increased sciatic pain, and parasthesia following lumbar epidural injections (150,151).

Seizures can result from cervical epidural injections. These seizures may be a result of anesthetic-, or cardiac-induced hypotension secondary to neuroblockade. Prolonged protracted seizures can result in brain injury if they last longer than 30 minutes (152).

DURAL PUNCTURE AND POSTDURAL PUNCTURE HEADACHE

The potential complication of entering the subarachnoid space by penetration of the dura exists in any spinal injection. This can occur in any region of the spine (cervical, thoracic, or lumbosacral). The incidence of an inadvertent dural puncture in lumbar epidural injections has been reported to be as low as 0.5% and as high as 5% (153,154). The incidence of spinal headache following dural puncture in the lumbar spine has been reported to be between 7.5% and 75% depending on the technique, experience, and the size of the needle used (155,156). These headaches may be from unrecognized dural puncture causing a leakage of CSF or they may result from inadvertent injection of air into the subarachnoid space (157,158).

When smaller-gauge needles are used in spinal anesthesia there is less incidence of postdural puncture headache. The incidence is approximately 40% with a 22-ga needle, 25% with a 25-ga needle (158–160), 2% to 12% with a 26-ga Quincke needle (161), and less than 2% with a 29-ga needle (162).

If a postdural puncture headache occurs, the headache will usually occur within three days of the procedure. Up to 66% of it begin within the first 48 hours. The headache can also present immediately following a dural puncture (163–165).

The pain associated with the headache is described as being a shearing and severe spreading pain. Distribution of the pain appears to be in the frontal and occipital areas, which can radiate into the neck and shoulders. There tends to be stiffness in the neck and the pain is exacerbated with head movements and relieved with lying down (165). Symptoms that can also appear in dural puncture headaches include nausea, vomiting, hearing loss, tinnitus, vertigo, dizziness, paresthesias of the scalp, and upper/lower limb pains. There have also been reports of visual disturbances such as diplopia or cortical blindness (166,167). There are also reports of intracranial subdural hematomas, cerebral herniation, and death (168).

Review of the literature has revealed that spontaneous rate of recovery from postdural puncture headache is that 85% of patients recover from postdural puncture headache within six weeks (169). However, owing to the severity of the headaches treatment be necessary. This treatment consists of assorted therapies such as rehydration, acetaminophen, nonsteroidal anti-inflammatory drugs, opioids, and antiemetics (170). Caffeine has been utilized in the treatment of postdural headache at a dose of 300 to 500 mg of oral or intravenous once or twice daily (171). The most definitive treatment is an epidural blood patch (172). This technique has a success rate of 70% to 98% if it is performed more than 24 hours after a dural puncture (173). The exact mechanism by which the epidural blood patch eliminates the headache is unknown. Cervical epidural blood patch with 7 ml of autologous blood has been shown to be effective in the treatment of cervical dural puncture headache (174).

Slipman et al. (175) reported that fluoroscopically guided cervical transforaminal epidural blood patch proved to be more effective than a cervical interlaminar blood patch in the treatment of a cervical interlaminar epidural postdural puncture headache. Lumbar epidural blood patch has been shown to be effective even in the treatment of a cervical postdural puncture headache (176).

Complications can arise from the epidural blood patch. Exacerbation of symptoms and radicular pain may occur (177). Pneumocephalus has also been described following epidural blood patch (178). An inadvertent subdural blood patch has been described resulting in a nonpositional persistent headache with resulting lower extremity discomfort (163). Contraindications for doing a blood patch include: sepsis, active neurologic disease, and local infection near the injection site.

Respiratory complications can arise in cervical epidural injections. These complications are very rare and can be the result of sedation, central nervous system trauma owing to needle puncture of the spinal cord or lung (pneumothorax).

Cervical spinal injections can injure the recurrent laryngeal nerve. A patient with such an injury may present with a reduction in their ability to protect their airway and may also have hoarseness. This condition is usually self-limiting and resolves. Dysphonia can result as well (179).

The most common urinary problem is urinary retention, which may follow injections of spinal anesthetic (180). The other possible cause of urological problems can result from an infection such as an epidural abscess or epidural hematoma, which can compromise the spinal cord and/or cauda equina.

PROCEDURE-SPECIFIC COMPLICATION STUDIES
Cervical Interlaminar Epidural Injections
Review of studies evaluating complications/adverse effects of cervical interlaminar epidural injections have been performed (35,37,38,147,181–183). There is one report of superficial infection at the injection site (181). Two studies have been performed to assess the incidence of complications utilizing fluoroscopic technique and reported no major complications (182,183).

Cervical Transforaminal Epidural Injections
Spinal cord infarction has been reported in cervical transforaminal epidurals, possibly through intravascular injection into a radicular artery (184). Brouwers et al. (185) described a cervical anterior spinal artery syndrome after a diagnostic block of the right C6 nerve. Similarly, Rosenkranz (186) described anterior spinal artery syndrome following a left C6-7 transforaminal epidural steroid injection.

A case of quadraparesis and brainstem herniation after a selective cervical transforaminal injection on the right at C5-6 has been reported by Tiso et al. (187). A case of death has been reported during a C7 nerve root block (188). Brady et al. (189) found two complications following 357 transforaminal epidural steroid injections. Both complications were transient loss of consciousness followed by nausea and vomiting. A study by Slipman et al. (190) reported no complications in 20 patients with cervical spondylitic radicular pain who underwent cervical transforaminal injection. Slipman et al. (190) in a prospective study of 89 cervical selective nerve root injections reported the following immediately after the procedure: 22.7% of injections resulted in increased pain at the injection site, 18.2% had increased radicular pain, 13% had light-headedness, 9.1% had increased spine pain, 4.5% had no specific headache, and 3.4% had nausea. Ninety-one percent experienced no complications or side-effects during the procedure. Ma et al. (191) showed no catastrophic complications in a series of 1036 fluoroscopically guided extraforaminal cervical nerve blocks.

Lumbar Transforaminal Epidural Injections
Botwin et al. (192) in their study of 322 lumbar transforaminal injections reported a 9.6% incidence of minor complications, which were entirely transient and resolved without morbidity. Complications included postprocedural back pain at the injection site, increased leg pain, and transient leg weakness.

Huston et al. (190) in a prospective study of 217 lumbosacral nerve root injections found no major complications but did report an immediate postprocedure incidence of 17.1% increased pain at injection site, 8.8% increased radicular pain, 6.5% light-headedness, 5.1% increased spine pain, 3.7% nausea, 1.4% nonspecific headache, and 0.5% vomiting per injection. The potential complications of lumbar transforaminal epidural injections include: infection, dural puncture, nerve injury and vascular infiltration, and hyperglycemia in patients with diabetes.

Fluoroscopically Guided Caudal Epidural Injections
Botwin et al. (193) reported a 15.6% incidence of minor complications in fluoroscopically guided caudal epidural injections. The most common minor complications observed was 4.7% insomnia on the night of injection, 3.5% nonpositional headache, 3.1% increased back pain at injection site, and 0.4% increased leg pain.

REFERENCES
1. Bogduk N, Christophidis N, Cherry D. Epidural use of steroids in the management of back pain. Report of working party on epidural use of steroids in the management of back pain. National Health and Medical Research Council, Canberra, Commonwealth of Australia, 1994, 1–76.
2. Bogduk N. Epidural steroids for low back pain and sciatica. Pain Digest 1999; 9: 226–227.
3. O'Neill C, Derby R, Kenderes L. Precision injection techniques for diagnosis and treatment of lumbar disc disease. Sem Spine Surg 1999; 11:104–118.
4. Bogduk N. The innervation of the lumbar spine. Spine 1983; 8:286–293.
5. Bromage PR. Anatomy. In: Bromage PR, ed. Epidural Analgesia. Philadelphia: WB Saunders, 1978:14.
6. Bowsher D. A comparative study of the azygous venous system in man, monkey, dog, cat, rat and rabbit. J Anat 1954; 88:400–406.

7. Woollam DHM, Millen JW. The arterial supply of the spinal cord and its significance J Neurochem 1955; 18:97–102.
8. Mathews JA, Mills SB, Jenkins VM, et al. Back pain and sciatica: controlled trials of manipulation, traction, sclerosant and epidural injections. Brit J Rheumatol 1987; 26:416–423.
9. Cheng PA. The anatomical and clinical aspects of epidural anesthesia. Curr Res Anesth Analg 1963; 42:398–415.
10. Ramsey RH. The anatomy of the ligamenta flava. Clin Orthop 1966; 44:129–140.
11. Ho PS, Sether L, Wagner M, Ho K, Haughton ZM. Ligamentum flavum; appearance on sagittal and coronal MR images. Radiology 1988; 168:469–472.
12. Blomberg RG, Joanivald A, Walther S. Advantages of the paramedian approach for lumbar epidural analgesia with catheter technique. A clinical comparison between midline and paramedian approaches. Anesthesia 1989; 44:742–746.
13. Blomberg RG. The dorsomedian connective tissue band in the lumbar epidural space of humans: an anatomical study using epiduroscopy in autopsy cases. Anesth Analg 1986; 65:747–752.
14. Hogan Q. Lumbar epidural anatomy: a new look by cryomicrotome section. Anesthesiology 1991; 75:767–775.
15. Schellinger D, Manzh Vidic B, Patronas N, Devekis J, Muraki A, Adbdulla HD. Disc Fragment Migration Radiology 1990; 175:831–836.
16. Hoyland JA, Freemont AJ, Jayson MIV. Intervertebral foramen venous obstruction. A cause of periradicular fibrosis? Spine 1989; 14:558–568.
17. Olmarker K, Rydevik B, Nordberg C. Autologous nucleus pulposus induces neurophysiologic and histologic changes in porcine cauda equina nerve roots. Spine 1993; 18:1425–1432.
18. Rydevik B, Brown MD, Lundborg G. Pathoanatomy and pathophysiology of nerve root compression. Spine 1984; 8:7–15.
19. Olmarker K, Rydevik B, Holan S. Edema formation in spinal nerve roots induced by experimental, graded compression. An experimental study on the pig cauda equina with special reference to differences in effects between rapid and slow onset of compression. Spine 1989; 14:569–573.
20. Olmarker K, Blomquist J. Stromberg J, Nannmark U, Thomsen P, Rydevik B. Inflammatogenic properties of nucleus pulposus. Spine 1995; 20:665–669.
21. Saal JS, Franson RC, Dobrow R, Saal JA, White AH, Goldthwhite N. High levels of phospholipase A2 activity in lumbar spine herniations. Spine 1990; 15:674–678.
22. Takahuski HM, Sugaro T, Okazima Y, Motegi M, Okada Y, Kakiuchi T. Inflammatory cytokines in the herniated disc of the lumbar spine. Spine 1996; 21:218–224.
23. Flower RJ, Blackwell GJ. Anti-inflammatory steroids induce biosynthesis of phospholipase A2 inhibitor which prevents prostaglandin generation. Nature 1979; 278:456–459.
24. Olmarker K, Byrod G, Cornefjord M. Effects of methylprednisolone on nucleus pulposus induced nerve root injury. Spine 1994; 19:1803–1808.
25. Bryan BM, Lutz C, Lutz GE. Fluoroscopic assessment of epidural contrastspread after caudal injection. Seventh Annual Scientific Meeting of the International Spinal Injection Society, Las Vegas, August 13–15, 1999, pg 57.
26. Johansson A, Hao J, Sjolund B. Local corticosteroid application blocks transmission in normal nociceptive C-fibers. Acta Anesthesiol Scan 1990; 34:335–338.
27. Kantrowitz F, Robinson DR, McGuire MB, et al. Corticosteroids inhibit prostaglandin production by rheumatoid synovia. Nature 1975; 258:737–739.
28. Fuxe K, Harfstrand A, Agnati LF. Immunocytochemical studies on the localization of glucocorticoid receptor immunoreactive nerve cells in the lower brain stem and spinal cord of the male rat using monoclonal antibody against rat liver glucocorticoid receptor. NeurosciLett 1985; 60:1–6.
29. Hua SY, Chen YZ. Membrane receptor-mediated electrophysiological effects of glucocortiocoid on mammalian neurons. Endocrinology 1989; 124:687–691.
30. Kang JD, Georgescu HI, McIntyre-Larkin L. Herniated lumbar intervertebral discs spontaneously produce matrix metalloproteinases, nitric oxide, interleukin-6, and prostaglandin E2. Spine 1996; 21:271–277.

31. Kawakami M, Tamaki T, Hashizume H. The role of phospholipase A2 and nitric oxide in pain related behavior produced by an allograft of intervertebral disc material to the sciatic nerve of the rat. Spine 1997; 22:1074–1079.

32. Lee HM, Weinstein JN, Meller ST. The role of steroids and their effect on phospholipase A2. An animal model of radiculopathy. Spine 1998; 23:1191–1196.

33. Minamide A, Tamaki T, Hashizume H. Effects of steroids and lipopolysaccharide on spontaneous resorption of herniated intervertebral discs. An experimental study in the rabbit. Spine 1998; 23:870–876.

34. Korovessis PG. The role of steroids and their effects on phospholipase A2. Spine 2000; 25:2004–2005.

35. Shulman M. Treatment of neck pain with cervical epidural steroid injections. Reg. Anesth 1986; 11:92–94.

36. Rowlingson JC, Kirschenbaum LP. Epidural analgesic techniques in the management of cervical pain. Anesth Analg 1986; 65:938–942.

37. Purkis IE. Cervical epidural steroids. The Pain Clinic. 1986; 1:3–7.

38. Warfield CA. Epidural steroid injection as a treatment for cervical radiculitis. Clin J Pain 1988; 4:201–204.

39. Cicala RS, Thoni K, Angell JJ. Long term results of cervical epidural steroid injections. Clin J Pain 1989; 5:143–145.

40. Proano FA. Cervical steroid epidural block for treatment of cervical herniated intervertebral discs. Pain 1990; 5:S87.

41. Mangar D, Thomas OPS. Epidural steroid injections in the treatment of cervical and lumbar pain syndromes. Corres Regional Anesthes 1991; 4:346.

42. Stav A, Ovadia L, Sternberg A, Kaadan M, Weksler N. Cervical epidural steroid injection for cervicobrachialgia. Acta Anaesthesiol Scand 1993; 37:562–566.

43. Ferrante FM, Wilson SP, Iacobo C, Orav EJ, Rocco AG, Lipson S. Clinical classification as a predictor of therapeutic outcome after cervical epidural steroid injection. Spine 1993; 18:730–736.

44. Castagnera L, Maurette P, Pointillart V, Vital JM, Erny P, Senegas J. Long term results of cervical epidural steroid injection with and without morphine in chronic cervical radicular pain. Pain 1994; 58:239–243.

45. Saal JS, Saal JA, Yurth EF. Nonoperative management of herniated cervical intervertebral disc with radiculopathy. Spine 1996; 21:1877–1883.

46. Slipman CW, Lipetz JS, Jackson HB, Rogers DP, Vresilovic EJ. Therapeutic selective nerve root block in the nonsurgical treatment of atraumatic cervical spondylotic radicular pain: a retrospective analysis with independent clinical review. Arch Phys Med Rehabil 2000; 81:741–746.

47. Klein GR, Vaccaro AR. Efficacy of cervical epidural steroids in the treatment of cervical spine disorders. Am J Anesthesiol 2000; 9:547–552.

48. Bush K, Hillier S. Outcome of cervical radiculopathy treated with periradicular/epidural corticosteroid injections: a prospective study with independent clinical review. Eur Spine J 1996; 5:319–325.

49. Cyteval C, Thomas E, Pecoux E, Sarrabere MP, Cottin A. Cervical radiculopathy: open study on percutaneous periradicular foraminal steroid infiltration performed under CT control in 30 patients. AJNR Am J Neuroradiol 2004; 25:441–445.

50. Kepes ER, Duncalf D. Treatment of backache with spinal injections for local anesthetics, spinal and systemic steroids. A review. Pain 1985; 22:33–47.

51. Rapp SE, Haselkorn JK, Elam K. Epidural steroid injection in the treatment of low back pain: a meta-analysis. Anesthesiology 1994; 78A:923–928.

52. Bogduk N. Epidural steroids for low back pain and sciatica. Pain Digest 1999; 9:226–227.

53. Watts RW, Silagy CA. A meta-analysis on the efficacy of epidural corticosteroids in the treatment of sciatica. Anaesth Inten Care 1995; 23:564–569.

54. Koes BW, Scholten RJ, Mens JM. Efficacy of epidural steroid injections for low back pain and sciatica: a systematic review of randomized clinical trials. Pain 1995; 63:279–288.

55. Koes BW, Scholten R, Mens JM. Epidural steroid injections for low back pain and sciatica. An updated systematic review of randomized clinical trials. Pain Digest 1999; 9:241–247.

56. vanTulder MW, Koes BW, Bouter LM. Conservative treatment of acute and chronic nonspecific low back pain. A systematic review of randomized controlled trials of the most common interventions. Spine 1997; 22:2128–2156.
57. McQuay HI, Moore RA. Epidural corticosteroids for sciatica. An Evidence-Based Resource for Pain Relief. New York: Oxford University Press, 1998:216–218.
58. Rosenberg S, Dubourg G, Khalifa P. Efficacy of epidural steroids in low back pain and sciatica: a critical appraisal by a French task force of randomized trials. Revue du Rhumatisme 1999; 66:79–85.
59. Vroomen PC, deKrom MC, Slofstra PD. Conservative treatment of sciatica: a systematic review. J Spinal Disord 2000; 13:463–469.
60. Nelmans PJ, deBie RA, deVet HC. Injection therapy for subacute and chronic benign low back pain. Spine 2001; 26:501–515.
61. Manchikanti L, Singh V, Kloth D. Interventional techniques in the mangement of chronic pain: Part 2.0. Pain Physician 2001; 4:24–98.
62. Manchikanti L, Staats P, Singh V. Evidence based practice guidelines for interventional techniques in the management of chronic spinal pain. Pain Physician 2003; 6:3–80.
63. Boswell MV, Hansen HC, Trescot AM, Hirsch JA. Epidural steroids in the management of chronic spinal pain and radiculopathy. Pain Physician 2003; 6:319–334.
64. Dilke TF, Burry HC, Grahame R. Extradural corticosteroid injection in the management of lumbar nerve root compression. Br Med J 1973; 2:635–637.
65. Snoek W, Weber H, Jorgensen B. Double blind evaluation of extradural methylprednisolone for herniated lumbar disc. Acta Orthop Scand 1977; 48:635–641.
66. Ridley MG, Kingsley GH, Gibson T. Outpatient lumbar epidural corticosteroid injection in the management of sciatica. Br J Rheumatol 1988; 27:1003–1007.
67. Carette S, Leclaire R, Marcoux S. Epidural corticosteroid injections for sciatica due to herniated nucleus pulposus. N Engl J Med 1997; 336:1634–1649.
68. Wilson-McDonald, J, Graham B, Griffin D, Glynn C. Epidural steroid injection for nerve root compression: a randomized controlled trial. JBJS (Br) 2005; 3:352–355.
69. Cuckler JM, Bernini PA, Wiesel SW. The use of epidural steroid in the treatment of radicular pain. J Bone Joint Surg 1985; 67:63–66.
70. Rogers P, Nash T, Schiller D. Epidural steroids for sciatica. Pain Clinic 1992; 5:67–72.
71. White AH, Derby R, Wynne G. Epidural injections for the diagnosis and treatment of low back pain. Spine 1980; 5:78–82.
72. Klenerman L, Greenwood R, Davenport HT. Lumbar epidural injections in the treatment of sciatica. Br J Rheumatol 1984; 23:235–238.
73. Helliwell M, Robertson JC, Ellis RM. Outpatient treatment of low back pain and sciatica by a single epidural corticosteroid injection. Br J Clin Pract 1985; 39:228–231.
74. Kolsi I, Delecrin J, Berthelot JM, Thomas L, Prost A, Maugars Y. Efficacy of nerve root versus interspinous injection of glucocorticoids in the treatment of disk related sciatica. A pilot prospective randomized, double blind study. Rev Rhum (Eng Ed) 2000; 67:113–118.
75. Lutz GE, Wisneski RJ. Fluoroscopic Transforaminal lumbar epidural steroid injection: outcome study. Arch Phys Med Rehabil 1998; 79:1362–1366.
76. Kraemer J, Ludwig J, Bickert U. Lumbar epidural perineural injection: A new technique. Eur Spine J 1997; 6:357–361.
77. Vad V, Bhat A, Lutz G. Transforaminal epidural steroid injections in lumbosacral radiculopathy; a prospective randomized study. Spine 2002; 27:11–16.
78. Riew KD, Yin Y, Giluyla L. The effect of nerve root injections on the need for operative treatment of radicular pain. A prospective, randomized, controlled double blind study. JBJS 2000; 82A:1589–1593.
79. Botwin KP, Gruber RD, Bouchlas CG, et al. Fluoroscopically guided lumbar transforaminal epidural steroid injection in degenerative lumbar spinal stenosis: an outcome study. Am J Phys Med Rehabil 2002; 81:895–905.
80. Rosenberg SK, Grabinsky A, Kooser C, Boswell MV. Effectiveness of transforaminal epidural steroid injections in low back pain: a one-year experience. Pain Physician 2002; 5:226–270.

81. Thomas E, Cytval C, Abiad L, Picot MC, Taurel P, Blotman F. Efficacy of transforaminal versus interspinous corticosteroid injection in discal radiculagia a prospective, randomized, double-blind study. Clin Rheumatol 2003; 22:299–304.

82. Karppinen J, Malimvaara A, Kunrunlahti M. Periradicular infiltration for sciatica: a randomized controlled trial. Spine 2001; 26:1059–1067.

83. Breivik H, Hesla PE, Molnar I, Lind B. Treatment of chronic low back pain and sciatica. Comparison of caudal epidural injections of bupivacaine and methylprednisolne with bupivacaine followed by saline. In: Bonica JJ, AlbeFesard D, eds. Advances in Pain Research and Therapy. Vol. 1. New York: Raven Press, 1976:927–932.

84. Helsa PE, Breivik H. Epidural analgesia and epidural steroid injection for treatment of chronic low back pain and sciatica. Tidsska Nor Laegeforen 1979; 99:936–939.

85. Bridenbaugh PO, Green NM. Spinal (subarachnoid) neural blockage. In: Cousins MJ, Bridenbaugh PO, eds. Neural Blockade in Clinical Anesthesia and Management of Pain. Philadelphia: J.B. Lippincott, 1998:213–251.

86. Bush K, Hillier S. A controlled study of caudal epidural injections of triamcinolone plus procaine for the management of intractable sciatica. Spine 1991; 16:572–575.

87. Revel M, Auleley GR, Alaoui S, et al. Forceful epidural injections for the treatment of lumbosciatic pain with post operative lumbar spinal fibrosis. Rev Rhum Engl Ed 1996; 63:270–277.

88. Meadeb J, Rozenberg S, Duquesnoy B, et al. Forceful sacrococcygeal injections in the treatment of postdiscectomy sciatica. A controlled study versus glucocorticoid injections. Joint Bone Spine 2001; 68:42–49.

89. McGregor AH, Anjarwalla NK, Stambach T. Does the method of injection alter the outcome of epidural injections? J Spinal Disord 2001; 14:507–510.

90. Abdi S, Datta, S, Lucas L. Role of epidural steroids in the management of chronic spinal pain: a systematic review of effectiveness and complications. Pain Physician 2005; 8:127–143.

91. Waldman SD, Greek CR, Greenfield MA. The caudal administration of steroids in combination with local anesthetics in the palliation of pain secondary to radiographically documented lumbar herniated disc a prospective outcome study with six month follow up. Pain Clinic 1998; 11:43.

92. Wilson WL, Waldman SD. Role of the epidural administration of steroids and local anesthetics in the palliation of pain secondary to vertebral compression fractures. Pain Digest 1992; 1:294–298.

93. Portenoy RK, Waldman SD. Managing cancer pain non-pharmacologically. Contemp OB/GYN 1994; 39:82–87.

94. Waldman SD. Acute herpes zoster and post-therapeutic neuralgia Intern Med 1990; 11:33–38.

95. Rosen CP, Kahanovitz N, Bernstein R. A retrospective analysis of the efficacy of epidural steroid injections. Clin Orthop 1988; 228:270–272.

96. Hoogmartens M, Morelle P. Epidural injection in the treatment of spinal stenosis. Acta Orthop Belg 1987; 53:409–411.

97. Ciocon JO, Galindo-Ciocon D, Amaranth L. Caudal epidural blocks for elderly patients with lumbar canal stenosis. J Am Geriatr Soc 1994; 42:593–596.

98. Botwin KP, Gruber RD. Lumbar epidural steroid injections in the patient with lumbar spinal stenosis. Phys Med Rehabil Clin N Am 2003; 14:121–141.

99. Botwin KP, Gruber RD, Bouchlas CG, et al. Fluoroscopically guided lumbar transforaminal epidural steroid injections in degenerative lumbar spinal stenosis. Am J Phys Med Rehabil 2002; 81:898–905.

100. Barre L, Lutz GE, Southern D, Cooper G. Fluoroscopically guided caudal epidural steroid injections for lumbar spinal stenosis: a retrospective evaluation of long term efficacy. Pain Physician 2004; 7:187–195.

101. Jamison RN, Boncouer T, Feriante FM. Low back pain patients unresponsive to an epidural steroid injection: identifying predictive factors. Clin J Pain 1991; 7:311–317.

102. Raj PP. Prognostic and therapeutic local anesthetic blockade. In: Cousins MJ, Bridenbaugh PO, eds. Neural Blockade in Clinical Anesthesia and Management of Pain. Philadelphia: J.B. Lippincott, 1988:899–934.

103. Swerdlow M, Sayle-Creer W. A study of extradural medication in the relief of the lumbosciatic syndrome. Anesthesiology 1970; 25:341–345.
104. El Khoury GY, Ehara S, Weinstein JN. Epidural steroid injection: a procedure ideally performed under fluoroscopic control. Radiology 1988; 2:554–557.
105. Derby R. Point of view cervical epidural steroid injections. Spine 1998; 23:2141.
106. Stewart HD, Quinnel RC, Dann N. Epidurography in the management of sciatica. Br J Rheumatol 1987; 26:424–429.
107. Manchikanti L, Bakhit CE, Pakanati RR. Fluoroscopy is medically necessary for the performance of epidural steroids. Anesth Analg 1999; 89:1330–1331.
108. Renfrew DL, Moore TE, Kathol MH. Correct placement of epidural steroid injections: fluoroscopic guidance and contrast administration. AJNR Am J Neuroradiol 1991; 12:1003–1007.
109. Mehta M. Extradural block. Confirmation of the injection site by x-ray monitoring. Anesthesia 1985; 40:1009–1012.
110. White AH. Injection techniques for the diagnosis and treatment of low back pain. Orthop Clin North Am 1983; 14:553–567.
111. Friedman B, Nun MB, Zohar E. Epidural steroids for treating "failed back surgery syndrome": is fluoroscopy really necessary? Anesth Analg 1999; 88:367–372.
112. Stojanovic MP, Vu TN, Caneris O, Slezak J, Cohen SP, Sang CN. The role of fluoroscopy in cervical epidural steroid injections: an analysis of contrast dispersal patterns. Spine 2002; 27:509–514.
113. Sullivan WJ, Willick SE, Chira-Adisai W, et al. Incidence of intravascular uptake in lumbar spinal injection procedures. Spine 2000; 25:481–486.
114. Furman MB, O'Brien EM, Zgleszewski TM. Incidence of intravascular penetration in transforaminal lumbosacral epidural steroid injections. Spine 2000; 25:2628–2632.
115. Cousins MJ, Bromage PR. Epidural neural blockage. In: Cousins MJ, Bridenbaugh PO, eds. Neural Blockade in Clinical Anesthesia and Management of Pain. Philadelphia: J.B. Lippincott, 1988:253–360.
116. Bridenbaugh PO, Greene NM. Spinal (subarachnoid) neural blockade. In: Cousins MJ, Bridenbaugh PO, eds. Neural Blockade in Clinical Anesthesia and Management of Pain. Philadelphia: J.B. Lippincott, 1988:213–251.
117. Cluff R, Mehio A, Cohen S, Chang C, Stojanovic M. The technical aspects of epidural steroid injections: a national survey. Anesth Analg 2004; 95:403–408.
118. Shenouda P, Cunningham B. Assessing the superiority of saline versus air for use in the epidural loss of resistance technique; a literature review. Reg Anesth Pain Med 2003; 28:48–53.
119. Usubiaga JE, Wikinski JA, Usubiaga LE. Epidural pressure and its relation to spread of anesthetic solutions in epidural space. Anesth Analg 1967; 46:440–446.
120. White AH. Injection techniques for the diagnosis and treatment of low back pain. Orthop Clin North Am 1983; 14:553–569.
121. Harley C. Extradural corticosteroid infiltration. A follow-up study of 50 cases. Ann Phys Med 1966; 9:22–28.
122. Cyriax JH. Epidural anesthesia and bedrest in sciatica. BMJ 1961; 1:20–24.
123. Bogduk N, Aprill C, Derby R. Precise localization of low back pain and sciatica. Presented at the International Spinal Injection Society Meeting, San Diego, 1993.
124. Bryan BM, Lutz C, Lutz G. Fluoroscopic assessment of epidural contrast spread after caudal injection. J Orthopaedic Med 2000; 22:38–41.
125. Botwin KP, Natalicchio J, Brown LA. Epidurography contrast patterns with fluoroscopic guided lumbar transforaminal epidural injections: a prospective evaluation. Pain Physician 2004; 7:211–215
126. Burn JM, Lang L. Duration of action of epidural methylprednisolone. Am J Phys Med 1974; 53:29–34.
127. Derby R, Baker R, Dreyfus P, Weinstein SM. Cervical radicular pain: transforaminal vs. interlaminar steroid injections. Spine Line 2004; July/August:16–21.
128. Chan ST, Leung S. Spinal epidural abscess following steroid injection for sciatica. Case report. Spine 1989; 14:106–108.
129. Goucke CR, Craziotti P. Extradural abscess following local anesthetic and steroid injection for chronic low back pain. Br J Anaesth 1990; 65:427–429.

130. Cooper AB, Sharpe MD. Bacterial meningitis and cauda equina syndrome after epidural steroid injections. Can J Anaesth 1996; 43:471–474.
131. Dougherty JH, Fraser RA. Complications following intraspinal injections of steroids. Report of two cases. J Neurosurg 1978; 48:1023–1025.
132. Roberts M, Sheppard GL, McCormick RC. Tuberculous meningitis after intrathecally administered methylprednisolone acetate. JAMA 1967; 200:894–896.
133. Tham E. Stoodley M, Macintyre P. Back pain following postoperative epidural analgesia: an indicator of possible infection. Anesth Intensive Care 1997; 25:297–301.
134. Groen RJM, Van Alphen HAM. Operative treatment of spontaneous spinal epidural hematomas: a study of the factors determining postoperative outcome. Neurosurgery 1996; 39:484–509.
135. Inoue K, Yokoyama M, Nakatsuka H. Spontaneous resolution of epidural hematoma after continuous epidural analgesia in a patient without bleeding tendency. Anesthesiology 2002; 97:735–737.
136. Abram SE, O'Connor TC. Complications associated with epidural steroid injections. Reg Anesth 1996; 21:149–162.
137. Williams KN, Jackowski A, Evans PJ. Epidural hematoma requiring surgical decompression following repeated cervical epidural steroid injections for chronic pain. Pain 1990; 42:197–199.
138. Reitman C, Watters W. Subdural hematoma after cervical epidural steroid Injection Spine 2002; 3:E174–E176.
139. Ng WH, Lim CC, Mg PY. Spinal epidural hematoma: MRI aided diagnosis. J Clin Neurosci 2002; 9:92–94.
140. Alexiadou-Rudolf C, Ernestus RI, Nanassis K. Acute nontraumatic spinal epidural hematomas. An important differential diagnosis in spinal emergencies. Spine 1998; 23:1810–1813.
141. DeLeon-Casasola OA, Lema MJ. Postoperative epidural bupivacaine-morphine therapy: experience with 4,227 surgical cancer patients. Anesthesiology 1994; 81:368–375.
142. Auroy Y, Narchi P, Messiah A. Serious complications related to regional anesthesia. Anesthesiology 1997; 87:479–486.
143. DeLeon-Casasola OA, Parker B, Lema MJ. Postoperative epidural bupivacaine-morphine therapy: experience with 4,227 surgical cancer patients. Anesthesiology 1994; 81:368–375.
144. Giebler RM, Scherer R, Peters J. Incidence of neurologic complications related to thoracic epidural catheterization. Anesthesiology 1997; 86:55–63.
145. Cicala RS, Westbrook L, Angel JJ. Side effects and complications of cervical epidural steroid injections. J Pain Symptom Manag 1989; 4:64–70.
146. Hodges SD, Castleberg RL, Miller T, Ward R, Thornburg C. Cervical epidural steroid injection with intrinsic spinal cord damage. Spine 1998; 23:2137–2142.
147. Chan ST, Leung S. Spinal epidural abscess following steroid injection for sciatica. Case report. Spine 1989; 14:106–108.
148. Oza RM, Oleson CV, Formal CS. Tetraplegia after cervical epidural steroid injection: a case report presented at Annual meeting of the Association of Academic Physiatrists, Las Vegas, Nevada, February 28–March 2, 2002. Am J Phys Med Rehabil 2002; 81:528.
149. Siegfried RN. Development of complex regional pain syndrome after a cervical epidural steroid injection. Anesthesiology 1997; 86:1394–1396.
150. Winnie AP, Hartman JT, Meyers HL. Pain clinic II. Intradural and extradural corticosteroids for sciatica. Anesth Analg 1972; 51:990–1003.
151. Warr AC, Wilkinson JA, Burn JMB. Chronic lumbosciatic syndrome treated by epidural steroid injection and manipulation. Practitioner 1972; 209:53–59.
152. Lacey DJ. Status epilepticus in children and adults. J Clin Psychiatry 1988; 49:S33–S36.
153. Bromage PR. Complications and contraindications. In: Bromage PR, ed. Epidural Analgesia. Philadelphia: WB Saunders, 1878:654–711.
154. Barry PJC, Kendall PH. Corticosteroid infiltration of the extradural space. Ann Phys Med 1962; 6:267–273.
155. Nishimura N. The spread of lidocaine and I-131 solution in the epidural space. Anesthesiology 1959; 20:785–789.

156. Boys JE. Accidental subdural analgesia. A case report, possible clinical implications and relevance to "massive extradurals". Br J Anesth 1975; 47:111–113.
157. Abram SE, Cherwenka RW. Transient headache immediately following epidural steroid injections. Anesthesiology 1979; 50:461–462.
158. Katz JA, Lukin R, Bridenbaugh, PO, Gunzenhauser L. Subdural intracranial air: an unusual cause of headache after epidural steroid injection. Anesthesiology 1991; 74:615–618.
159. Barker P. Headache after dural puncture. Anaesthesia 1989; 44:696–697.
160. Flaatten H, Rodt S, Rosland J, Vamnes J. Postoperative headache in young patients after spinal anesthesia. Anesthesia 1987; 42:202–205.
161. Flaatten H, Rodt SA, Vamnes J, Rosland J, Wisborg T, Koller ME. Postdural puncture headache. A comparison between 26 and 29 gauge needles in young patients. Anaesthesia 1989; 44:147–149.
162. Geurts JW, Haanschoten MC, vanWijk RM, Kraak H, Besse TC. Post-dural puncture headache in young patients. A comparative study between the use of 0.52 mm (25 gauge) and 0.33 mm (29 gauge) spinal needles. Acta Anaesthesiol Scand 1990; 34:350–353.
163. Reynolds AF, Jr., Hameroff SR, Blitt CD, Roberts WL. Spinal subdural epiarachnoid hematoma: a complication of a novel epidural blood patch technique. Anesth Analg 1980; 59:702–703.
164. Leibold RA, Yealy DM, Copppola M, Cantees KK. Post-dural puncture headache: characteristics, management, and prevention. Ann Emerg Med 1993; 22:1863–1870.
165. McGrady EM, Freshwater JV. "Spinal" headache—with no headache. Anaesthesia 1991; 46:794–797.
166. Lybecker H, Anderson T. Repetitive hearing loss following dural puncture treated with autologous epidural blood patch. Acta Anaesthesiol Scand 1995; 39:987–989.
167. Schabel JE, Wang ED, Glass PS. Arm pain as an unusual presentation of postdural puncture intracranial hypotension. Anesth Analg 2000; 91:910–912.
168. Eerola M, Kaukinen L, Kaukinen S. Fatal brain lesion following spinal anesthesia. Report of a case. Acta Anaesthesiol Scand 1981; 25:115–116.
169. MacArthur C, Lewis M, Knox EG. Accidental dural puncture in obstetric patients and long term symptoms. BMJ 1992; 304:1279–1282.
170. Ostheimer GW, Palahniuk RJ, Shnider SM. Epidural blood patch for post lumbar puncture headache. Anesthesiology 1974; 41:307–308.
171. Jarvis AP, Greenawalt JW, Fagraeus L. Intravenous caffeine for post-dural puncture headache. Anesth Analg 1986; 65:316–317.
172. Digiovanni A. Epidural injection of autologous blood for post lumbar puncture headache. Anesth Analg 1979; 49:268–271.
173. Abouleish E, Vega S, Blendinger I, Tio TO. Long term follow up of epidural blood patch. Anesth Analg 1975; 54:459–463.
174. Waldman SD, Feldstein GS, Allen ML. Cervical epidural blood patch for treatment of cervical dural puncture headache. Anesthesiol Rev 1987; 14:23–25.
175. Slipman CW, Ed Abd OH, Bhargava A, DePalma MJ, Chin KR. Transforaminal cervical blood patch for the treatment of post-dural puncture headache. Am J Phys Med Rehabil 2005; 84(1):76–80.
176. Colonna-Romano P, Linton P. Cervical dural puncture and lumbar extradural blood patch. Can J Anesth 1995; 42:1143–1144.
177. Woodward WM, Levy DM, Dixon AM. Exacerbation of postdural puncture headache after epidural blood patch. Can J Anaesth 1994; 41:628–631.
178. Kawamata T, Omote K, Matsumoto M, Toriyabe M, Ito T, Namiki A. Pneumocephalus following an epidural blood patch. Acta Anaesthesiol Scand 2003; 47:907–909.
179. Bhat AL, Chow DW, DePalma MJ, et al. Incidence of vocal cord dysfunction after fluoroscopically guided steroid injection in the axial skeleton. Arch Phy Med Rehabil 2005; 86:1330–1332.
180. Armitage EN. Lumbar and thoracic epidural. In Wildsmith JAW, Armitage EN, eds. Principles and Practice of Regional Anesthesia. New York: Churchill Livingstone, 1987:109.

181. Waldman SD. Complications of cervical epidural nerve blocks with steroids: a prospective study 790 consecutive blocks. Regional Anesthesia 1989; 3:149–151.
182. Johnson BA, Schellhas KP, Pollei SR. Epidurography and therapeutic epidural injections: technical considerations and experience with 5334 cases. AJNR 1999; 20:697–705.
183. Botwin KP, Castellanos R, Raos, et al. Complications of fluoroscopically guided interlaminar cervical injections. Arch Phys Med Rehabil 2003; 84:627–633.
184. Baker R, Dreyfus P, Mercer S. Cervical transforaminal injection of corticosteroids into a radicular artery: a possible mechanism for spinal cord injury. Pain 2003; 103:211–215.
185. Brouwers PJ, Kottink EJ, Simon MA. A cervical anterior spinal artery syndrome after diagnostic blockade of the right C5 nerve root. Pain 2001; 91:397–399.
186. Rosenkranz M, Grzyska U, Niesen W. Anterior spinal artery syndrome following periradicular cervical nerve root therapy. J Neurol 2004; 251:229–231.
187. Tiso RL, Cutler T, Catania JA, Whalen K. Adverse central nervous system sequelae after selective transforaminal block: the role of corticosteroids. Spine J 2004; 4:468–474.
188. Rozin L, Rozin R, Koehler SA, et al. Death during transforaminal epidural steroid nerve root block (C7) due to performation of the left vertebral artery. Am J Forensic Med Pathol 2003; 24(4):351–355.
189. Brady RD, Wolff MW, Lagattuta FP. Complications of transforaminal cervical epidural steroid injections. Presented at North American Spine Society 14th Annual Meeting, p. 142–143.
190. Huston CW, Slipman CW, Garvin C. Complications and side effect of cervical and lumbosacral selective nerve root injections. Arch Phys Med Rehabil 205; 86:277–283.
191. Ma DJ, Gilula LA, Riew KD. Complications of fluoroscopically guided extraforaminal cervical nerve blocks. An analysis of 1036 injections. JBJS 2005; 87:1025–1030.
192. Botwin KP, Gruber RD, Bouchlas CG, et al. Complication of fluoroscopically guided transforaminal lumbar epidural injections. Arch Phys Med Rehabil 2003; 81:1045–1050.
193. Botwin KP, Gruber RD, Bouchlas CG, et al. Complications of fluoroscopically guided caudal epidural injections. Am J Phys Med and Rehab 2001; 80:416–424.
194. Browning DHJ. Acute retinal necrosis following epidural steroid injections. American Journal of Opthalmology 2003; 136:192–194.

14 Techniques and Indications of Cervical Discography

Michael J. DePalma

Department of Physical Medicine and Rehabilitation, Virginia Commonwealth University/Medical College of Virginia, Richmond, Virginia, U.S.A.

Curtis W. Slipman

Department of Physical Medicine and Rehabilitation, and The Penn Spine Center, Hospital of the University of Pennsylvania, Philadelphia, Pennsylvania, U.S.A.

INTRODUCTION

Epidemiological reports have sometimes clustered neck and limb pain, but neck complaints are ubiquitous. The prevalence of neck pain with or without upper limb pain ranges from 9–18% of the general population (1–4), and one out of three individuals can recall at least one incidence of neck pain in their lifetime (1). Cervical pain is more frequently encountered in clinical practice than low back pain (5), and traumatic neck pain becomes chronic in up to 40% of patients, with 8% to 10% experiencing severe pain (6). The occurrence increases in the workplace, with a prevalence of 35% to 71% among Swedish forest and industrial workers (7,8). The frequency of occupational cervical complaints increases with age. Approximately 25% to 30% of workers less than 30 years of age report neck stiffness, and 50% of workers over 45-years-old report similar complaints (2,3,9).

Cervical radiculopathy occurs less commonly, with an annual incidence of 83.2 per 100,000, and peaks at 50 to 54 years of age (10). Five to ten percent of workers less than 30-years-old complain of pain referring into the upper limb, whereas 25% to 40% of those over 45 years experience pain in the upper limb (9). Overall, 23% of working men have experienced at least one episode of upper limb pain (9). Neck pain and/or cervical radicular pain are common complaints across different patient profiles.

The cervical intervertebral disc can become a source of chronic cervical pain (11–13). Internal disc disruption (IDD) was first described by Crock over 30 years ago, and is defined by an intervertebral disc that has lost its normal internal architecture, but maintains a preserved external contour, in the absence of nerve root compression (Fig. 1) (14). In traumatically induced chronic neck pain, 20% of patients may be suffering from cervical internal disc disruption (CIDD), and another 41% may be suffering from CIDD and a concomitant facet joint injury at that level (15). Physical examination findings may be underwhelming (16), and imaging studies typically do not discriminate symptomatic from asymptomatic cervical intervertebral discs (17–20). A significant proportion of patients experiencing chronic cervical axial pain will have persistent symptoms despite conservative care (12,21,22). Functional diagnostic testing, such as provocative discography, in which subjective feedback from the patient is mandatory helps clarify the source of these chronic symptoms, and helps to guide surgical intervention (16).

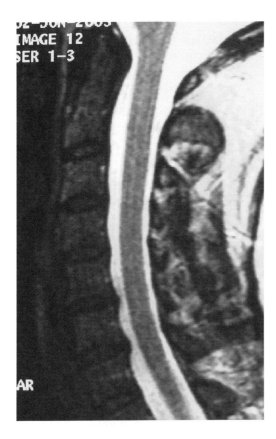

FIGURE 1 Sagittal magnetic resonance imaging (MRI) of cervical spine illustrating relatively normal disc countour with mild loss of disc height and mild to moderate disc desiccation of the upper three cervical discs.

In the late 1950s, Smith (23), and subsequently Cloward (24) independently developed a similar cervical disc injection technique to evaluate patients complaining of cervical and shoulder girdle pain. Each investigator found that injection of symptomatic discs reproduced the patients' axial complaints enabling the clinician to identify which segmental level should be targeted with more aggressive therapeutic intervention. Smith and Cloward utilized discography to select the appropriate cervical levels for their interbody fusion techniques, which are practiced till date (25,26).

In 1964, Holt studied 148 cervical intervertebral discs in 50 asymptomatic penitentiary inmates, concluding that "cervical discography is a painful and expensive procedure and is without diagnostic value" (27). However, Holt completed the procedures using an irritating contrast agent, without fluoroscopic guidance (27,28), and utilizing an injection technique that has been described as suspect regarding mechanical performance, discometric data, and imaging results (29). Despite Holt's disparaging claims, cervical discography has been widely studied playing a viable role as a diagnostic tool to discriminate painfully deranged intervertebral discs from nonpainful adjacent level discs (13,30–34).

INDICATIONS

Painful cervical intervertebral discs manifest clinically as axial cervical pain, sometimes associated with referred pain into the occipital, scapular, upper limb, head, and chest regions (11,35). Therefore, indications for cervical discography include: (*i*) chronic and intractable cervical pain of several months duration despite medical rehabilitation and interventional spine care (32,36); (*ii*) cervical radicular pain, positive root tension signs, and equivocal imaging studies (33); (*iii*) the evaluation of discs adjacent to levels facing impending fusion for spondylolisthesis, fractures, instability, postlaminectomy kyphosis, or myelopathy (36); and (*iv*) prior to therapeutic intradiscal procedures, such as disc decompressive techniques (37). The treating spine specialist should thoroughly rule out the cervical joint pain or radicular pain as the cause of persistent symptomatology to increase the pretest probability of discogenic pain (38).

CONTRAINDICATIONS

Cervical discography must not be performed in the presence of certain structural spinal abnormalities. Incomplete cervical myelopathy could progress to complete tetraplegia upon disc stimulation in the presence of a large disc protrusion (39). Therefore, absolute contraindications to discography include spinal infection, bacteremia, local cellulis or ulceration, neoplasms, central canal stenosis, uncontrolled coagulopathy (28), and symptoms of myelopathy (40). Anticoagulant therapy and contrast dye allergy represent relative contraindications (41). Patients can be covered on low molecular weight heparin after stopping their coumadin, both decisions would need to be medically cleared by the patient's treating physician. Gadolinium followed by magnetic resonance imaging (MRI) may be substituted for omnipague contrast dye in patients allergic to the latter (42).

TECHNIQUE

Prophylactic antibiotics may be administered, but may only be necessary in patients with facial hair, diabetes mellitus, or mitral valve prolapse (40). Typically, 1 g of cefazolin is administered intravenously within an hour prior to the procedure. If a patient is allergic to cephalosporins or penicillins, 600 mg of clindamycin is substituted intravenously for cefazolin (43). Cefazolin (0.5 mL of 10 mg/5 mL) or clindamycin (0.5 mL of 6 mg/5 mL) may be combined with the nonionic contrast medium (300 mg I/mL) to maximize the concentration of antibiotic within the disc space where the infection is likely to occur (43).

The patient is placed in the supine position with two folded sheets placed under his or her shoulders in order to position the neck in mild extension (23). Alternatively, a shallow triangle (28) can be utilized to achieve extension of the cervical spine (Fig. 2). The head is rotated slightly away approximately 10° (23) from the discographer (Fig. 2) (28). After the anterolateral neck is prepped and draped with betadine, or a noniodine-based solution in patients with an allergry to iodine or betadine, and sterile towels, a segmentation count is performed using a cross-table lateral fluoroscopic view (28). Typically, each segmental level is counted sequentially from the C2-3 level down to one level caudad to the last level to be studied (Fig. 3) (28). Longitudinal distraction of both upper limbs may be necessary to adequately visualize C5-6 through C7-T1, as the overlying shoulder girdles can attenuate the X-ray beam obscuring the cervical bony anatomy. This initial survey will allow the physician to judge the orientation of each intervertebral disc space and adjust needle trajectory in order to place the needle tip within the nucleus.

Under a straight posteroanterior view, the targeted disc space is visualized, and the right uncinate process is identified as a landmark (Fig. 4). The fluoroscope

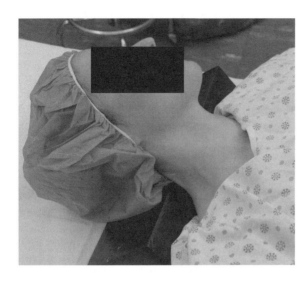

FIGURE 2 A small triangular pillow is placed under the cervical spine to place it into mild extension.

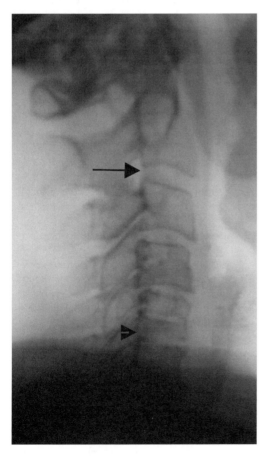

FIGURE 3 Lateral fluoroscopic view of the cervical spine obtained for segmental level count. *Black arrow* depicts the C2-3 disc space and the *arrowhead* highlights the C5-6 disc space.

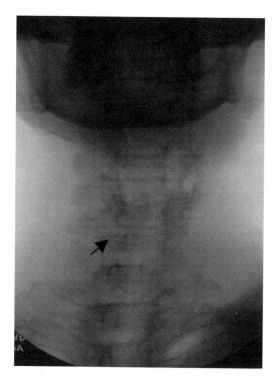

FIGURE 4 A coronal view of the cervical spine allows detection of the uncinate processes (*arrow*).

is rotated ipsilaterally approximately 30° to 45° depicting the proper view for initial needle placement. The skin overlying the medial sternocleidomastoid muscle is infiltrated with 1% lidocaine. A 23- to 25-gauge, 2- to 3.5-inch spinal needle is then advanced under intermittent fluoroscopy into the targeted intervertebral disc. The spinal needle is introduced approximately 30° to 45° obliquely from the midline and slightly below the target disc (23). The left index finger is used to push the carotid artery laterally and the esophagus medially away from the projected needle tract (Fig. 5) (23,24,28) providing a safe path for accessing the disc, at the same time as avoiding the great vessels, larynx, thyroid, and esophagus (44). The carotid pulsations should be felt by the finger tips as the carotid artery is displaced laterally, and deeper digital pressure will approximate the anterolateral surface of the spine in thin patients (24). The 25-gauge needle is held in the dominant hand between the index finger and thumb, and advanced medial to the uncinate process and into the central portion of the disc (23,24,28). The needle tip encounters the superior edge of the caudad vertebral body at which point it is walked superiorly until it enters the cephalad intervertebral disc space (23). The novice discographer should learn to abut the subjacent vertebral endplate with the needle tip to confirm proper depth prior to advancing superiorly and puncturing the annular fibers. The patient will experience a sudden, but transient, moment of cervical and/or shoulder girdle pain upon needle piercing of the annulus (28,35). Occasionally, anterior spondylotic spurs partially obstruct entry into the disc space and must be circumvented by the spinal needle. Although the medial border of the sternocleidomastoid serves as a relative skin surface entry mark, a more lateral approach may be required to avoid the hypopharynx at the

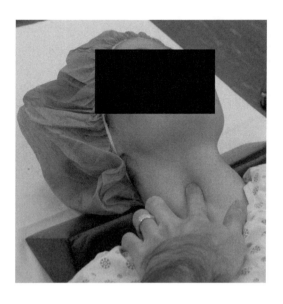

FIGURE 5 The left index finger of the examiner displaces the trachea and esophagus medially and the carotid artery laterally.

C2-3 and C3-4 levels, whereas a more medial entry may be necessary to avoid the apex of the lung at the C7-T1 level (28). The spinal needle will enter the nucleus of the disc if it is directed toward the central third of the disc past the medial border of the uncinate process of the caudal vertebrae. Caution must be exercised to avoid advancing the needle tip through the disc into the spinal cord. Needle position must be examined in both the posteroanterior and lateral views to ensure proper height and depth, confirming needle placement within the central third in both planes.

Upon successful needle placement, nonionic contrast dye is injected under live fluoroscopy in the lateral view. Intraoperative measurements have demonstrated that intact cervical discs will maintain high intradiscal pressures at the same time as accepting 0.2 to 0.4 mL of solution (45). In contrast, discs that permitted posterior extension of contrast dye accommodated 1.5 mL of volume at low, wavering pressures (45). Yet, herniated or degenerated discs with intact outer annular fibers accepted intermediate volumes of 0.5 to 1.5 mL at sustained, yet intermediate, intradiscal pressures (45). Cervical intervertebral discs that accept more than 0.5 ml of contrast dye typically extravasated dye from the posterolateral annular regions (46). Form these data, it is apparent that intact cervical intervertebral discs hold less than 0.5 mL of contrast dye at which point in time, a firm end point is encountered (23,24,28).

Injection of contrast medium within the cervical nuclear confines reveals the integrity of the nuclear–annular interface, known as a nucleogram. Similar to their lumbar counterparts, cervical nucleograms may adopt a variety of configurations, including spherical, disc-shaped, or lobular patterns (Fig. 6). Extension of contrast material beyond the nuclear region denotes annular disruption. However, the fleeing of contrast material from the nucleus into the uncinate recesses can occur with aging, and may reflect maturation of the disc's internal architecture (28,47). Disruption of the annular fibers allows extension of nuclear material into the outer third of the annulus sensitizing annular nociceptive nerve fibers (48) producing pain. A cervical intervertebral disc can only be judged to be a source

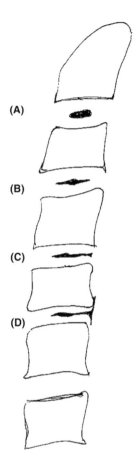

FIGURE 6 Schematic illustration of lobular (**A**), irregular (**B**), fissured (**C**), and ruptured (**D**) nucleograms.

of chronic neck pain if it produces the patient's symptoms, even as demonstrating annular disruption in the axial plane. Hence, postdiscography computed tomography (CT) must be performed to allow analysis of the nucleogram in the axial plane.

Transverse imaging of the cervical intervertebral disc can be challenging owing to the small volume of contrast agent injected and the sparse nuclear dispersal pattern (28). High resolution, thin-section computed axial tomography (CT) can capture postdiscography nuclear detail not revealed by magnetic resonance imaging (MRI) or CT alone (28). Sections are obtained at 1.5-mm slices at a gantry angle parallel to each intervertebral disc space (28).

INTERPRETATION

Despite the early contention questioning cervical discography's diagnostic value (27,49), cervical discography has become a useful diagnostic tool to help guide further therapeutic intervention (13,30–34). However, as with any diagnostic test, the pretest probability influences the test results, and errors must be minimized to improve the test's accuracy. The utility of cervical discography lies in its ability to reveal which intervertebral disc is responsible for the patient's symptoms. Discography represents a functional diagnostic test by virtue of the fact that the patient's subjective response is integral in the outcome of the test. Conversely, visual anatomic testing, such as imaging evaluations can capture diagnostic information, regardless of the patient's report of symptomatology.

Discography requires the diagnostician to assign clinical significance to structural abnormalities, revealed by nucleogram patterns. The patient's response to stimulation of the intervertebral disc is evaluated as the contrast medium is injected under lateral fluoroscopic monitoring. Typically, the patient is instructed to notify the examiner if he or she experiences any cervical pain or pressure as the contrast solution is injected. The sensation of pressure does not indicate a symptomatic intervertebral disc. If the patient complains of pain, the examiner immediately identifies, via targeted questioning, the precise location of the pain, its quality, and severity on a scale of 0 to 10. We then verify if this pain is the patient's exact pain in location and character, and confirm that we are provoking their usual symptomatology. Furthermore, we assess for whether or not the disc stimulation produced all of the patient's usual pain or just a portion of it. During the procedure for each level interrogated, we record the pain location, its character, severity, and whether it was concordant or partially concordant with their typical symptoms.

As we monitor the patient's response, it is imperative to evaluate the nuclear pattern as the contrast dye is injected. At each segmental level, in addition to the aforementioned criteria, the nulceogram pattern, the volume of dye injected to reach this pattern, and the endpoint resistance are recorded as well. If the dye reaches the outer annular fibers concurrently with the patient's report of concordant pain, and the severity of this pain is rated at least 7/10 or higher by the patient, that segmental disc is probably the source of the patient's neck pain. However, the spread of the contrast pattern must be assessed in the axial plane by postdiscography CT. Extension of the contrast to the outer annular fibers or beyond into the epidural space indicates a structurally incompetent disc, providing evidence of internal derangement responsible for the concordant pain described by the patient. Partially concordant pain would implicate that the segmental level is responsible for a piece but not all the symptoms of the patient, or that every portion of the internal derangement was not adequately stimulated to provoke every aspect of the pain location (50). The need to systematically and meticulously collect specific and precise information from the patient during the intervention requires that the patient remain cognizant to respond to our inquiries. It is for this reason that sedation should be avoided unless absolutely necessary. In our experience, however, performance of provocative, cervical discography without sedation has been proven tolerable by patients undergoing the examination.

The physiologic status of the cervical intervertebral disc can be assessed to confirm the nucleogram. The hydrodynamic biomechanics of the disc will typically corroborate what the clinician is witnessing under lateral fluoroscopy. If the cervical disc accepts more than 0.5 mL of contrast, annular disruption is likely to be present (45). The endpoint will help indicate whether the outer annular fibers are completely disrupted. In the scenario of complete annular dysfunction, the discographer will likely observe morphologic evidence of this as dye escapes posteriorly into the anterior epidural space. An endpoint may never be encountered if contrast volumes of 1.0 to 1.5 mL are infused. Conversely, a herniated or degenerate cervical disc that still contains intact outer annular fibers may demonstrate a soft yet still definable endpoint upon injection of 0.5 to 1.0 mL of contrast without evidence of epidural spread. Therefore, it is imperative that each of these data is meticulously collected and quickly audited to assign clinical meaning to the preliminary outcome of the diagnostic intradiscal procedure.

Examination of the nuclear contrast pattern in the axial plane via postdiscography CT will validate extension of contrast material into circumferential or radial annular tears, which may not be fully appreciated during fluoroscopy. Contrast material may reside within the uncinate recesses of the posterolateral regions of the cervical intervertebral disc. On posterioanterior fluoroscopic view, this pattern appears bulbous, and on corresponding lateral views, this dye pattern appears to indicate a posterior protrusion (28). However, postdiscography CT in this instance would reveal contrast within the nucleus and uncinate recesses solely. The apparent protrusion on the lateral fluoroscopic view was created by extension of contrast material into the posterolateral-oriented uncinate recesses (28). Observation of a relatively firm endpoint at a volume at or near 0.5 mL would have suggested to the discographer the fallacy of the seemingly abnormal dye pattern on the lateral fluoroscopic view.

Intervertebral discs that do not demonstrate encroachment of the outer annular fibers by contrast material have been observed to seemingly produce cervical pain during discography. In these instances, a relatively mildly degenerate disc with a relatively firm endpoint close to 0.5 mL of contrast dye may be associated with partially concordant neck pain. The adjacent, caudal disc probably would reveal annular disruption and concordant symptomatology. When we encounter this scenario, we will subsequently anesthetize the painful disc that demonstrated the abnormal nucleogram with 0.5 mL of 2% xylocaine and repeat stimulation of the cranial level after 10 minutes have elapsed. If no pain is reproduced upon repeat stimulation of the normal nucleogram disc after anesthetization of the abnormal level, the initially painful response of the more cranial level was a false positive response. This occurrence might be explained by a pressure-transduction phenomenon, but this postulate has not been further evaluated in a systematic manner.

A positive level is defined therefore, as an intervertebral disc that produces severe, concordant or partially concordant pain upon injection of contrast material that reaches the outer annular fibers, at the time of pain provocation, as demonstrated during fluoroscopy, and confirmed with axial postdiscography CT. Additionally, an adjacent control level must not produce pain upon stimulation. If the discogram reveals one or two contiguous levels producing concordant pain, then the patient might be a surgical candidate, provided conservative care has failed. If three or more levels are concordant, two levels are noncontiguous, or any concordantly painful discs are lobular, then the patient requires a comprehensive chronic pain modulation program.

COMPLICATIONS

Discitis, subdural empyema, spinal cord injury, vascular injury, and prevertebral abscess have all been reported as complications of provocative cervical discography (31,39,51–55). Infection of the disc space is the most widely recognized complication associated with diagnostic cervical discography (31,40,52,54–55). A variety of causes have been postulated, including inadequate skin preparation (55), needle contamination (39), and contamination from esophageal contents owing to improper needle placement (24). Epidural, subdural, or retropharyngeal abscess may occur as sequelae of disc space infection or as the primary source of infection after penetration of the esophagus or hypopharynx (53). Yet, the incidence of discitis per patient is low ranging from 0.1% to 1% with a per disc incidence of 0.15 to 0.2% (31,40,52,54,55). Risk factors for infectious complications appear to include beards, thick or short necks, and male gender (40). Preprocedure prophylactic antibiotics may not always prevent infectious complications after cervical discography (40). Intradiscal antibiotics are most likely sufficient to ward against disc-space infections related to discography, and may obviate the need for systemic antibiotic prophylaxis (56).

Spinal cord compression and myelopathy are rare complications of cervical discography (39). However, this has occurred in a cervical spine with significant preprocedure cord compromise. Although potential intervertebral disc injury from nuclear distension has been suggested (57), possibly explaining cord involvement, no subsequent experimental studies have corroborated such speculation. The overall incidence of significant complications associated with cervical provocative discography in the largest published report that has been observed to be 0.6% per patient, all of which were infectious (40). These findings corroborate our experience in performing 3500 diagnostic or therapeutic cervical intradiscal procedures during which no infections were noted. Only one case of a cervical hematoma was encountered that resolved without airway compromise. We must highlight that these low rates of serious complications related to cervical discography can only be expected in the hands of experienced and well-trained interventional spine specialists.

UTILITY OF CERVICAL PROVOCATIVE DISCOGRAPHY

The only surgical treatment for CIDD or symptomatic cervical degenerative discs is fusion (58–60), which can be accomplished by anterior cervical discectomy and fusion or by posterior fusion. The rationale is that by fusing the bony vertebral elements, motion is eliminated, thereby reducing discogenic pain. The utility of provocative discography to determine the level(s) to fuse is controversial. Some authors have reported "good or excellent" results in 70% to 96% of patients after cervical fusion of levels determined by discography (13,31,34,61). Siebenrock (34) observed a pain reduction of greater than 75% in 96% of 27 patients who underwent cervical fusion of a total of 39 levels. The review was retrospective, and the authors might have included some patients who had primarily radicular complaints. Garvey et al. (32) found that 82% of 87 patients reported their self-perceived outcome as good, very good, or excellent at a mean of 4.4 years after fusion. Ninety-three percent of these patients reported greater than 50% reduction in their pain rating postsurgically. Interestingly, a statistically significant difference was obtained for patients who were treated based on a truly positive discogram.

CONCLUSION

Diagnostic cervical provocative discography is a useful diagnostic intervention to aid the spine care specialist in determining the best way to treat chronic cervical and shoulder girdle pain. When performed correctly by experienced physicians, cervical discography poses minimal risk of significant complications. Despite controversy surrounding the utility of cervical discography, when performed attentively employing meticulous fluoroscopic guidance, nonionic contrast agents, knowledge of disc biomechanics and pathology, and appropriate imaging modalities, it is a valuable adjunct in determining which segmental levels to surgically fuse.

REFERENCES

1. Lawrence JS. Disc degeneration: its frequency and relationship to symptoms. Ann Rheum Dis 1969; 28:121.
2. Westerling D, Jonsson BG. Pain from the neck-shoulder region and sick leave. Scand J Soc Med 1980; 8:131–136.
3. Takala J, Sievers K, Klaukka T. Rheumatic symptoms in the middle-aged population in southwestern Finland. Scand J Rheumatol (suppl) 1982; 47:15–29.
4. Makela M, Heliovara M, Sievers D, et al. Prevalence, determinants, and consequences of chronic neck pain in Finland. Am J Epidemiol 1991; 134:1356–1367.
5. Ylinen J, Ruuska J. Clinical use of isometric neck strength measurement in rehabilitation. Arch Phys Med Rehabil 1994; 75:465–469.
6. Deans G, Magalliard J, Kerr M, et al. Neck pain: a major cause of disability following car accidents. Injury 1987; 18:10–21.
7. Hult L. Cervical, dorsal, and lumbar spinal syndromes. Acta Orthop Scand (suppl) 1954; 17:39–102.
8. Hult L. The munkfors investigation. Acta Orthop Scand (suppl) 1954; 17:1–38.
9. Hult L. Frequency of symptoms for different age groups and professions. In: Hirsch C, Zotterman Y, eds. Cervical Pain. New York: Pergamon Press, 1971:17–20.
10. Radharkrishnan K, Litchy WJ, O'Fallon WM, et al. Epidemiology of cervical radiculopathy. A population-based study from Rochester, Minnesota, 1976–1990. Brain 1994; 117(Pt 2):325–335.
11. Cloward RB. Cervical discography: a contribution of the etiology and mechanism of neck, shoulder and arm pain. Ann Surg 1959; 150:1052–1064.
12. DePalma AF, Rothman RH, Levitt RL, et al. The natural history of severe cervical disc degeneration. Acta Orthop Scand 1972; 43:392–396.
13. Whitecloud TS III, Seago RA. Cervical discogenic syndrome. Results of operative intervention in patients with positive discography. Spine 1987; 12:313–316.
14. Crock HV. A reappraisal of intervertebral disc lesions. Med J Aust 1970; 1:983–989.
15. Bogduk N, Aprill C. On the nature of neck pain, discography and cervical zygapophysial joint blocks. Pain 1993; 54:213–217.
16. DePalma MJ, Slipman CW. Treatment of common neck problems. In: Braddom R, ed. Physical Medicine and Rehabilitation. 3rd ed., Philadelphia: Elsevier; 2006:797–824.
17. Teresi LM, Lufkin RB, Reicher MA, Moffit BJ, et al. Asymptomatic degenerative disk disease and spondylosis of the cervical spine: MR imaging. Radiology 1987; 164:83–88.
18. Boden SD, McCowin PR, Davis DO, et al. Abnormal magnetic resonance scans of the cervical spine in asymptomatic subjects: a prospective investigation. J Bone Joint Surg 1990; 72(8):1178–1184.
19. Matsumoto M, Fujimura Y, Suzuki N, et al. MRI of cervical intervertebral discs in asymptomatic subjects. J Bone Joint Surg 1998; 80(B):19–24.
20. Zheng Y, Liew S, Simmons E. Value of magnetic resonance imaging and discography in determining the level of cervical discectomy and fusion. Spine 2004; 29(19):2140–2145.
21. DePalma AF, Subin DK. Study of the cervical syndrome. Clin Orthop 1965; 38:135–141.
22. Robertson JT, Johnson SD. Anterior cervical disectomy without fusion: long-term results. Clin Neurosurg 1979; 27:440–449.
23. Smith GW, Nichols P. The technique of cervical discography. Radiology 1957; 68: 718–720.

24. Cloward RB. Cervical discography. Technique, indications and use in the diagnosis of ruptured cervical disks. AJR 1958; 79:563–574.
25. Cloward RB. The anterior approach for removal of ruptured cervical disks. J Neurosurg 1958; 15:602–617.
26. Smith GW, Robinson RA. The treatment of certain cervical spine disorders by anterior removal of the intervertebral disc and interbody fusion. J Bone Joint Surg 1958; 40A:607–623.
27. Holt EP. Fallacy of cervical discography. Report of 50 cases in normal subjects. JAMA 1964; 188(9):799–801.
28. Fortin JD. Cervical discography with CT and MRI correlations. In: Lennard TA, ed. Physiatric Procedures. Philadelphia, PA: Hanley and Belfus, 1995.
29. Aprill CN III. Diagnostic disc injection. In: Frymoyer JW, ed. The Adult Spine. New York: Raven Press, 1991:403–442.
30. Riley LH Jr, Robinson RA, Johnson KA, et al. The results of anterior interbody fusion of the cervical spine: review of 39 consecutive cases. J Neurosurg 1969; 30:127–133.
31. Simmons EH, Segil CM. An evaluation of discography in the localization of symptomatic levels in discogenic disease of the spine. Clin Orthop 1975; 108:57–69.
32. Garvey TA, Transfeldt EE, Malcolm JR, et al. Outcome of anterior cervical discectomy and fusion as perceived by patients treated for dominant axial mechanical cervical spine pain. Spine 2002; 27(17):1887–1895.
33. Kikuchi S, Macnab I, Moreau P. Localisation of the level of symptomatic cervical disc degeneration. J Bone Joint Surg 1981; 63-B(2):272–277.
34. Seibenrock KA, Aebi M. Cervical discography in discogenic pain syndrome and its predictive value for cervical fusion. Arch Orthop Trauma Surg 1994; 113:199–203.
35. Slipman CW, Plastaras C, Patel R, et al. Provocative cervical discography symptom mapping. Spine J 2005; 5(4):381–388.
36. Grubb SA, Kelly CK. Cervical discography: clinical implications from 12 years of experience. Spine 2000; 25(11):1382–1389.
37. Knight MTN, Goswami A, Patko JT. Cervical percutaneous laser disc decompression: preliminary results of an ongoing prospective outcome study. J Clin Laser Med Surg 2001; 19(1):3–8.
38. Slipman CW, Chow DW, Isaac Z, et al. An evidence-based algorithmic approach to cervical spinal disorders. Crit Rev Phys Rehabil Med 2001; 13(4):283–299.
39. Laun A, Lorenz R, Agnoli AL. Complications of cervical discography. J Neurosurg Sci 1981; 25:17–22.
40. Zeidman SM, Thompson K, Ducker TB. Complications of cervical discography: analysis of 4400 diagnostic disc injections. Neurosurgery 1995; 37(3):414–417.
41. Slipman CW, Palmatier RA. Diagnostic selective nerve root blocks. Crit Rev Phys Med Rehabil 1998; 2:1–24.
42. Slipman CW, Rogers DP, Isaac Z, et al. MR lumbar discography with intradiscal gadolinium in patients with severe anaphylactoid reaction to iodinated contrast material. Pain Med 2002; 3(1):23–29.
43. Endres SM, Bogduk N. International spinal injection society practice guidelines and protocols: lumbar disc stimulation. ISIS 9th Annual Scientific Meeting Syllabus, 2001.
44. Bonaldi G, Minonzio G, Belloni G, et al. Percutaneous cervical diskectomy: preliminary experience. Neuroradiology 1994; 36:483–486.
45. Kambin P, Abda S, Kurpicki F. Intradiskal pressure and volume recording: evaluation of normal and abnormal cervical disks. Clin Orthop 1980; 146:144–147.
46. Saternus KS, Bornscheuer HH. Comparative radiologic and pathologic-anatomic studies on the value of discography in the diagnosis of acute intervertebral disc injuries in the cervical spine. Rofo Fortschr Geb Rontgenstr Neuen Bildgeb Verfahr 1983; 139:651–657.
47. Hirsch C, Schajowicz R, Galante J. Structural changes in the cervical spine: a study on autopsy specimens in different age groups. Acta Orthop Scand Suppl 1967; 109:7–77.
48. DePalma MJ, Slipman CW. Non-endoscopic percutaneous disc decompression as treatment of discogenic radiculopathy. In: Lewandrowski LE, ed. Innovations in Spinal Reconstruction: Clinical Examples of Basic Science, Biomechanics, and Engineering. New York: Taylor and Francis Group (in press).

49. Holt EP. Further reflections on cervical discography. JAMA 1975; 231(6):613–614.
50. Slipman CW, Patel RK, Zhang L, et al. Side of symptomatic annular tear and site of low back pain: is there a correlation? Spine 2001; 26(8):E165–E168.
51. Agnoli A, Laun A. Komplikationen bei ossovenographie und discographie im halsbereich. Roentgen-Blatte 1977; 30:616–620.
52. Guyer RD, Collier R, Stith WJ, et al. Discitis after discography. Spine 1988; 13:1352–1354.
53. Lownie SP, Ferguson GG. Spinal subdural empyema complicating cervical discography. Spine 1989; 14:1415–1417.
54. Roosen C, Bettag R, Fiebach O. Komplikationen der cervikalen diskographie. Rofo Fortschr Geb Roentgenstr Neuen Bildgeb Verfahr 1975; 122:520–527.
55. Schaerer J. Cervical discography. J Int Coll Surg 1964; 42:287–296.
56. Klessig HT, Showsh SA, Sekorski A. The use of intradiscal antibiotics for discography: an in vitro study of gentamicin, cefazolin, and clindamycin. Spine 2003; 28(15): 1735–1738.
57. Smith GW. The normal cervical diskogram with clinical observations. AJR 1959; 81:1006–1010.
58. Gore DR, Sepic SB, Gardner GM, et al. Neck pain: a long-term follow up of 205 patients. Spine 1987; 12:1–5.
59. Hunt WE. Cervical spondylosis: natural history and rare indications for surgical decompression. Clin Neurosurg 1980; 27:466–480.
60. White III AA, Southwick WO, Deponte RJ, et al. Relief of pain by anterior cervical spine fusion for spondylosis. A report of sixty-five patients. J Bone Joint Surg [Am] 1973; 55A:525–534.
61. Gore DR, Sepic SB. Anterior cervical fusion for degenerated or protruded discs. A review of one hundred forty-six patients. Spine 1984; 9(7):667–671.

15 Lumbar Discography

Syed A. Hasan
Department of Physical Medicine and Rehabilitation, and The Penn Spine Center, Hospital of the University of Pennsylvania, Philadelphia, Pennsylvania, U.S.A.

Michael J. DePalma
Department of Physical Medicine and Rehabilitation, Virginia Commonwealth University/Medical College of Virginia, Richmond, Virginia, U.S.A.

Curtis W. Slipman
Department of Physical Medicine and Rehabilitation, and The Penn Spine Center, Hospital of the University of Pennsylvania, Philadelphia, Pennsylvania, U.S.A.

INTRODUCTION

The intervertebral disc is now recognized as a common source of chronic axial pain (1–3). They are endowed with necessary innervation to be a source of pain (4,5). Cases of ruptured intervertebral discs have been reported as early as 1896 (6). In 1911, Middleton and Treacher of the United Kingdom (7) and J.E. Goldwait of Boston (8) independently described the entity known as the ruptured intervertebral disc. In 1929, studies by Dandy (9) and Schmorl (10) provided evidence of the possible clinical significance of the ruptured disc. In 1934, a widespread interest was created in the disc as a source of pain (11). This mechanical model by Mixter and Barr became the central model of spine pain, which preoccupied the medical community and diverted attention from other possible causes. The question of the existence of an intradiscal pain mechanism arose in 1984 when Hirsch (12) injected procaine into a herniated disc and reported relief of sciatica. It was Roofes' description of annulus fibrosus innervation in 1940 that provided an alternative model of the disc as a pain generator independent of a neurocompressive paradigm (13). The clinical validation of Roofes' discovery came from Vanharanta et al. (14). This paper demonstrated that only an annular fissure which extends from the mid to outer annular region significantly correlates with pain with a provocative injection. Since then, several studies have identified the existence of irritant chemical substances within the disc that could cause sensitization of the disc annulus with mechanical loading (15,16). This sensitivity has been documented both by eliciting the axial pain by pressing on the posterior annulus during lumbar surgery in awake patients (1) and with low pressure (chemical) activation of annular nociceptors (17). The rich innervation of the mid to outer annular layers has been substantiated by four independent studies (18–21) using sophisticated staining and magnification studies.

The internal disc disruption syndrome has been the most comprehensively understood cause of low back pain. Clinical studies have determined the internal disc disruption syndrome as a pain source in as many as 40% of patients with chronic low back pain (20). This is a condition in which the disc has an intact perimeter, but an internal disc derangement (21). The initiating factor is a fatigue failure of the vertebral end plate (22). This endplate fracture is caused by a product of degree of compression load which could be tolerated by the ultimate end-plate tensile strength and number of repetitions (23,24), encountered during daily heavy work activities. The endplate fatigue failure results in a series of bio-chemical, biophysical, and morphological features (21). These biochemical, biophysical, and morphological features have all been shown to correlate with the discogenic pain. The biochemical features as studied in animal studies (25) include de-aggregation of proteoglycans in the nucleus, a reduction in water content, and annular delamination. The biophysical features comprise reduced and irregular stress in the nucleus pulposus, and an increased posterior annular stress. This is in contrast to the uniform stress seen with axial loading on these structures (22), as evidenced on stress profilometry, a technique in which internal stresses within a disc can be measured. The depressurization of the nucleus and consequent increase in posterior annular stress results from a decrease in the water content of the nucleus. The morphological features of the internal disc disruption syndrome are characterized by the degradation of nuclear matrix and radial fissures, which penetrate the annulus fibrosus without actually breaking the outer lamella. These radial fissures are graded according to the extent that they penetrate into the annular lamella: inner one-third (grade I), middle one-third (grade II), outer one-third (grade III), and circumferential (grade IV) (26,27).

Multiple studies have shown that multidisciplinary and behavioral therapy programs may not succeed in completely alleviating the pain; this implies a source of persistent pain (21). The morphological features of the internal disc disruption syndrome cannot be demonstrated by plain radiology or computed tomography (CT) (21). Although magnetic resonance imaging (MRI) can show morphological abnormalities of the disc, they are of limited value in demonstrating which structure is painful. Discography remains the only test that provides physio-logical information whether or not a given intervertebral disc is painful (28). It is employed as a presurgical diagnostic tool by numerous physicians (29–31).

HISTORICAL BACKGROUND

In 1944, Lindblom (32) demonstrated radial annular fissures by injecting red dye into the nucleus, and then observing the contrast leak into the annulus in cadavers. However, he did not apply disc injections clinically because of Peases' study (33), which demonstrated disc damage with inadvertent disc penetration upon attempted lumbar thecal puncture in children with purulent meningitis. Subsequently, Hirsch et al. (34) used intraoperative disc distention with saline, and noted concordant pain without secondary disc damage. In 1948, Lindblom reported nucleographic patterns of 15 discs in 13 patients. By early 1960s, discogra-phy appeared to have the potential of replacing myelography as the premier disc-imaging study. This trend ended following the demonstration of a 37% false-positive rate by Holt in 1964 and 1968 (35). A recent critical review found Holts' methods of dubious validity because of poor selection criteria, high technical failure rate, lack of sophisticated technology, and the use of hypaque, a known neurotoxic contrast material (36). In 1968, Wiley et al. (37) found a viable role for discography in the diagnostic evaluation of patients with axial pain and no definite disc prolapse on myelography. However, until recently, their work had been over-shadowed by Holts' studies. A recent well-controlled prospective study by Walsh et al. (38) disproved Holts' data in a group of asymptomatic volunteers by using stringent criteria of radiological abnormality and reproduction of patients' pain pattern. With a false-positive rate of 0%, they found discography to be a highly reliable and specific method of distinguishing symptomatic versus asymptomatic discs. Other investigators have also attempted to estimate the possible false-positive rate by studying discography in asymptomatic volunteers. The available data provided by these studies is conflicting, but also confounded by other variables. Massie and Steven (39) found discography to be only occasionally positive, and Carragee et al. (40,41) found a 10% false-positive in subjects without a history of low back pain.

INDICATIONS

Most of the current literature (42–44) supports the use of discography in select situations. According to the position statement by the North American Spine Society diagnostic and therapeutic committee, indications for discography include, but are not limited to:

1. Patients with unremitting severe symptoms in whom the other diagnostic tests, including CT, MRI, and/or myelography have failed to reveal clear confirmation of a suspected disc as a source of pain.
2. Further evaluation of demonstrably abnormal discs to help assess the extent of the abnormality or correlation of abnormality with the clinical symptoms, including recurrent pain from a painfully operated disc and lateral disc herniation.
3. Postsurgical fusion assessment. Patients who have failed to respond to posterior fusion to determine if there is painful pseudoarthrosis versus symptomatic disc as a source of pain in the fused segment and to help evaluate for possible recurrent disc herniation.
4. Presurgical planning for fusion. To assess the integrity of the disc(s) in the proposed fusion segment and the adjacent discs.
5. Confirm a contained disc herniation as a part of the work-up for minimally invasive intradiscal procedures.

CONTRAINDICATIONS

Discography is contraindicated (44) in patients with a neoplastic, infectious, or infilterative process, and uncontrolled coagulopathy. Anticoagulant therapy and contrast dye allergy represent relative contraindications. In the setting of patients with iodine contrast allergy, gadolinium discography (45) has been used as a safe, viable alternative to the conventional discography. Postdiscography CT scans adequately visualize intradiscal gadolinium in a more timely and costeffective manner than MRI.

MAGNETIC RESONANCE IMAGING CORRELATES OF PAIN RESPONSE

Typical MRI findings that correlate with concordant pain (46,47) at discography include:

1. *Moderate to severe disc degeneration (grades 4 and 5)*: Grade 4 disc degeneration implies moderate disc degeneration, a loss of differentiation of the nucleus pulposus from the annulus, and moderately decreased nuclear signal with a hypointense zone. Grade 5 disc degeneration is characterized by severe degeneration, a loss of nuclear and annular differentiation, and hypointense

signal of the nucleus pulposus with or without a horizontal hyper intense band. Grades 1 and 2 are normal and grade 3 implies mild disc degeneration.

2. *Disc height*: An association was found with positive pain response by Millet et al. (47), but not in a study carried out by Chae-Hun et al. (46).
3. *High-intensity zone (HIZ)*: This a hyperintense signal contained within the posterior annulus seen on the T2-weighted sagittal and axial images. It has an estimated sensitivity of 45% and specificity of 84% (48), and its presence renders, more likely than not, that the affected disc is a source of pain.
4. *Modic type I and II changes*: There are two studies in which endplate changes have not been shown (46,47) to significantly correlate to concordant pain seen with provocative discography.

TECHNIQUE
Patient Positioning
Prior to appropriate patient positioning, a careful evaluation of the approach is made. This is based on factors such as patient size, patient compliance, disc space height, pelvic configuration, presence of transitional segments and prior lumbar surgery. The patient's skin is then carefully prepped using betadine if the patient is not allergic to iodine. This is followed by draping using sterile towel.

Two-Needle Technique
A two-needle technique is employed with 18- or 20-gauge introducer needle. As this needle does not enter the disc space, the risk of placement of skin flora into the nucleus is minimized. The inner 22- or 25-gauge needle is placed into the nucleus.

Care is taken to avoid penetration into the end plate as this will create pain during the insertion and the injection of contrast. This may result in a false-positive result.

Lumbar discography can be accomplished via three approaches:

1. *Posterolateral approach with the patient resting in the prone-oblique position.* A right-sided entrance site is typically employed, thereby requiring that the patient rest on the left side. The right hip is flexed and slightly abducted, whereas the right knee is flexed. Pillows are placed under the distal medial aspect of the thigh to support the right leg. This leg position relaxes the right L5 nerve root, thereby minimizing the chance of needle contact during an attempt to enter the L5-S1 disc. A bolster is placed under the left flank, which would slightly tilt the pelvis and open the entrance to the L5-S1 disc. The inner needle can be curved prior to insertion into the introducer needle. This technique is reserved for the L5-S1 disc space. This curve allows the needle to hug the S1 superior articular process pass by and not into the L5 nerve, and reach the nucleus.
2. *Posterolateral approach with the patient prone.* In contrast to the aforementioned posterolateral approach, this technique requires biplanar imaging with each advance of the needle when performed by novices.
3. *Transdural approach with the patient prone.* A paramedian needle entrance point is used. Extra care is taken when aligning the guide needle, as the second needle would pierce the dural membrane twice before entering the disc space. If the alignment is not accurate, repeat attempts to advance the needle will be

required, with each trial causing not one, but two dural punctures. Therefore, the risk of headache, nerve root injury, meningitis, and meningocele formation is theoretically increased. Consequently, a transdural approach should be reserved for instances in which the L5-S1 disc cannot be entered with the two other techniques.

COMPLICATIONS

The reported complication rate of provocative lumbar discography is low, ranging from 0 to 2.5% (49). The potential complications of provocative lumbar discography include:

1. *Discitis:* This is the most widely recognized complication; patients may be more prone to this complication because of the large avascular space within the disc. The incidence, however, is only 0.1–1.3% (37,50–54). Isolation of staphylococcus and *Escherichia coli* suggests the role of skin surface contaminants and bowel flora, respectively (51,55,56). There are a variety of ways to retrieve disc tissue for gram stain and culture. At The Penn Spine Center, we have found the safest and most rapid technique to extract an adequate amount of disc material by using the dekompressor. Technologies, such as coblation or auto-mated percutaneous lumbar discectomy are not helpful. In the former instance, nuclear material is evaporated, and in the latter, the material retrieved is extensively lavaged by normal saline. Even when sufficient tissue is obtained, it may be difficult to isolate the organisms. A possible explanation is that there is rapid immunological attenuation caused by the natural course of organisms with subsequent neovascularization from the endplate tributaries (51,52). Another possibility is the involvement of indolent organisms of low virulence (57). Others have postulated (58–60) an aseptic or chemical form of discitis caused by aseptic disc necrosis by concentrated iodine product. A dramatic increase in pain and stiffness or a change in the character of symptoms should raise a high index of suspicion warranting obtaining a C-reactive protein and a sedimentation rate as a screening tool. If either of these acute phase reactants are elevated, then an MRI is essential (61,62). Without timely intervention, a discitis can result in an epidural abscess (53).
2. *Nerve root injury:* This could result from impalement of the nerve root caused by direct needle trauma if careful technique is not employed (44).
3. *Thecal puncture headache:* The L5-S1 level is most vulnerable for this complication which could result from malpositioning of the outer needle with excessive bending of the inner needle. A transdural approach can also result in headaches (44).
4. *Discography-induced acute lumbar disc herniation:* Poynton et al. (49) reported a series of five cases of acute lumbar disc herniation precipitated by discography. All patients developed an acute exacerbation of radicular leg pain following multilevel provocation lumbar discography with one patient actually developing foot drop. Comparison of the MRI before and after the procedure revealed either a new herniated disc fragment or an increase in the size of a pre-existing disc herniation in all cases. An annular deficiency was considered an obvious predisposing factor to discogram-related disc herniation.
5. *Long-term back symptoms:* Carragee et al. (63) reported significant back pain one year after discogram. This occurred in patients with emotional and chronic pain

problems. The patients with normal psychometric test profile had no reports of significant long-term back symptoms after discography.

INTERPRETATION

Since its introduction in 1948, lumbar discography has been practiced without any well-defined operational criteria. This has resulted in a high false-positive rate, which has led to a debate on its validity. For a test to be valid, it should have a low rate of false-positive responses. These false-positive responses could be reduced by using unambiguous operational criteria.

Several studies have shown a high false-positive rate of discography, although the results of these studies have been confounded by other variables. Carragee et al. (40,41) studied three sets of patients: patients who had no symptoms, patients with chronic pain which was not back pain, and patients with a diagnosis of somatization disorder; the imputed false-positive rates in these categories were 10, 20, and 75%, respectively. However, these results have been criticized (21) for lack of adherence to the recommended disc stimulation criteria, including anatomic and manometric controls, although intradiscal pressures were recorded in their study. The patient population in the study was also small, resulting in a wide confidence interval. It has been shown (21) that by using the criteria of anatomic and manometric control, the false-positive rate in their study could be reduced to as low as 10% and 25–50%, respectively.

In a separate study, Carragee et al. (64) also questioned the ability of the discography to differentiate spinal from nonspinal source of pain. In their study, lumbar discogram was carried out in 24 discs in eight subjects without a previous history of low back pain, approximately two to four months after the harvesting of iliac bone graft for nonspinal reasons. Four out of eight subjects (50%) were regarded to have positive discogram experiencing concordant painful sensations with their usual gluteal area pain.

The influence of emotional and psychological factors, chronic pain behavior and ongoing compensation claim on the discogram outcome has also been demonstrated (65). In their study of 72 patients, Block et al. (66) showed the influence of personality, as assessed by Minnesota Multiphasic Personality Inventory, on discography-induced pain. Patients with elevated scores on hypochondriasis, hysteria, and depression scales tend to over-report pain during discography.

Studies have been conducted in an attempt to define operational criteria with respect to the limit of the stimulation intensity and degree of response. In their study on 13 volunteers, Derby et al. (67) were able to derive a receiver–operator curve to demonstrate combination of pain intensity and pressure below which the probability of a response was zero or less than 10%. They demonstrated that false-positive responses occur only above certain pressures and pain scores. Combining their data with that of Carragee (40,41), they concluded that if the operational criteria for a positive discography is set as pressures not greater than 50 psi, and the intensity of evoked pain is greater than 4, then the false-positive rate would be less than 10%. A false-positive rate of 0 could be achieved if the required pain score is held at 4, and the threshold pressure of injection lowered to 30 psi. Conversely, if the required pressure is 50 psi, the pain score would need to be raised to 6. In this study, they were also able to demonstrate that not all normal discs could be rendered painful. Some 56% of the discs in their study were not painful on provocative discogram. If the normal disc were made painful, the pain was mild and it required higher pressures.

The false-positive rate could be further reduced using findings on the CT discogram. In their study, Chae-Hun et al. (46) demonstrated that typical findings on CT discogram with concordant pain were fissured/ruptured discs and contrast extending into/beyond the outer annulus. In another study of 279 discs that underwent pressure-controlled discography, Derby et al. (68), showed that 88 out of 93 painful discs (94.6%) had annular disruption greater than a grade 3.

Based on these studies, the International Spine Intervention Society (ISIS) has provided guidelines (69) for the diagnostic criteria of internal disc disruption syndrome on discography. These criteria are:

- Reproduction of the patients' pain by stimulation of the affected disc.
- Evoked pain must have an intensity of at least 7 on a 10-point scale.
- Pain is reproduced at a low pressure of stimulation—15 psi.
- Stimulation of adjacent discs does not reproduce pain.
- Postdiscography CT should demonstrate a grade III or IV fissure.

If these stringent operational criteria are applied, the false-positive rate could be effectively reduced to zero or at least to an acceptable level of less than 10% in asymptomatic individuals and patients with chronic low back pain. In patients with emotional problems, pain behavior, and somatization, false-positive rates would remain high. In the latter patient population, discogram results should be applied carefully in clinical decision-making, particularly when considering discography as part of preoperative evaluation for surgical fusion.

UTILITY

Precise prospective categorization of positive discographic diagnoses may predict outcome from treatment, surgical or otherwise, and thereby facilitate therapeutic decision making. Derby et al. (70) used pressure-controlled manometric discography to isolate highly (chemically) sensitive discs which achieved significantly better long-term outcomes with interbody/combined fusion than with intertransverse fusion. Patients without disc surgery had the least favorable outcome.

For optimal results with intradiscal electrothermal therapy, Bogduk (21) describes the appropriate placement of the electrodes crossing the radial fissure and lying peripheral or parallel to the circumferential fissure. This necessitates the precise identification of the annular fissure on CT discogram before contemplating the procedure.

CONCLUSION

The controversy about discography as a diagnostic tool because of false-positive results has been secondary to ambiguous operational criteria in the past. Recently, the criteria have been re-evaluated, and the findings have been incorporated in the guidelines provided by ISIS. Using stringent operational criteria, the rate of false-positive results in provocative lumbar discography can be reduced to an acceptable level of less than 10% or even to zero. In this setting, provocative lumbar discography can be a useful diagnostic tool to confirm the intervertebral disc as a pain generator. It can provide valuable precise anatomic details required for minimally invasive intradiscal procedures, and help to predict the outcome of spinal fusion surgery. However, the results should be carefully interpreted in patients with emotional, chronic pain, and somatization disorders.

REFERENCES

1. Copps MH, Marani E, Thomeer RtWM, Groen GJ. Innervation of "painful" Lumbar discs. Spine 1997; 22:2342–2350.
2. Kuslich SD, Ahern JW, Garner MD. An in-vivo, prospective analysis of tissue sensivity of lumbar spinal tissues. Proceedings of the 12th Annual Meeting of the North American Spine Society, New York, October 22–25, 1997.
3. Schwarzer AC, Aprill CN, Derby R, Fortin J, Kine G, Bogduk N. The prevalence and clinical features of internal disc disruption syndrome with chronic low back pain. Spine 1995; 20:1878–1883.
4. Bogduk N, Tynan W, Wilson AS. The nerve supply to the human lumbar intervertebral discs. J Anat 1981; 132:39–56.
5. Bogduk N. The innervation of intervertebral discs. In: Ghosh P, ed. The Biology of Intervertebral Discs. Vol. 1. Boca Raton, FL: CRC Press, 1988:135–149.
6. Kocher T. Die Verletzungen der Wirbelsaule zugleich als Beitrag zur physiologie des mensch-lichen Ruckenmarks. Mitt az Grenzgeb d Med u Chir 1896; 1:415–480.
7. Middleton GS, Treacher JH. Injury of spinal cord due to rupture of an intervertebral disc during muscular effort. Glasgow Med J 1911; 76:1–6.
8. Goldwait JE. The lumbosacral articulation: an explanation of many causes of "lumbago", "sciatica" and paraplegia. Boston Med Surg J 1911; 164:365–372.
9. Dandy WE. Loose cartilage from intervertebral disc simulating tumor of spinal cord. Arch Surg 1929; 19:660–662.
10. Schmorl G. Ueber Knorpelknotchen an der Hinterflache der Wirbelsbandscheiben. Fortshr a.d Geb.d Rontgenstraheln 1929; 40:629–634.
11. Mixter WJ, Barr JS. Ruptures of the intervertebral discs with involvement of the spinal canal. N Engl J Med 1934; 211:210.
12. Hirsch C. An attempt to diagnose level of disc lesion clinically by disc puncture. Acta Orthop Scand 1948; 18:131–140.
13. Roofe PG. Innervation of the annulus fibrosus and posterior longitudinal ligament. Arch Neurol Psych 1940; 44:100–103.
14. Vanharanta H, Sach BL, Ohnmeiss DD, et al. Pain provocation and disc deterioration by age. A CT/discographic study in low back pain population. Spine 1989; 14:420–423.
15. Saal JS, Franson RC, Dobrow R, Saal JA, White AH, Goldthwaite N. High levels of inflammatory phospholipase A2 activity in lumbar disc herniation. Spine 1990; 15:674–678.
16. Weinstein JN. Mechanism of spinal pain. The dorsal root ganglion and its role as a mediator of low back pain. Spine 986; 11:999–1001.
17. Derby R. Lumbar discometry. Newsletter Int Spinal Inject Soc 1993; 1:8–17.
18. Groen G, Baljet B, Drukker J. The nerves and nerve plexuses of human vertebral column. Am J Anat 1990; 188:282–296.
19. Malinsky J. The ontogenetic development of nerve terminations in the intervertebral discs of man. Acta Anat 1959; 38:96–113.
20. Yoshizawa H, O'Brien JP, et al. The neuropathology of intervertebral discs removed for low back pain. J Path 1980; 132:95–104.
21. Nikolai Bogduk. Why I pursue discogenic pain. Synopsis of the case for, in a debate on discogenic pain conducted at the annual scientific meeting of the German Pain Society, held in Bremen on October 20, 2005.
22. Adams Ma, McNally DS, Wagstaff J, Goodship AE. Abnormal stress concentrations in lumbar intervertebral discs following damage to the vertebral bodies: a cause of disc failure? Eur Spine J 1993; 1:214–221.

23. Hansson TH, Keller TS, Spengler DM. Mechanical behavior of human lumbar spine. II. Fatigue strength during dynamic compressive loading. J Orthop Res 1987; 5:479–487.
24. Liu YK, Njus G, et al. Fatigue response of lumbar intervertebral joints under axial cyclic loading. Spine 1983; 8:857–865.
25. Holm S, Kaigle-Holm, Ekstrom L, et al. Experimental disc degeneration due to endplate injury. Spinal Disord Tech 2004; 17:64–71.
26. Sachs BL, Vanharanta H, Spivey M A, et al. Dallas discogram description; a new classification of CT/discography in low-back disorders. Spine 1987; 12:287–294.
27. Aprill C, Bogduk N. High-intensity zone: a diagnostic sign of painful lumbar disc on magnetic resonance imaging. Dr J Radiol 1992; 65:361–369.
28. Anderson MW. Lumbar discography: an update. Semin Roentgenol 2004 Jan; 39(1): 52–67.
29. Brinckmann P, Frobin W, et al. Deformation of the vertebral end-plate under axial loading of the spine. Spine 1983; 8:851–856.
30. Brodsky AE, Binder WF. Lumbar discography. Spine 1079; 4:110–120.
31. Crock HV. Internal disc disruption. Spine 1986; 11:650–653.
32. Lindblom K. Protrusions of disc and nerve compression in the lumbar region. Acta Radiol Scand 1944; 25:195–212.
33. Pease CN. Injuries to the vertebrae and intervertebral discs following lumbar puncture. Am J Dis Child 1935; 49:849–860.
34. Hirsch C, Schajowicz R, Galante J. Structural changes in cervical spine. A study in autopsy specimens in different age groups. Acta Orthop Scand 1967; (suppl 109):7–77.
35. Holt EP Jr. The question of lumbar discography. J Bone Joint Surg [Am] 1968; 50:720–726.
36. Simmons EH, Segil CM. An evaluation of discography in the localization of symptomatic levels in discogenic disease of spine. Clin Orthop Rel Res 1975; 108:57–69.
37. Wiley J, McNab I, Wortzman G. Lumbar discography and its clinical applications. Can J Surg 1968; 11:280–289.
38. Walsh T, Weinstein J, et al. The question of discography revisited. A controlled prospective study of normal volunteers to determine the false positive rate. J Bone Joint Surg [Am] 1990; 72:1081–1088.
39. Massey WK, Stevens DB. A critical evaluation of discography. J Bone Joint Surg 1967; 49A:1243–1244.
40. Carragee EJ, Tanner CM, Khurana S, et al. The rates of false positive discography in select patients without low back symptoms. Spine 2000; 25:1373–1381.
41. Carragee EJ, Alamin TF. Discography: a review. Spine J 2001; 364–372.
42. Richard D Guyer, Donna D Ohnmeiss, Alexander Vaccaro. Lumbar discography. Spine J 2003; 3(3):11–27.
43. Guyer RD, Ohnmeiss DD. Lumbar discography. Position statement from the North American Spine Society diagnostic and therapeutic committee. Spine 1995; 20(18):2048–2059.
44. Zeidman SM, Thompson K, Ducker TB. Complications of cervical discography: analysis of 4400 diagnostic disc injections. Neurosurgery 1995; 37(3):414–417.
45. Slipman CW, Rogers DP, Isaac Z, et al. MR lumbar discography with intradiscal gadolinium in patients with severe anaphylactoid reaction to iodinated contrast material. Pain Med 2002; 3(1):1–7.
46. Chae-Hun Lim, Won-Hee Jee, et al. Discogenic lumbar pain; association with MRI imaging and CT discography. Eur J Radiol 2005; 54:431–437.
47. Milette PC, Fontaine S, Lepanto L, et al. Differentiating lumbar disc protrusions, disc bulges and discs with normal contour but abnormal signal intensity. Magnetic resonance imaging with discographic correlations. Spine 1999; 24(1):44–53.
48. Carragee EJ, Paragoudakis SJ, Khurana S. Lumbar high intensity zone and discography in subjects without low back problems. Spine 2000; 25:2987–2992.
49. Poynton AR, Hinman A, Lutz G, Farmer JC. Discography-induced acute lumbar disc herniation: a report of five cases. J Spinal Disord Tech 2005; 18(2):188–192.
50. Roosen K, Betag W, Fiebach O. Komplikationen der cervikalen discographie. ROFO 1975; 122:520–527.

51. Fraser RD, Osti OL, Vernon-Roberts B. Discitis after discography. J Bone Joint Surg [Br] 1987; 69:26–35.
52. Fraser RD, Osti OL, Vernon-Roberts B. Discitis following chemonucleolysis. An experimental study. Spine 1986; 11:679–687.
53. Lownie SP, Ferguson GG. Spinal subdural empyema complicating cervical discography. Spine 1089; 14:1415–1417.
54. Milette PC, Melanson D. A reappraisal of lumbar discography. Journal De L' Association Canadienne Des Radiologists 1982; 11:176.
55. Guyer RD, Collier R, et al. Discitis after discography. Spine 1988; 13:1352–1354.
56. Agre K, Wilson RR, Brim M, et al. Chymodiactin post-marketing surveillance. Demographic and adverse experience data in 29,075 patients. Spine 1984; 9:479–485.
57. Scofferman L, Schofferman J, Zucherman J, et al. Occult infections causing persistent low back pain. Spine 1989; 14:417–419.
58. Crock H. Practice of spinal surgery. New York: Springer-Verlag, 1983.
59. DeSeze S, Levernieux J. Les Accidents de la discographie. Rev Rheum 1952; 19: 1027–1033.
60. Smith MD, Kim SS. A herniated cervical disc resulting from discography: an unusual complication. Spinal Disord 1990; 3(4):392–395.
61. Fernand R, Lee CK. Postlaminectomy disc space infection. A review of the literature and report of three cases. Clin Orthop 1986; 209:215–218.
62. Thibodeau AA. Closed space infection following removal of intervertebral disc. J Bone Joint Surg [Am] 1968; 50:400–410.
63. Carragee EJ, Chen Y, Tanner CM, et al. Can discography cause long-term back symptoms in previously asymptomatic subjects? Spine 2000; 25(14):1803–1808.
64. Carragee EJ, Tanner CM, et al. False positive findings on lumbar discography. Reliability of subjective concordance assessment during provocative disc injection. Spine 1999; 24(23):2542–2547.
65. Carragee EJ. Is lumbar discography a determinate of discogenic low back pain: provocative discography reconsidered. Curr Rev Pain 2000; 4(4):301.
66. Block AR, Vanharanta H, Ohnmeiss DD, Guyer RD. Discographic Pain Report. Influence of Psychological factors.
67. Derby R, Lee S-H, Kim BJ, Chen Y, Aprill C, Bogduk N. Pressure-controlled Lumbar discography in volunteers without low back symptoms. Pain Med 2005; 6:213–221.
68. Derby R, Kim BJ, Chen Y, et al. The relationship between annular disruption on computed tomographic scan and pressure controlled discography. Arch Phys Med Rehabil 2005; 86:1534–1538.
69. International Spine Intervention Society. Lumbar disc stimulation. In: Bogduk N, ed. Practice Guidelines for Spinal Diagnostic and Treatment Procedures. San Francisco: International Spine Intervention Society, 2004:20–46.
70. Richard D, Mark HW, Joseph GM, John J, van Peteghem PK, Ryan Deaglan P. The ability of pressure controlled discography to predict surgical and nonsurgical outcomes. Spine 1999; 24:364–371.

Intradiscal Electrothermal Therapy and Other Percutaneous Disc Procedures

Zach Broyer

Rothman Institute, Thomas Jefferson University Hospital, Philadelphia, Pennsylvania, U.S.A.

INTRODUCTION

The intervertebral disc is the cause of chronic back pain in up to 40% of patients (1). The treatments available today for discogenic low back pain range from the less invasive treatments, including modalities, rest, oral medications, and physical therapy, to the more aggressive epidural injections, fusion and disc replacement. Several treatments have been proposed to prevent the need for surgery in patients with continued low back pain in spite of conservative management. The most commonly performed procedure is intradiscal electrothermal therapy (IDET). Less common options include nucleoplasty and percutaneous discectomy. "Internal disc disruption," as first described by Crock (2), is discogenic low back pain without necessarily having pain symptoms into the lower extremity. Traditional imaging studies do not reveal the segments which are painful. Imaging studies, such as magnetic resonance imaging (MRI) demonstrate anatomic changes of the disc, but only provocative discography can prove which disc is generating the patient's pain. This chapter will focus on IDET.

PROCEDURE

Intradiscal electrothermal therapy is a trademarked technique. The equipment and technique is Federal Drug Administration (FDA) approved as of 1998 for intradiscal electrothermal annuloplasty (3). Under fluoroscopic guidance, a trocar is placed into the disc using a posterolateral approach similar to standard discogram practice. Once the trocar is placed, the catheter is advanced through the trocar and across the nucleus to the inner anterolateral annulus. The catheter is then advanced along the area between the inner annulus and nucleus. The catheter has a heating element that conducts electricity using radiofrequency energy converted to thermal energy. The heating is done using a radiofrequency generator that heats the distal 50 mm by 1° every 30 seconds up to 90° by 12 minutes, and then maintains the 90° for another 4.5 minutes. This regimen is thought to be enough energy to denature collagen and cause coagulation (4).

INDICATIONS

Intradiscal electrothermal therapy is done on patients with axial low back pain that has lasted for more than six months. The disc should be evaluated by discography after other causes of pain have been ruled out. One must rule out disc herniations, spinal stenosis, the sacroiliac joint or the facet joint as the etiology of pain. Discs must be greater than 50% of their normal height (5).

MECHANISM OF ACTION

There are several theories as to why IDET decreases lumbar disc pain. One possible explanation is that IDET denatures collagen in the annulus fibrosis and shrinks the nucleus or seals the annulus (6). The other notion is that IDET ablates the nociceptive fibers within the posterior aspect of the disc. The recurrent sinuvertebral nerve forms the nerves that innervate the posterior annulus (7). The posterior third of the normal outer annulus contains the A delta and C sensory fibers. In the degenerated disc, there is an ingrowth of these nerve fibers (8). Studies done to monitor the effectiveness of IDET to ablate nerve fibers or to denature collagen to yield shrinkage have had varying results.

Kleinstuck used cadaveric lumbar discs to measure the temperatures achieved during IDET. The catheter was placed within the 19 cadaveric lumbar discs with intact anterior and posterior longitudinal ligaments. After completion of the IDET protocol, the measured temperatures ranged from 37°C to 65°C. The highest temperature was noted 1 mm from the catheter tip and the lowest temperatures were noted 10 to 15 mm from the catheter. In this study, the catheter was positioned 10 to 15 mm from the posterior annulus. There was insufficient change in temperature to denature collagen except at the IDET catheter itself. Histologically, there was no significant difference in the annular fibers from the heated and nonheated areas of the disc. Kleinstueck concluded that IDET did not change the biomechanical or histological properties of the disc (9).

Klienstueck again studied the temperature effects of IDET in 2003. He placed the catheter 10 to 15 mm from the outer annulus and used the IDET heating protocol. This time, the spines were placed in a 37°C water bath to mimic body temperature. He concluded that temperatures high enough to cause coagulation of collagen are achieved in a 2-mm area surrounding the catheter, and temperatures high enough for nerve ablation are achieved in an area 6 mm around the catheter. He also concluded that temperature increases during the final minutes of the protocol require exact placement of the catheter to be effective, and may require an increase in the heating time to further extend the area that would reach effective temperatures (10).

Freeman et al. did stab incisions into two discs of Merino sheep without penetrating the nucleus pulposus. Twelve weeks following the incision, the animals underwent IDET with thermocouples anterior and posterior to the catheter. Intradiscal electrothermal therapy was then performed on the cut and uncut discs. The animals were sacrificed, and their discs were then assessed. At 12 weeks, even without IDET, there was abundant granulation tissue with neoinnervation in the periannular and outer annular region of the cut discs. Collagen denaturation requires a temperature of 60°C, and nerve destruction requires 45°C. This study was able to demonstrate that at 90°C, the nucleus and most of the annulus reached a temperature high enough to cause denaturation and coagulation of the inner annulus and nucleus. The nuclear temperature was higher than that of the annulus in 25 of the 40 discs. The mean annular temperature was 63.6°C and the mean nuclear temperature was 67.8°C. The nuclear temperature exceeded 60°C in 35 of the 40 discs. At all discs, the temperatures achieved were greater than the 45°C needed to cause neural ablation. The posterior annular temperature exceeded 60°C in 28 of the 40 discs. There was no difference in the temperature achieved in the noncut discs compared with the cut discs. At the very least, the study demonstrates that the temperatures achieved were adequate to cause neural ablation. Surprisingly, immunohistochemical analysis did not demonstrate a difference in the innervation of the IDET and non-IDET discs. Thermal necrosis was noted from the inner annulus to the nucleus, but thermal necrosis was not noted in the outer annulus. Freeman (11) concluded that the mechanisms that cause a decrease in pain following IDET are not the result of annular collagen denaturation or nerve ablation.

Pollintine et al. performed stress tests on cadaveric discs to mimic physiologic pressures pre- and post-IDET. Compression stress profiles on flexion and extension were assessed. Stress testing was done after catheter placement, and once again after heating of the element using the standard IDET protocol. Sham IDET caused no change in stress profile in the neutral position. Intradiscal electrothermal therapy reduced nucleus pressure by 10% and posterior annulus pressure by 40%. Annular stress peaks were reduced by more than 8% in 12 of the IDET discs. Nuclear stress was decreased by 6% in the flexion group and by 13% in the extension group. Intradiscal electrothermal therapy consistently seemed to increase the width of the nucleus, but inconsistently decreased nucleus pressures. He concluded that there may be an inconsistent mechanism of action of IDET that decreases the disc pressure and leads to patient relief (12).

Bono studied nine cadaveric discs with beef strips surrounding the area to mimic body tissue. The temperature readings within the disc were allowed to equalize with the 37°C water temperature bath. Heating of the catheter using the IDET protocol was then performed. The study demonstrated that within 3 mm of the catheter, the temperatures achieved are greater than 60°C, and that within 10 mm of the catheter, the temperatures achieved are at least 50°C. Unlike Klienstuecks' study where the catheter was placed in the anterolateral annulus, in this study the catheter was placed in the posterior annulus. In the outer loop area, temperatures of 60°C or more were noted in 13 of 14 discs, whereas only two discs reached above 65°C. Hence, in the posterior annulus represented by the outer loop area, it may be possible to get collagen denaturation up to 4 mm from the catheter. Neural ablation temperatures were reached up to 14 mm from the catheter within the inner loop. However, the outer loop temperatures only reached 45°C in 10 discs and 40°C in 13 discs. He concluded that not all discs will reach temperatures great enough to cause collagen denaturation or nerve ablation, and that maintaining the proper location of the catheter is extremely important (13).

COMPLICATIONS

The complication rate of IDET is low. In Cohen's study of 108 IDET discs, only 10% had a complication and the majority of these were self-limited and transient (14). Saal and Saal (15) had a complication rate of 0.7% in their study of 1675 patients. The highest complication rate reported was 16% in Freedman's study. As in the other studies, the complications were transient (16).

Transient problems, such as transient burning dysesthesias and nondermatomal numbness and parasthesias have been reported. L4 weakness, associated with the catheter insertion site, with accompanying foot drop has been described in the literature. This resolved six weeks after surgical treatment. One patient with a migraine history had a nonpositional headache that was different from her usual headache. This resolved after five days of hospitalization (16).

Increased disc protrusion has been reported after IDET. A patient with a small L5/S1 herniation developed increased back and thigh pain with MRI findings of a very large herniation requiring surgery (17). Two cases of avascular necrosis of the vertebral body and one case of cauda equina were also reported following IDET. Avascular necrosis following IDET at L4/5 and L5/S1 presented with worsening low back pain and leg dysesthesias. All blood work was negative, but MRI demonstrated edema at both the L5 and S1 vertebral bodies. Biopsies of the vertebral body and disc done at the time of an anterior–posterior fusion with instrumentation demonstrated necrotic bone and disc material (18). Osteonecrosis may have been the result of the rise in the endplate temperature, as demonstrated by Yentkilner and Brandt (19). They proved, in rabbits, that heating of the vertebral body to more than 70°C causes histologic changes consistent with osteonecrosis (20).

The case of cauda equina syndrome involves a 56-year-old woman who developed urinary retention, bowel incontinence, loss of sensation, and weakness in her leg following IDET. Intradiscal electrothermal therapy was performed at the L5/S1 level without incident. The patient had IDET at the L4/5 level, and developed burning pain radiating from her left buttock to her foot and the posterior leg. It was noted under fluoroscopy that the catheter was in the spinal canal, rather than within the disc. The catheter was then repositioned correctly. Following the procedure, she presented with the aforementioned symptoms (21). This complication was not directly secondary to IDET, but rather to technical error. Prior to heating the catheter, placement is supposed to be checked in both the anteroposterior and lateral views to ensure proper intradiscal placement (22).

CONTRAINDICATIONS

Intradiscal electrothermal therapy cannot be performed on patients with sepsis, osteomyelitis, cellulitis, discitis, bleeding diathesis, cauda equina syndrome, vertebral fractures, and segmental instability as determined by flexion extension roenterograms. Severe disc space narrowing, sequestered disc herniations and large disc herniations are contraindications. The presence of hardware should lead to extreme caution for fear of heating fusion hardware, spinal cord stimulator, or intrathecal pump. One must also be wary of patients with psychological issues, such as somatization or conversion disorders and patients with potential secondary gain (4).

The other relative contraindication to IDET may be obesity. Although not statistically significant, and of a small sample size, Cohen was able to show that obese IDET patients had a higher failure rate. Of the 15 smokers in his study, five of the obese smokers failed IDET, whereas only four of the 10 nonobese smokers had poor outcomes. The lone risk factor for failure in this study was obesity. Of the 10 obese patients, only one had a good outcome and two of the 10 had worsening of the treated disc. The one patient that developed a herniation post-IDET was obese. The mechanism of collagen reformation and immediate weakening postprocedure may have led to the herniation (23). Although obesity itself is a risk factor for back pain (24), obese patients may have other factors that predispose them to fail IDET. Some of these factors include inability to wear the brace or perform adequate rehabilitation, and a failure of the annulus to heal because of increased pressure owing to patient body weight (23).

OUTCOMES

There have been a few outcome studies on IDET. Initial prospective studies by Saal and Saal showed promise for IDET to alleviate low back pain. Saal and Saal studied 1116 patients who had back pain for more than three months. Sixty-two patients that did not improve after six months of conservative treatment were treated with IDET. Pain concordance was then established using discography. Success was based on a change of 7 points in the SF-36 and a 2-point change in the Visual Analog Scale (VAS). Thirty patients underwent IDET at one level and 32 patients underwent IDET at multiple levels. Mean change of the VAS at one year was 3.4 in the single-level group and 2.6 in the multilevel group. Scores in the SF-36 scale improved in 44 of the patients (71%), 24 of the 30 single-level patients and 20 of the 32 multilevel patients. Ninety-seven percent of the private pay patients and 83% of the compensation patients returned to work. All but one of the previously working patients returned to work. Patients with preserved disc height undergoing multilevel procedures did better than those with decreased disc height. Single-level IDET procedures did not show statistical difference in outcomes based on disc height. Disc space narrowing of less than 30% was associated with less favorable outcomes in the multilevel group, but not in the single-level group. Those patients with heavier labor jobs returned to work in four to six months, and patients with lighter duty jobs returned to work in one to three months. No difference was noted between the compensation patient and the private pay patient outcomes. At the one-year follow up, there were no complications or worsened outcomes reported (25).

At the two-year follow-up, Saal and Saal demonstrated sustained improvement from the procedure. Only one patient went on to fusion. At 24 months, 72% of the patients maintained a 2-point improvement on the VAS, and 50% of the patients maintained at least a 4-point VAS reduction. There was improvement in the SF-36 of 7 points in 78% of patients and 14 points in 59% of patients. At this point, the change post-IDET between the single and multilevel patients was equivalent (26).

Karasek studied 53 patients as a prospective case control study using the insurance-denied patients as controls. At three months post-IDET, 23 of the 35 patients noted improvement. Changes persisted at six and 12 months. The author reported partial benefit in 60% and complete relief in 23% of IDET patients (27).

Using a manufacturer-sponsored registry, Thompson found that following IDET, there was an improvement in the VAS and SF-36 scores at six and 12 months. Gender was not shown to be predictive of the level of improvement. However, multiple-level procedures were associated with greater levels of pain at six and 12 months with no difference in overall level of improvement post-IDET. The compensation group was noted to have lower physical function scores with less improvement following IDET (28). Webster used worker's compensation records of 142 IDET cases to track outcomes. Poor results were noted when the same physician did the discogram and subsequent IDET procedure. In addition, patients using narcotics in the three months prior to IDET and patients in litigation had poorer outcomes (29).

The first randomized, placebo-controlled trial of IDET, was undertaken by Pauza. Patients were selected for the study following six weeks of unsuccessful nonoperative care. Further criteria included no surgery within three months of the procedure, and disc height narrowing could not exceed 20%. Compensation patients were deliberately excluded. Following discography to determine concordance patients were randomized and blinded to the procedure. The investigator learned which patient would undergo treatment and which would undergo sham once the introducer had been placed to the level of the outer annulus. In the IDET group, the procedure was performed, but in the sham group, the patients watched fluoroscopic images of catheter placement and heard noises mimicking actual procedure noises. Patients wore a lumbar corset for six weeks in both groups, and underwent a spine stabilization program with progression to an independent program by the twelfth week. All interactions were with blinded staff members.

Outcomes were assessed using the VAS, SF-36, and the Oswestry Disability Index. These were scored before treatment and at the six-month point. Sixty-four patients were enrolled, of which 37 underwent IDET and 27 underwent the sham procedure. The patients did have relatively high SF-36 scores with little disability prior to IDET. Five patients from the IDET group and three sham patients had to be rejected for violating the protocol. One IDET patient had to be removed owing to improper electrode placement. Eventually, there were 32 IDET-randomized patients and 24 sham patients. In the treatment group, 78% thought they had undergone treatment, and in the sham group, 74% thought they had been treated. Both groups demonstrated improvements in pain scores, but the IDET improvements were higher. Statistical significance was met in the VAS for absolute and relative pain changes. Intradiscal electrothermal therapy was shown to be more effective in patients with pain scores less than 70 and for patients with poorer function prior to procedure. It was not significantly better than the sham procedure in those with low disability and good physical function.

In this study, only 40% of patients treated had greater than 50% relief. Intradiscal electrothermal therapy was significantly more effective in patients with poor physical function and greater disability, but not more effective in the healthier subset. Visual Analog Scale scores were reduced from 6.6 to 4.2, which is similar to the Saal study. Interestingly, 33% of the sham patients reported greater than 50% relief, with one getting complete relief. Because of the high level of improvement in the sham group, Pauza concluded that nonspecific factors may be a major factor in improvement, but that this is not the complete reason for IDET efficacy (30).

At this time, the most recently published study was the prospective, randomized, double-blinded, placebo-controlled trial of Freeman et al. (31) A total of 57 patients were enrolled. All patients had chronic discogenic low back pain with marked disability, degenerative disc disease on MRI, and failure of conservative management. All patients had symptomatic discogenic pain at either one or two levels as proven by provocative discography. Computed tomography (CT) scan was then used to determine internal disc disruption. Of the 57 patients in the study, 38 randomized to IDET and 19 to placebo. The catheter was placed to cover 75% of the posterior annulus or 75% of the annular tear as demonstrated on postdiscography CT scan. An independent technician covertly connected the catheter or did not connect the catheter according to a randomized schedule. Both the surgeon and the patient were blinded to this. Standard heating protocol was used with antibiotic administration postcatheter removal followed by a Pilates-based exercise program. Subjects were then re-evaluated at six weeks and six months by a third party. Successful outcome required no neurologic deficit caused by the procedure, improvement in the Low Back Pain Outcome Score of

7 or more and an improvement in the subscales of the SF36 greater than 1 standard deviation from the mean.

Patients were questioned using the Low Back Pain Outcome Score, the Oswestry Disability Index, the Zung Depression Index, and the modified Somatic Perception Questionnaire. Two of the patients were removed. One left the study because of technical failure and one patient with increased low back pain chose to withdraw at three months. Radiculopathy was reported in four patients who underwent IDET and one patient who had the sham procedure. No patient met the criteria set for improvement. Freeman et al. (31) concluded that highly selected patients show marginal benefit and the majority of patients with chronic discogenic low back pain do not get demonstrable benefit from IDET.

OTHER PERCUTANEOUS DISC PROCEDURES

Nucleoplasty uses radiofrequency energy to shrink the nucleus pulposus and alleviate low back pain. By using coblation, a field generated around the electrode, the disc material is ablated in channels and then coagulated on withdrawal of the Perc-D Spine Wand. Chen, (32) in three cadavers, was able to show that coblation reduced intradiscal pressure in healthy cadaver discs. The pressure dropped by only 5% in degenerated cadaver discs. He concluded that nucleoplasty significantly reduces pressures in the nondegenerated disc, but has minimal effect on the degenerated disc.

Sharps (33) has demonstrated that nucleoplasty may be of some promise in alleviating back pain. However, Cohen (34) showed that nucleoplasty should have a limited role in patient care. In his study of active duty patients that underwent nucleoplasty and IDET, or nucleoplasty alone, only one patient had greater than 50% reduction in pain. Two patients had new neurologic symptoms for which work up was negative. He determined that adding nucleoplasty to IDET does not lead to further patient benefit and that nucleoplasty should not be used as a treatment for axial low back pain. He also concluded that its role should be limited to patients with radicular pain, intact outer annulus, and disc protrusion less than 6 mm.

Removal of nucleus material using the dekompressor, a rotatory motored probe, has been used as well. In Amoretti's study, (35) eight of the 10 patients had greater than 70% improvement on VAS, but one patient had a disc extrusion following the procedure with recurrence of radicular symptoms. He concluded that the dekompressor may have benefits over other percutaneous discectomy methods owing to ease of placement of the trocar, rotatory action of the motor allowing for aspiration of disc material, and the potential decrease in pressure caused by the disc material removal.

Automated percutaneous lumbar discectomy (APLD) has been used to remove disc material to decrease back pain. Teng performed APLD in 1474 patients with an 83% success rate and only a 0.06% complication rate. Patients with disc extrusions, sequestered disc herniations, long-term symptomology, old age, calcified longitudinal ligament, and previous discectomy had poorer outcomes (36).

However, Sahlstrand (37) demonstrated no change in the disc protrusion at six weeks post-APLD. There was appreciable change in the straight leg raise, but not in back or leg pain. He concluded that APLD was ineffective. Furthermore, seven patients had results that were poor enough to necessitate surgery. In total, the failure rate approached 60%.

Percutaneous laser discectomy has been used to reduce the size of disc hernia-tions by ablating the nucleus pulposis. This was improved upon by adding an endoscope to the Nd:YAG laser. There have been a small number of percutaneous endoscopic laser discectomy case studies with short follow-up periods. Currently, most laser procedures in the United States are done without endoscopy, and endo-scopic skill level affects clinical outcomes (38). Choi (39) demonstrated irreversible matrix alteration, by the Nd:YAG laser, causing a drop in nucleus volume and changes in the shape of bovine discs.

Choy (40) performed 2400 percutaneous endoscopic laser disc decompression (PELD) procedures in a 17-year series. His overall success rate was 89% with a recurrence rate of 5%. The only major complication was discitis, which occurred at a rate of 0.4%. McMillan et al. (41) showed in a three-month follow-up study after PELD that 80% of patients had improvement in symptoms at the three-month point. On an average, the improvement was noted to be 44% based on the American Academy of Orthopedic Surgery Symptom Scoring Scale.

CONCLUSION

Several percutaneous disc procedures have been developed. All have had initial promise, but most have not been able to stand up to further rigorous training. Although IDET has been shown to be a procedure with minimal long-term compli-cations, the mechanism of action is uncertain and the outcomes are minimally beneficial. Although earlier prospective studies demonstrated effectiveness of the procedure, more recent blinded randomized studies have not been able to demonstrate a definite benefit. Until further double-blinded randomized studies demonstrating efficacy are done, one should exercise caution in proposing the IDET procedure or any of the other percutaneous disc procedures.

REFERENCES

1. Schwarzer AC, Aprill CN, Derby R, et al. The prevalence and clinical features of internal disc disruption in patients with chronic low back pain (comment). Spine 1995; 20(17):1878–1883.
2. Crock HV. A reappraisal of intervertebral disc lesions. Med J Aust 1970; 1(20):983–989.
3. Heary RF. Intradiscal electrothermal annuloplasty: the IDET procedure. J Spinal Disord 2001; 14(4):353–360.
4. Chou LH, Lew HL, Coelho PC, et al. Intradiscal electrothermal annuloplasty. Am J Phys Med Rehabil 2005; 84(7):538–549.
5. Derby R, Eck B, Chen Y, et al. Intradiscal electrothermal annuloplasty (IDET): a novel approach for treating chronic discogenic back pain. Neuromodulation 2000; 3:69–75.
6. Shah RV, Lutz GE, Lee J, et al. Intradiscal electrothermal therapy: a preliminary histo-logic study. Arch Phys Med Rehabil 2001; 82(9):1230–1237.
7. Bogduk N, Tynan W, Wilson AS. The nerve supply to the human lumbar intervertebral discs. J Anat 1981; 132(1):39–56.
8. Freemont AJ, Peacock TE, Goupille P, et al. Nerve ingrowth into diseased intervertebral disc in chronic back pain. Lancet 1997; 350(9072):178–181.
9. Kleinstueck FS, Diedrich CJ, Nau WH, et al. Acute biomechanical and histological effects of intradiscal electrothermal therapy on human lumbar discs. Spine 2001; 26(20): 2198–2207.
10. Kleinstueck FS, Diedrich CJ, Nau WH, et al. Temperature and thermal dose distributions during intradiscal electrothermal therapy in the cadaveric lumbar spine. Spine 2003; 28(15):1700–1708.

11. Freeman BJ, Walters RM, Moore RJ, et al. Does intradiscal electrothermal therapy denervate and repair experimentally induced posterolateral annular tears in an animal model? Spine 2003; 28(23):2602–2608.
12. Pollintine P, Findlay G, Abrams MA. Intradiscal electrothermal therapy can alter compressive stress distributions inside degenerated intervertebral discs. Spine 2005; 30(6):E134–E139.
13. Bono CM, Iki K, Jalota A, et al. Temperatures within the lumbar disc and endplates during intradiscal electrothermal therapy: formulation of a predictive temperature map in relation to distance from the catheter. Spine 2004; 29(10):1124–1129.
14. Cohen SP, Larkin T, Abdi S, et al. Risk factors for failure and complications of intradiscal electrothermal therapy: a pilot study. Spine 2003; 28(11):1142–1147.
15. Saal JA, Saal JS, Wetzel FT, et al. IDET related complications: a multi-center study of 1675 treated patients with a review of FDA MDR Data Base. 16th Annual Meeting of North American Spine Society, Seattle, Washington October–November, 2001. North American Spine Society, 2001.
16. Freedman BA, Cohen SP, Kukio TR, et al. Intradiscal electrothermal therapy (IDET) for chronic low back pain in active-duty soldiers: 2 year follow-up. Spine J 2003; 3(6):502–509.
17. Cohen SP, Larkin T, Polly DW. A giant herniated disc following intradiscal electrothermal therapy. J Spinal Disord Tech 2002; 12(6):537–541.
18. Djurasovic M, Glassman SD, Dimar JR, et al. Verterbral osteonecrosis associated with the use of intradiscal electrothermal therapy: a case report. Spine 2002; 27(13):E325–E328.
19. Yetkinler D, Brandt L. Interval disc temperature measurements during nucleoplasty and IDET. 9th Meeting of the International Spinal Injection Society, Boston, Massachusetts, September 14–16, 2001, International Spine Injection Society, 2001.
20. Berman A, Reid J, Yanicke D, et al. Thermally induced bone necrosis in rabbits: relation to implant failure in humans. CORR 1984; 186:284–292.
21. Hsia A, Isaac K, Katz J. Cauda equina syndrome from intradiscal electrothermal therapy. Neurology 2000; 55(2):320.
22. Wetzel FT. Cauda equina syndrome from intradiscal electrothermal therapy (comment). Neurology 2001; 56(11):160.
23. Cohen SP, Larkin T, Abdi S, et al. Risk factors for failure and complications of intradiscal electrothermal therapy: a pilot study. Spine 2003; 28(11):1142–1147.
24. Leboeuf-Yde C. Body weight and low back pain: a systematic literature review of 56 journal articles reporting on 65 epidemiologic studies. Spine 2000; 25:225-237.
25. Saal JA and Saal JS. Intradiscal electrothermal treatment for chronic discogenic low back pain: a prospective outcome study with minimum 1-year follow-up. Spine 2000; 25(20):2622–2627.
26. Saal JA and Saal JS. Intradiscal electrothermal treatment for chronic discogenic low back pain: a prospective outcome study with minimum 2-year follow-up. Spine 2002; 27(9):966–973.
27. Karasek M, Bogduk N. Twelve-month follow-up of a controlled trial of intradiscal thermal anuloplasty for back pain due to internal disc disruption. Spine 2000; 25(20):2601–2607.
28. Thompson K, Eckel T. IDET nationwide registry preliminary results: 6-month follow-up data on 170. 15th Meeting North American Spine Society, New Orleans, Louisiana, October 25–28, 2000. North American Spine Society, 2000.
29. Webster BS, Verma S, Pransky GS. Outcomes of worker's compensation claimants with low back pain undergoing intradiscal electrothermal therapy. Spine 2004; 29(4):435–441.
30. Pauza KJ, Howell S, Dreyfuss P, et al. A randomized, placebo-controlled trial of intradiscal electrothermal therapy for the treatment of discogenic low back pain. Spine J 2004; 4(1):27–35.
31. Freeman BJC, Fraser RD, Cain CMJ, et al. A randomized, double-blind, controlled trial: intradiscal electrothermal therapy versus placebo for the treatment of chronic discogenic low back pain. Spine 2005; 30(21):2369–2377.
32. Chen YC, Lee S, Chen D. Intradiscal pressure study of percutaneous disc decompression with nucleoplasty in human cadavers. Spine 2003; 28(7):661–665.

33. Sharps LS, Isaac Z. Percutaneous disc decompression using nucleoplasty. Pain Physician 2002; 5(2):121–126.
34. Cohen S, Williams S, Kurihara C, et al. Nucleoplasty with or without intradiscal electro-thermal therapy (IDET) as a treatment for lumbar herniated disc. J Spinal Disord Tech 2005; 18(1):S119–S124.
35. Amoretti N, Huchot F, Flory P, et al. Percutaneous nucleotomy: preliminary communication on a decompression probe (Dekompressor) in percutaneous discectomy. Ten case reports. Clin Imaging 2005; 29(2):98–101.
36. Teng G, Jeffrey RF, Guo J, et al. Automated percutaneous lumbar discectomy: a prospective multiinstitutional study. J Vasc Interv Radiol 1997; 8(3):457–463.
37. Sahlstrand T, Lonntoft M. A prospective study of preoperative and postoperative sequential magnetic resonance imaging and early clinical outcome in automated percutaneous lumbar discectomy. J Spinal Disorders 1999; 12(5):368–374.
38. Singh K, Ledet E, Carl A. Intradiscal therapy: a review of current treatment modalities. Spine 2005; 30:s20–s26.
39. Choi JY, Tenenbaum BS, Milner TE, et al. Thermal, mechanical, optical and morphologic changes in bovine nucleus pulposus induced by Nd:YAG (lamba = 1.32 micron) laser irradiation. Lasers Surg Med 2001; 28(3):248–254.
40. Choy DS. Percutaneous laser disc decompression: an update. Photomed Laser Surg 2004; 22:393–406. Choy DS. Percutaneous laser disc decompression: a 17-year experience. Photomed Laser Surg 2004; 22(5):407–410.
41. McMillan MR, Patterson PA, Parker V. Percutaneous laser disc decompression for the treatment of discogenic lumbar pain and sciatica: a preliminary report with 3-month follow-up in a general pain clinic population. Photomed Laser Surg 2004; 22(5):434–438.

Index